Anna Brus, Michi Knecht, Martin Zillinger (eds.)
The Post/Colonial Museum

Redaktionen

ZfK – Zeitschrift für Kulturwissenschaften

Hg. von Karin Harrasser und Elisabeth Timm

Begründet und herausgegeben (2007 bis 2012) von Thomas Hauschild und Lutz Musner

Anna Brus, Michi Knecht, Martin Zillinger (eds.)

The Post/Colonial Museum

ZfK – Zeitschrift für Kulturwissenschaften 2|2021

Die Zeitschrift für Kulturwissenschaften erscheint zweimal jährlich. Wir senden Ihnen Ihr Exemplar gerne portofrei zu (innerhalb Deutschlands).

Sie können die Zeitschrift für Kulturwissenschaften als Jahresabonnement direkt über den Verlag abonnieren.

Das Abonnement beginnt mit dem aktuellen Heft und verlängert sich automatisch um jeweils ein Jahr, wenn es nicht bis zum 1. Februar eines Jahres beim Verlag gekündigt wird. Die Zusendung der abonnierten Exemplare erfolgt unmittelbar nach Erscheinen.

Weitere Informationen finden Sie unter: www.transcript-verlag.de/zeitschriften-abonnements

Selbstverständlich ist die Zeitschrift für Kulturwissenschaften auch über jede Buchhandlung erhältlich.

Gefördert durch die Deutsche Forschungsgemeinschaft (DFG) – Projektnummer 262513311 – SFB 1187, aus Mitteln des Postcolony-Lab, WoC-Worlds of Contradiction, Universität Bremen und des GSSC - Global South Studies Centre, Universität Köln.

Die ZfK wird außerdem mitgetragen von der Abteilung Kulturwissenschaft der Kunstuniversität Linz und dem Institut für Kulturanthropologie/Europäische Ethnologie der Westfälischen Wilhelms-Universität Münster.

Alle Beiträge in der ZfK durchlaufen ein *editorial review*. Wenn einzelne Artikel zudem das von der ZfK angebotene *double-blind-review* durchlaufen haben, ist dies am Ende des jeweiligen Textes dokumentiert.

Bibliographische Information der Deutschen Nationalbibliothek:
Die Deutsche Nationalbibliothek verzeichnet diese Publikation in der Deutschen Nationalbibliografie; detaillierte bibliographische Daten sind im Internet über https://dnb.d-nb.de abrufbar.
Indexiert in EBSCOhost-Datenbanken.

Redaktionsassistenz: Moritz Pisk
Layoutentwurf: Leonie Lehner
Satz und Layout: Hana Oprešnik
Covergraphik: Post-Museen, Anna Habaschy aka Minaechx, Wien 2021 (www.minaechx.at)
Produktion: Die Produktion – Agentur für Druckrealisation GmbH, Düsseldorf
Printed in Europe
ISBN: 978-3-8376-5397-7
ISBN PDF: 978-3-8394-5397-1
ISSN: 2197-9103
eISSN: 2197-9111

Gedruckt auf alterungsbeständigem Papier mit chlorfrei gebleichtem Zellstoff.

Besuchen Sie uns im Internet: http://www.transcript-verlag.de
Bitte fordern Sie unser Gesamtverzeichnis und andere Broschüren an unter:
info@transcript-verlag.de

https://zeitschrift-kulturwissenschaften.de

Table of Contents

Subject

Transforming the Post/Colonial Museum

Anna Brus and Martin Zillinger

Much has been said in recent years about the colonial origin and enduring legacy of former ›anthropological‹ or imperial museums. Programmatic attempts to decolonize them by opening up (Snoep 2020, 2021), worlding (Modest et al. 2019; de Cesari et al. 2020), mobilizing (Oforiatta-Ayim 2015ff.), unlearning (Azoulay 2019), repairing (Attia 2014), and restituting (Sarr/Savoy 2018) have multiplied in the museum sector. At the same time, new centers of museum work have emerged, especially on the African continent; be it in Dakar, Accra, Cape Town, or Nairobi, artists and curators have been working successfully to redefine the museum and to establish new hotspots of an increasingly globalized art scene. This issue of the *Zeitschrift für Kulturwissenschaften* invited museum practitioners and curator-activists from the African continent who have been working together with these influential and highly visible initiatives. Situated in the archives, depots, and museums of formerly colonial institutions, Nelson Abiti, Mary Mbewe, Paul Tichmann, and Lynn Abrahams take the challenge to rethink ›ethnographic collections‹ and undo the problematic category of the ›ethnographic object‹ in their day-to-day work. Their contributions are supplemented by papers by Richard Fossi and Bernard Müller that deal with the historical conditions and surviving memories of colonial collectivism and violence. These conditions and memories continue to shape the work in and on colonial collections and bring about this sense of urgency that characterizes the ongoing museum debate. A third focus is on the historical trajectories, contemporary challenges, and utopian designs of museum work on the continent. To this end, Sabrina Moura looks at the long history of the Museum of Black Civilizations in Dakar. Conversations with the former Director of the Musée des Civilisations, Abidjan, and currently Directrice Générale de la Culture de Côte d'Ivoire Sylvie Memel-Kassi and the director of the art space Bandjoun Station, Barthélémy Toguo, then explore transformative in(ter)ventions on the continent, and the contours of a future museum take shape. The thematic section ends with a close reading of the exhibition *Beyond Compare. Art from Africa in the Bode Museum in Berlin* by Helen Verran, who reflects on the challenges of a decolonizing curatorial practice. Last but not least, the *Adapter* was designed by the activist-artist Catarina Simão and contains a meticulous reflection about her long-term project on the German-Portuguese researchers Margot and Jorge Dias. Her compilation of text and images explores the production of

ZfK – Zeitschrift für Kulturwissenschaften 2|2021
urn:nbn:de:hbz:6:3-zfk-2021-41916

anthropological knowledge and the afterlife of images across space and time, unraveling violent encounters and forms of resistance in the ethnographic archive that question concepts such as ›authenticity‹ and ›coloniality‹. Distancing herself from the intended use of Margot and Jorge Dias' photographs of Makonde culture as an object of scientific studies, she excavates invisible micro-histories on the reverse side of the official narrative.

All of the contributions engage with objects and object practices in order to reach out to people. They can be read as part of the struggle to find new ways of »federat[ing] around a conversation« that researchers and artists such as Kader Attia and Felwine Sarr have identified at the actual core of the restitution debate (Attia/Möntmann 2021). We are therefore grateful that the authors of this issue help us widen the focus of the heated debate in Europe and thus remind us to not turn it into another form of navel-gazing. Instead of adding to the debate on the (im-)possibilities of addressing the colonial specters within collections in Europe, their contributions zoom in on this other phantom of the colonial past, the anthropological museum as it was implemented on the African continent as part of colonial governance and control. Nelson Abiti in Kampala (Uganda), Mary Mbewe in Mbala (Zambia), and Paul Tichmann and Lynn Abrahams in Cape Town (South Africa) have not only dug deep into colonial archives and unraveled the history of the collections for which they have taken responsibility, they have also engaged with different stakeholders and communities that relate to the objects (Karp/Kratz 2014), or rather, as Erika Lehrer and Michael Rothberg would have it, that find themselves related »by implication« (Lehrer 2018; Rothberg 2009). To be sure, as Tichmann/Abrahams (in this volume) acknowledge, as insiders to the very institution they want to transform, they cannot avoid some sort of complicity and continuously risk reproducing some of the institutional knowns ingrained in the institutions' postcolonial histories. But their work testifies that and how anthropological museums can turn into what Helen Verran (in this volume) describes as sites of »multiversal relationality« – by creating spaces for »epistemic incommensurability« and »ontological happenings« – in terms of what objects »are«, how they are categorized or »known«, and what they allow for, once they cease to be merely modern »lumps of matter with particular attributes and qualities« (Verran in this volume, p. 149), that illustrate and characterize ›ethnographic cases‹ (cf. Ingold 2017).

The Post/Colonial Museum

We decided to call this issue *The Post/Colonial Museum* to emphasize the difficulties and obstacles that come with the museums' colonial legacy and that remain part and parcel of a transforming museum. The violence and racism, the history of dislocation and loss that underlie their collections continue to spawn conflicts and to create phantom pains up to the very present, as Bernard Müller describes in recounting oral histories of severed thumbs from Togo and as Silvie Kassi and her project *La Collection Fantôme* in the Ivory Coast remind us (Müller; Kassi/Snoep/Zillinger, in this volume). The injustice and trauma that is imbricated in these collections cannot be easily addressed, let alone undone in the different postcolonial contexts at stake. With Helen Verran, we contend that, to envision a postcolonial museum, it is necessary to describe its colonial modalities and search for a postcolonial impulse that consists of and enables »different epistemics and their practicalities [to] come together to abut and abrade, to interrupt or to offer affordances« in past and present (Verran 2019: n.p.). Such impulses create a museum that is not only transforming, but that may also incite transformation well beyond its walls, as Abiti, Mbewe and Tichmann/Abrahams (all in this volume) demonstrate by engaging communities and their object practices in their museum work. We speak of a *Post/Colonial* museum to mark these and other attempts and ongoing struggles to deal with and ultimately oppose the colonial make-up of former anthropological museums and to interrupt the musealized epistemic, ontological, and social orders they embody.

›White Spaces‹: Museums as Citadels of Colonialism

While the papers collected for this issue deal with museums on the continent, it would be misleading to speak of an ›African museum‹. The historical, political, and economic contexts of the various museums, collections, and curatorial practices vary, as do the ways they remain entangled in the bequeathed transnational history of dominance and control, but also of cooperation (cf. Laely/Meyer/Schwere 2018). All of them, however, struggle with colonial legacies and the continuous purification work of modernity that has separated ›art‹ from ›ethnographic artifact‹, ›culture‹ from ›nature‹, ›subject‹ from ›object‹, and ›matter‹ from ›spirit‹ (see also Moura and her discussion of the Museum of Black Civilizations, Dakar, in this volume). Built and run by white colonialists, anthropological museums on the continent served to define the ›Other‹ within and, for a long time, have presented the deprived communities and their material culture in an everlasting ethnographic present (Fabian 1983), classified, ordered, and controlled by the invention of categories such as ethnicity, tribe, and tradition (Abiti; Tichmann/Abrahams, both in this volume). By transplanting the modern museum into colonized regions, the administrators and missionaries translated European imperial discourse on the ›Other‹ into the societies they had to control. As we learned from Tony Bennett in Europe, the public museum served to provide »objects lessons in power« to allow people »to know rather than be known« (Bennett 1988: 76), and to thus interiorize the regulating regime of modernity and modern statehood. While object lessons in power were pursued by museum practitioners-cum-colonialists on the continent, too (cf. Abiti; Mbewe, both in this volume), in many ways, the museums they founded remained until very recently spaces of being known and were, for good reasons, perceived as the »museums of the whites« (Kassi/Snoep/Zillinger, in this volume). The local communities were well aware that the objects were taken from them with the intention to store them out of reach and out of sight for most of them. Other collectors, such as the French-Canadian priest Jean Jacques Corbeil among Bemba communities, envisioned the museum as a place of knowledge transaction among and towards the communities they worked in and integrated the »salvaging« and displaying of artifacts in their proselytizing activities (Mbewe, in this volume). Both forms of museum work were part of technologies to turn people into colonial subjects that needed to be »civilized« (Simão, in this volume) and adapted to the needs and constraints of extractivist colonial regimes.

Europeans implementing the extractivist policies were often aware of the destruction they caused, but saw this as inevitable accompaniments of their civilizing mission.

As Richard Tsogang Fossi elaborates in detail in his analysis of diary entries of the German ›explorer‹ Zintgraff in Cameroon (in this volume), the colonial matrix did not include African communities' rights to their own material culture. Artifacts were either gathered by the colonizers to become objects of culture, and thus precious for anthropology and the colonial administrators, or they were not only not worth being preserved, but often, in a gesture of brutal demonstration of power, demolished and smashed.

With independence, the museums of the colonizers passed into the hands of the postcolonial states. The racist and modernist regimes that structured the archives, the collections, the display, and the architecture of these citadels of colonialism have endured into the present and have long continued to prevent the appropriation of the holdings by the very people whose former »subject-objects« (Sarr 2019) they hold and whose histories and futures they claim to administer. The *Post/Colonial Museum* is therefore marked by a painful and paradoxical relation to the social place it inhabits. For the visitors, who often encounter objects from and histories of a past they have been deprived of, the museum experience oscillates between total alienation and intense affinity.

Resisting the Alienating Museum

The colonial archive and the enduring categorizations of objects and people twists and erases memory and leads to forms of »unremembering« (Tichmann/Abrahams, in this volume) that are difficult to undo. Modernity's epistemic framework reached out far beyond the museum walls and distorted African knowledge practices and cosmologies, erasing, for example, histories of women, arts, and technologies from the public record until today (see Phiri Chitungu 2021). With the founding of museums, scientists and administrators implemented infrastructures that produced what they sought to describe: an Africa in the image of the »colonial library« (Mudimbe 1991) through which colonial officials, anthropologists, and missionaries, but in extension also art historians, geographers, political and social scientists, and economists have invented, essentialized, and continuously reproduced African identities that fitted seamlessly into the differentiation narratives of modernity. The political, religious, and scientific performance of dominance and control has pervaded museums on the continent and continues to draw its authority from the intellectual fields and colonial imaginaries that shaped their foundations, as Mudimbe lucidly noted (ibid.: 8). As Felwine Sarr (2019: 18) reminded us recently, the »hideous face of the Other« (Césaire 2001) has thus not only become constitutive of its epistemic orders and curatorial displays, it also evokes a form of Du Boisian double consciousness (cf. Du Bois 1903), through which societies on the continent perceive themselves in a distorting mirror. Museums have been instrumental in alienating communities from their past and material culture and were part and parcel of the overall imperial project to disseminate the idea of white supremacy.

This have never gone unchallenged, however. Orders of knowledge and the making of colonial truth have met with resistance, as we know through the work of anti-racist and anti-colonial thinkers such as W.E.B. Du Bois, Aimé Césaire, and Frantz Fanon. Apart from the work of these and other anti-colonial authors, resistance came to the fore in manifold ways – through non-hegemonic epistemic, social, and artistic practices engaging with the violent present and memories of colonialism (see Bernard Müller and Catarina Simão, in this volume). With her multi-layered juxtaposition of photos, documents, and films, the artist Catarina Simão unearths histories excluded from the colonial narrative. She explores the work of the German-Portuguese anthropologists Dias, who headed an ethnographic mission to the Macondes. While their work is deeply enmeshed in the colonial matrix of applied anthropology of the time, Simão regards the collection generated by their mission as an »original creative act«. Although the photographic inventory fostered concepts such as »authenticity« (sought by the anthropologists) and accounted for »coloniality« (enacted through their work), she uncovers seeds of resistance in the documents of their cooperation with research assistants and translators, and particularly in art practices they encountered. Collected as »Makonde sculpture«, these artworks from colonial contact zones turn our gaze back to the colonizers. They oscillate between sarcasm and resisting humor – or so it seems as suggested by the varying emotional reactions that range from loud laughter (in today's Mozambique) to embarrassed silence (in today's Portugal). Simão's experiments with different audience reactions to the sculptures of white Portuguese colonizers demonstrate that, today, the »ethnographic object« cannot be perceived in any way near to the way its originators or its collectors saw it. The responses to the art works are situated in space and time, they differ from setting to setting and are part and parcel of the different ways a historical »truth« is remembered.

Bernard Müller leaves the colonial archives and engages with memories of colonialism that are pursued, lived, and handed down outside of it, if that is possible at all. He visited regions in Togo that were renowned for their fierce resistance to German and French armies and traced the widespread rumors of severed thumbs that, according to oral history, were taken by colonizing militias to disable young men from operating the bow and joining the armed resistance. On their journey through the former colony »Togoland«, Müller and the Togolese writer Kangni Alem traced and documented an oral history that is told and retold against the grain of the official records. What has been called local knowledge reverses the clear-cut redistribution of agency and passivity in the bequeathed history of dominance and control and can complicate narratives of victimization. Müller and Alem met schoolchildren strolling around neglected graveyards of colonial soldiers, who turned memories of resistance and defeat into compassion with the fallen colonial soldiers – and with their families, who, as their young interlocutors see it, have failed to connect with their past and take care of their dead children. Forgetting and remembering, Müller states with Jorge Luis Borges, are equally inventive and carry the seed of resistance.

Resistance can also take the form of disinterest, when local communities ignore the museum as an inaccessible elitist place or a space that may be good enough to entertain tourists (cf. Kassi/Snoep/Zillinger, in this volume). Indeed, the effects of the physical (cf. in particular Fossi; Müller, both in this volume) and epistemic violence (cf. Abiti; Mbewe; Tichmann/Abrahams, all in this volume) of the colonial endeavor are mirrored in uncanny ways in local perceptions of museums as zones of danger, as »burial grounds« for »objects« – at times discarded in the religious register as cemeteries of fetishes (Silvie Kassi, personal communication, cf. Kassi 2020) or as places of black magic, as reported by Barthélémy Toguo (in this volume; for a discussion of the emergence of iconoclastic movements on the continent, see Brus/Knecht/Zillinger 2020). These perceptions and forms of resistance relate to a white historiography and its underlying evolutionism that manifests in alienating museum spaces. The damage these narratives and institutionalized orders have caused and the recklessness with which they were enforced finds its perhaps cruelest manifestations in human remains, thousands of which have been shipped as trophies and scientific material to museums and repositories in Europe, but were also stored across the continent (cf. Legassick/Rassool 2000; Förster/Stoecker 2016; cf. Sattler 2018). The »unfinished business of the dead« (Rassool 2015) continues to pervade the international networks of anthropological museums, natural history museums, and so-called scientific collections alike, testifying to the dehumanizing history of colonial collections that more often than not combined artifacts, specimen of nature, and the bodies or body parts of dead persons. As Paul Tichmann and Lynn Abrahams describe in their contribution to this issue, post-Apartheid museums such as the Iziko Museum in Cape Town have inherited these human remains and struggle to find a way »to restore dignity and humanity to these remains as well as to the descendants« (in this volume, p. 49), inciting a new dialogue between institutions, communities, and families, who try to regain the dead bodies of their lost loved ones.

The Transforming Museum

Museums are also perceived as spaces of death for the objects they draw together and for the social functions and practices these objects symbolize and contain. The dynamics of ritual practice and the delegation of authority, the memorizing of events, genealogies, and tradition, and the transmission and reinvention of knowledge constitute material objects as relational objects (cf. Küchler/Carroll 2021) and stand in stark contrast to the frozen and static storage of museum depots and the ethics of preservation that characterize the material culture in Europe's imperial museums. Much of the current debate on decolonizing the museum centers on how the immobilized and devitalized objects confined within museum walls (see for example the renewed interest in the film »Les statues meurent aussi« by Marker/Resnais/Cloquet, 1953) can regain an agentive quality and help rebuild the social fabric that has been distorted and disfigured by colonial and postcolonial violence.

In their contributions, Abiti, Mbewe, and Tichmann/Abrahams describe how objects in museums can be known, be enacted, and come to the fore differently from the way they were »known«, preserved, and practiced in the long history of their colonialized, institutionalized, and museumized existence.

Nelson Abiti describes how, after the civil war that ravaged Northern Uganda ended in 2006, the team of the National Museum of Uganda reached out to communities that had suffered from experiences of extreme violence. By bringing a double-headed, royal spear to the communities that no longer have these regalia in their possession, they enabled mediation and reconciliatory rituals during ceremonies of reburial for those who died far away from their ancestral lands. During the rituals, Abiti notes, these spears »are transformed from an artefact into a spirit« and become the medium of ancestral authority (in this volume, p. 41). In a situation in which communities have time and again been disconnected from their past through colonialism and civil war, that mourn the disappearance of their members and struggle to locate the remains of their beloved, but that also have to face profound social frictions that extend into each family, artifacts from the museum depots helped to reach out to chiefs, elders, and religious leaders. With the help of these objects, community memorials can be organized. Used in rituals to overcome the deficiencies, violence, and cleavages of the postwar and postcolonial social fabric, the artifacts gain a new power, a new form of agency, and the ability to enable cooperation. Reintegrating perpetrators of violence and enabling grief as much as forgiveness, this ritual cooperation ultimately becomes a cooperation for ›life‹, as Arthur M. Hocart (1970) put it once, by establishing mechanisms of justice and reconciliation. As Abiti emphasizes, the life of the artifacts brought to the villages was renewed in this process, as it renewed the life of the village. What was known as an artifact of warfare and stood in for a history of tribal wars in the colonial narrative became an object of memorialization, a medium for delegating ancestral authority, and a subject that performed »repair« (Attia 2014) and »healing« (Abiti, in this volume).

Mary Mbewe explores a collection that was used by the missionary Jean Jacques Corbeil in his proselytizing activities to gain knowledge of secret initiation rites for girls. As she emphasizes, these rites prepared girls for womanhood and were »at the heart of ensuring the health and progress of society« (in this volume, p. 62). By putting pressure on a woman of standing, Corbeil gained access to information that he was not entitled to as a foreigner, as a representative of the colonizing West as much as of the Catholic Church, and as a man. Mbewe situates Corbeil's activities within a wider field of ethnographic work produced by missionaries such as the White Fathers, to whom the priest belonged. Ethnographizing in this context, guised as a way to protect and preserve indigenous practice, she argues, also meant classifying, fixating, and controlling dynamic, centuries-old practices and devaluing them in order to spread the Gospel and prove the superiority of Christianity. Moreover, the collection of sacred objects, the recording and archiving of sacred songs, and the incremental pervasion of the traditional transmission of knowledge through which women defined and maintained their authority in society over time, are all examples of the epistemic violence enacted through ethnography that helped not only the colonial, but also the postcolonial governments to exercise control over women's bodies and sexuality (in this volume, p. 68). Corbeil used his ethnographic collection and the Moto Moto Museum he established to create knowledge about women's rituals and their place in society, but he also tried to train the people of his parish to become »modern knowers« by developing an ethnographic gaze onto their own culture, as the (self-)documentary on Corbeil and the Moto Moto museum clearly demonstrates (Owens/Corbeil n.d., see minute 27:50ff.). Until today, the Moto Moto Museum is an educational institution, and Mary Mbewe lucidly describes how its colonial legacy finds repercussions in the modernizing agendas of transnational actors and funding agencies forging new forms of cooperation between the museum, educational experts, and development workers with the so-called traditional authorities and the local population. While the devaluation of local knowledge and practice continues under various guises, these new forms of cooperation also provoke new conversations that escape the modernizing narratives of health education and development work and that can reinvest the *chisungu* collection with new meaning. The museum collection is thus folded into various attempts to change and improve the situation of women in terms of HIV/AIDS, gender relations, and reproductive health. Once knowledge transaction multiplies around collections, the question whether epistemic incommensurability and a multiversal relationality can emerge may be less a question of educational programs and, ultimately, control (e.g. through funding institutions) than of practices and conversations that unfold – and, therefore, of perspective.

Paul Tichmann and Lynn Abrahams turn to another form of community engagement in the museum. The colonial South African Museum had collected objects, photographs, and human remains since the 1820s, and the collection represents a colonial epistemology that was thrust on groups like the Khoi/San and/or ›Bushmen‹ – designations that are themselves a controversial part of this history. The Khoi-Boesman-Nguni Coalition successfully campaigned to close the ethnographic gallery that had remained part of what are today the Iziko Museums in Cape Town. One of the problems the gallery had perpetuated since colonial times was the representation of Khoi/San history as natural history, placing the communities outside of culture. As Tichmann and Abrahams describe, the controversy that unfolded around this campaign involved actors with very different backgrounds, opinions, and interests and accounted for what Erika Lehrer called »communities of implication« as »those mutually constitutive entanglements […] with ›significant Others‹ whose own experiences of and reaction to us make up the other half of the dialogue that always co-constitute our identities« (Lehrer 2020: 307). In discussing access to and the significance of the objects in the collection, representatives of the Khomani and San communities, the Khoi-Boesmann-Nguni Coalition, and the museum created a space to address the colonial violence the communities had to endure and the misrepresentation they have had to face in the encounter with white settler societies. At the same time, the complex relations between historical impositions of and contemporary claims to ethnic identity, land issues, and language policies came to the fore. During this process, the interests, perspectives, and concerns did not necessarily coincide. The museum representatives, for example, saw the conversation as part of a broader endeavor to rethink the colonial epistemic order and to reframe the collection from Khoi/San communities within the wider museum setting. The Khomani representatives, on the other hand, evaluated the objects as part of their ongoing struggle for political recognition and the rebuilding of their communities. The diverging viewpoints remained to a certain extent incommensurable and created uncomfortable insights into the inevitable epistemic violence enacted through any form of categorization and the »orders of justification« (Boltanski/Thévenot 2006) they invoke. The »awkward objects« (Lehrer 2020: 307) from the collection, with their painful histories and controversial present, draw together actors who and groups that are affected in different ways by their sheer presence in the museums, the histories they embody, and the controversies that unfold around them. They not only bring about »communities of implication« (Lehrer 2018; 2020) and »spark publics into being« (cf. Marres 2005); perhaps even more importantly, the objects foster forms of care from museum professionals and the Khomani communities for the deceased depicted on colonial photographs and their memory, but also for the specific knowledge that was articulated and the cultural practices that were reconstructed in the encounters and conversations.

A decolonized and decolonizing museum takes shape, then, when objects are allowed to »happen« (Verran, in this volume) in new ways. All three contributions explore pathways of a transforming museum that moves out of the depot, forges new forms of cooperation, and creates new forms and formats of knowledge. A transforming museum as described by Abiti and Tichmann/Abrahams allows emotions and memories to set in where colonial knowledge is deconstructed and enables forms of care and healing where epistemic and spatial control is relinquished. As Mbewe demonstrates, working towards a transforming museum demands foregrounding practice and resituating knowledge outside the classificatory regimes of colonial, national, or transnational institutions that perpetuate modernity's predicaments of extractivism, development, and control. This ›outside‹ ceases to be the ›other‹ of a universalizing Western episteme. It enables to confront the »colonial difference« (Mignolo 2002) and forms a space from which to undermine the systematic subalternation of epistemic, material and social practices by repositioning the very practices itself and their colonized histories in a pluralizing present (cf. Hammoudi 2021: 289). As Mbewe makes poignantly clear, this is an arduous task, full of pitfalls and drawbacks, since it upends the world of acting subjects, on the one hand, and objects that are acted upon, on the other (cf. Mbembe 2021: 371).

Decolonizing Knowledge and the Post/Colonial Museum

Salvage anthropology and the museumification of culture have put the »colonial library« into practice and helped establish access to people and artifacts, rendering them controllable in the post/colonial order of things. For people, signs, and things to become agentive in new, unprecedented ways and a source of resistance, epistemic practices need to run at cross purposes to the institutionalized routines and normative classifications that have tamed and controlled them. This is why Helen Verran rightly insists (in this volume) on the necessity to create moments of epistemic incommensurability in order to decolonize the museum and, by extension, our post/colonial world.

Anthropological museums – and by extension anthropology as a discipline – have produced knowledge that continues to be in dire need of decolonization, as critical social and anthropological work has emphasized for decades (see, among many others, Assad 1973; Restrepo/Escobar 2005; Fabian 1983; Ganslmayr/Paczensky 1984; Harms 1984; Leclerc 1972; Owusu 1979; Rabinow 1977). But it is perhaps not by chance that museums are currently both: hot spots of political and social controversies over colonialism and its afterlife, and spaces where initiatives are drawn together that work towards decolonizing knowledge. These spaces can perhaps emerge whenever anthropology is pursued in a mode of mutual learning that aims at generating »knowledge with«, instead of generating »knowledge of« (Ingold 2017), at establishing »partial connections« (Strathern 2004) rather than universalizing classifications, and at decentering established orders of knowledge rather than legitimizing them (cf. Schüttpelz 2005; see also Kramer 2018, 2019; Schüttpelz 2017a and 2017b). Foucault famously saw anthropology as forming this »perceptual principle of dissatisfaction, of calling into question, of criticism and contestation« (Foucault 2002: 407). Do not be mistaken, neither is this principle often realized in anthropological museums, nor does it come straightforwardly with the more far reaching plea for epistemic incommensurability. What we can see is that, today, not least due to the digitalization and the increasingly »unbounded historical resources, [which] swirl in abundance around the global public domain« (Edwards 2016: 53), expertise and epistemic practices are diversified, and awareness of the multiplying, problematic legacies of colonialism is growing.

The contributions to this issue make it clear that the challenge of decentering cannot be confined to colonial knowledge orders of the West. Already in the early days of postcolonial theory, criticism of its own blinders and white spots emerged from within the postcolonial movement itself. Recently, Abdellah Hammoudi noted that the postcolonial critique of anthropology as it developed in the Global North after Said's *Orientalism* (1978) left him »rather little in the manner of how postcolonial societies may generate knowledge about themselves« (Hammoudi 2021: 288) when he was working in and on Morocco. Evoking and rethinking the notion of »double critique« from the work of Abdelkebir Khatibi and Abdallah Laroui from the 1970s, who stressed the colonial legacies for both, colonizers and the formerly colonized, he makes a plea for generating knowledge from outside the European canon »besides«, but also »in critical exchange« with the Western episteme. Going beyond the deconstruction of colonial histories, as they appear from the perspective of European metropoles, this critical exchange re-appropriates the »massive colonial knowledge« (ibid.) and its ambiguous engagement of local life-worlds. As Kader Attia (2014) has reminded us, this re-appropriation can turn into an act of resistance, which creates a critical distance not only from the colonial past, but also from the postcolonial present.[1]

Restitution is crucial in this regard, precisely because it enables control to be relinquished and permits »ontological happenings« to change the way objects, persons, and epistemic things are »known«. But since this comes with a profound delegitimization of the expert culture of the museum, and may even call for an ethics of de-collecting, as Simão remarks, restitution does not come easy. Museum representatives, academics and politicians have fielded many arguments why restitution demands cannot or should not be met. What the contributions by Abiti, Mbewe, and Tichmann/Abrahams unanimously show is that the importance of restitution is neither established nor negotiated solely in the conference halls of academics, politicians, and curators. It is vital to all those groups, small communities, and often marginalized actors that struggle to revisit the past in order to build a future. As we infer from Hammoudi's recent intervention, the recirculation and re-appropriation of colonial collections can help to create this productive »outside«, that allows social, material and discursive practices to ›happen‹ differently and thus to work for multidirectional forms of decolonization. The production of knowledge »besides« the European episteme is crucial for decolonization, but no less crucial is the engagement with

1 Writing in Germany, we stress this point, since the at times fierce public debates in Europe too easily project the history of colonialism and its ongoing violent effects onto ethnology in disciplinary terms, onto former anthropological museums in institutional terms, and onto the past in temporal terms, as Elizabeth Edwards lucidly noted (2016). The current upswing of postcolonial activism and public scrutiny of enduring forms of racism has disturbed this comforting creation of an »elsewhere« that, as Edwards rightly observed, has denied the relevance of colonial legacies for knowledge formations other than in anthropology, and relegated it to past academic and social realities in Europe. The distance and distancing Hammoudi proposes is a productive one, that does not prevent, but helps to perform critique.

forms of knowledge generated in the colonial archive, and in the long and bequeathed history of transcultural encounter. Hammoudi situates the »outside« that is needed to decenter dominant knowledge orders in the very confrontation between non-Western knowledge traditions and local epistemes, on the one hand and Western knowledge, on the other. Decolonization, then, is not a break with colonialism, »when a particular ›us‹, who are not ›them‹, suddenly coalesces as opposition to colonizers« as Helen Verran noted some 20 years ago (2001: 38), reflecting on the possibility of critique in postcolonial times and places. It can be performed only in and through »the ambiguous struggling through and with colonial pasts in making different futures« (ibid.). Decolonizing knowledge emerges, then, in the reflection of the epistemological and methodological conditions of knowledge production in contact zones of the post/colonial encounter. These encounters take place in the former colonies as much as in the former centers of colonial empires – and the »disconcertment« (Verran this volume) that currently (or shall we say: finally) seizes curators, administrators and visitors in exhibitions and depots of anthropological museums in Europe as well as in Africa may indeed nurture »other« knowledge and epistemic practices than those that have been remade and institutionalized in museum spaces for decades.

Restitution and the Future Museum

Claims for restitution have been made throughout the colonial and postcolonial history in order to regain and re-appreciate what was not only robbed and bartered, gifted and exchanged within the colonial matrix, but also devalued and alienated. The current demands for restitution are far from novel and have been preceded by recurring efforts to bring lost regalia and important ceremonial objects back to the continent. One of the first official claims directed at Germany to regain looted royal objects was made as early as 1935 by the Oba Akenzua II, who tried in vain to buy back from the Völkerkunde Museum in Berlin two throne stools that had been in his ancestors' possession (Peraldi 2017). With the independence of the postcolonial states and the growing resistance to Western political and economic domination and interference, a new awareness of the importance of rebuilding a sense of cultural dignity emerged and ignited a debate on restitution that, particularly in Germany, came to a peak in the 1960s and 1970s (see Ganslmayr/Paczensky 1984; and for the meticulous reconstruction of these debates, Savoy 2021).

Particularly in Europe and North America, today the renewed upswing of the debate is fueled by a critical reassessment of colonial history and its afterlife in persisting forms of structural racism and, as discussed in this issue, diverging interaction orders of race across postcolonial settings (see Duck/Rawls, in this volume; cf. Brus/Knecht/Zillinger 2021). Despite the often-heard critique that restitution will most likely amount to a neo-colonial endeavor, since actors from the so-called Global North will continue to impose the terms, conditions, and results of this process, all the authors in this issue strongly support restitution. They stress that African communities are intellectually, politically and emotionally highly invested in African objects currently based in Europe, and they clearly formulate the challenges that come up when the communities, the curators and all other actors involved try to come to terms with these objects and their colonial histories.

It is noteworthy that the role of the museum in future restitution processes is discussed controversially. As the artist and director of the art space Bandjoun station, Barthélémy Toguo, emphasizes (in this volume),

> »If an object arrived and it was an object from Batcham or Bangangté or Foumban, which was used for a ceremony, it [...] should not return to a closed, glassed-in space, such as a museum, because from the outset it was not intended for museums. Such an object was intended for ceremonies, for practices, for acknowledgements by a chief who wanted to appreciate the arrival of his host, offer him a stool and ask him to sit. So put the stool back there, in the chiefdom. That's what [the people from the communities] think, they don't think about returning these objects to museums, they want them to be able to return to their usual functions in society« (Toguo/Brus/Müller, in this volume, p. 145).

For Silvie Kassi, a postcolonial museum that is run by Côte d'Ivorians instead of European colonizers has the obligation to offer communities the possibility to partake in and to write themselves into the museum space – by actively choosing objects to be safeguarded in the museum and by providing the information they want to see archived together with the objects. She vividly describes the challenges and problems she encountered as director of the Museum of Civilizations in Abidjan, but also the hopes and aspirations she and the various actors involved have had for building a contemporary museum of local as much as transnational importance. By turning the »embattled terrain, in which those who are being represented and those conceptualizing the representation seem to perform very different claims and very different interests« (Rogoff 2002: 64) into a space of dialogue and cooperation, her work also translates a history of loss and violence into the ongoing histories of communities and the equally ongoing nation-building process of Côte d'Ivoire.

As Tichmann and Abraham note, a transforming museum should depart from established conventions and be pursued not by filling gaps and providing ever more add-ons, but by the performance of loss that extends to the museum and its predicaments itself (cf. Rogoff ibid.). The efforts described in this volume to re-humanize collections by engaging anew with individuals and communities and by using the museum as a site of debate and education, of reconciliation and hospitality, are indicative of broader political and social processes. They shed light on transformative museum dynamics on the continent, which are part of a transnational conversation that, to paraphrase Latour (2005), is local at all points and thus manifests differently in different social settings. Barthélémy Toguo's Bandjoun Station is a case in point: a center for art and culture he founded in Cameroun's Western Region, it was built as a nonprofit organization that brings contemporary artists and experts in various fields into exchange with the local population. It explicitly sets itself apart from the Western concept of the museum. Bandjoun Station goes beyond the museum by offering a space for festivities, education, and sustainable agriculture. Performing the inversion of modernity and the modern separation of art from life and of culture from nature, the center fosters communities of practice in forms of mutual inspiration and assistance that are provided for and emerge through cooperation in fields such as arts, techniques and technologies, and health care. In this way, a museum turns into a platform for conversations about histories different from those told by the colonial archive (see Müller, in this volume), and it enables visitors to confront experiences of violence and military destruction (see Fossi) by translating them into new forms of agency and transnational cooperation.

In her paper on the history of the making of the Museum of Black Civilizations in Dakar, Sabrina Moura describes the various attempts to build a museum that »refuses to uphold a subaltern position regarding its Western counterparts« (in this volume, p. 111). In a transnational conversation, curators, researchers, and artists have tried to reassess the epistemologies of art history, ethnography, and the like and struggle to define – in the words of the philosopher Souleymane Bachir Diagne – a »mutant museum« (see ibid., p. 113) that escapes Eurocentric classification work and representation. As Moura's critical reading of the debates about the museum demonstrates, the making of a transformed museum needs to engage both with the transnational history and entangled present of African art as art and with the various cultural traditions of which art and artifacts have been part – be it craftsmanship, ritual, or ruling – and which, throughout the history of colonialism, have been continuously reinvented. A close analysis of the exhibitions after the opening of the museum, their presentation, and their reception shows a museum space that is first and foremost designed and celebrated as mobilizing. Reflecting the past and reassessing the present, it opens a »look toward the future« that has always been »a key principle for the different expressions of Black emancipation« (in this volume, p. 117), as Moura emphasizes.

As we noted at the outset of this introduction, programmatic attempts to decolonize have multiplied in the museum sector. At the core of all of these attempts is cooperation, the willingness to listen, to find new means to interact, to elaborate new procedures, and to decenter and rethink institutional, collective, and individual positionalities. The museum has become a privileged space for experimenting with new epistemic practices and for allowing the emergence of new publics, characterized by multiplying connections instead of differentiation and exclusion. As we learn from the contributions to this issue, the post/colonial museum has evolved out of entangled histories of dominance and control, but bears the seeds of resistance and, perhaps even more important, of other histories and creative futures that are written by the communities themselves (cf. Mbembe 2002). Given the dynamics in the African museum landscape, museums in Europe will evolve towards those on the African continent and elsewhere in the Global South, if they are to pave the way for a future, decolonized museum (cf. Jean and John Comaroff 2012). While the current attempts to bring about a radical change in transnational museum cooperation are impressive, it remains to be seen whether this process will put an end to the long history of self-assuring forms of remembrance and forgetting in the post/colonial museum, and successfully contribute to decolonize knowledge and institutions on the continent as much as in Europe.

This issue of the *Zeitschrift für Kulturwissenschaften* has been made possible by the generous support of the German Research Foundation (DFG), Collaborative Research Centre (CRC) »Media of Cooperation« – Project number 262513311. It unfolds a conversation that started during the conference »Museum Collections in Motion. Colonial and Postcolonial Encounters«, which the editors organized together with Larissa Förster

(Deutsches Zentrum Kulturgutverluste), Ulrike Lindner (University of Cologne), and Nanette Snoep (Rautenstrauch-Joest Museum, Cologne) in 2019. This conference brought together scholars, museum experts, and activists from Europe, the U.S., Australia and the Pacific, South America, and Africa and was realized in cooperation between the Global South Studies Center (GSSC) and the Rautenstrauch-Joest Museum, Cologne. We gratefully acknowledge the financial support from the Museumsgesellschaft, the Foreign Office of Germany, the GSSC, and the research platform »Worlds of Contradiction« (Bremen). We would like to express our deep gratitude to all of these institutions, as well as to our colleagues from the editorial board of the *boasblog DCNtR*: Carl Deussen (Rautenstrauch Joest Museum), Bernard Müller (École des Arts, Avignon), Gabriel Schimmeroth (Museum am Rothenbaum, Hamburg), and Ciraj Rassool (University of Western Cape) for true intellectual companionship over the last years. For comments on the introduction, the authors wish to thank Michi Knecht and the editors of the ZfK, Karin Harrasser and Elisabeth Timm, who never lost patience or faith in the project despite various delays. We also wish to thank Mitch Cohen for his meticulous copy-editing, and first and foremost our student colleagues Teresa Ellinger, Paula Linstädter, Fabian Lüke, Annette Steffny, Lennert Wendt, and Christine Dietze. Without their passion and dedication to this project, which evolved between two universities and brought together contributions from four continents in four languages, its completion would not have been possible.

Literature

Asad, Talal (ed.) (1973): *Anthropology and the Colonial Encounter*, London: Ithaca Press.

Attia, Kader (2014): *The Repair from Occident to Extra-Occidental Cultures*, Berlin: The Green Box.

Attia, Kader/Möntmann, Nina (2021): »The Decolonizing Agency of Repair. Objects, Epistemologies and the Neoliberal Value System«. In: *Museums in Motion Workshop Series*, https://boasblogs.org/dcntr/the-decolonizing-agency-of-repair/ (23.07.2021).

Azoulay, Ariella A. (2019): *Potential History. Unlearning Imperialism*, London, New York: Verso.

Bennett, Tony (1988): »The Exhibitionary Complex«. In: *new formations* 4:1, 73–102.

Boltanski, Luc/Thévenot, Laurent (2006): *On Justification: Economies of Worth*, Princeton: Princeton University Press.

Brus, Anna/Knecht, Michi/Zillinger, Martin (2020): »Iconoclasm and the Restitution Debate«. In: *HAU: Journal of Ethnographic Theory* 10:3, 919–927.

Césaire, Aimé (2001) [1989]: *Notebook of a Return to the Native Land*, trans. and ed. by Annette Smith and Clayton Eshleman, Middletown: Wesleyan University Press.

Comaroff, Jean/Comaroff, John (2012): *Theory from the South, Or, How Euro-America is Evolving Toward Africa*, London: Taylor and Francis.

De Cesari, Chiara/Goodwin, Paul/Juneja, Monica/Modest, Wayne/Tiampo, Ming (2020): *Trans-Atlantic Platform – Social Innovation (T-AP-SI) Grant – Worlding Public Cultures: The Arts and Social Innovation.*

Du Bois, William E.B. (1903): *The Souls of Black Folk*, London: Longmans, Green & Co.

Fabian, Johannes (1983): *Time and the Other: How Anthropology Makes its Object*, New York: Columbia University Press.

Edwards, Elizabeth (2016): »The Colonial Archival Imaginaire at Home«. In: *Social Anthropology/Anthropologie Sociale* 24: 1, 52–66.

Förster, Larissa/Stoecker, Holger (2016): *Haut, Haar und Knochen. Koloniale Spuren in naturkundlichen Sammlungen der Universität Jena*, Laborberichte, Vol. 9, Weimar: Verlag und Datenbank für Geisteswissenschaften.

Foucault, Michel (2002) [1966]: *The Order of Things*, London, New York: Routledge.

Ganslmayr, Herbert/Paczensky, Gert von (1984): *Nofretete will nach Hause. Europa – Schatzhaus der ›Dritten Welt‹*, Munich: Bertelsmann Verlag.

Hammoudi, Abdellah (2021): »Decolonizing Anthropology at a Distance. Some Thoughts«. In: *HAU: Journal of Ethnographic Theory* 11:1, 281–290.

Harms, Volker (1984) (ed.): *Andenken an den Kolonialismus. Ausstellungskataloge der Universität Tübingen Nr. 117*, Tübingen: Attempto.

Hocart, Arthur M. (1970) [1936]): *Kings and Councillors: An Essay in the Comparative Anatomy of Human Society*, Chicago: Chicago University Press.

Ingold, Tim (2017): »Anthropology contra Ethnography«. In: *HAU: Journal of Ethnographic Theory* 7:1, 21–26.

Karp, Ivan/Kratz, Corinne A. (2014): »The Interrogative Museum«. In: *Museum as Process: Translating Local and Global Knowledges*, ed. by Raymond A. Silverman, London, New York: Routledge, 279–298.

Kassi, Silvie M. (2021): »Iconoclasm and restitution. Between denial and cultural realism«, In: *HAU. Journal of Ethnographic Theory 10 (3)*: 962-966.

Kramer, Fritz (2018): »Anthropological Collections. Not an Apology, but an Amendment«, https://boasblogs.org/dcntr/anthropological-collections/ (19.08.2021).

Kramer, Fritz (2019): »Koloniales Erbe. Afrikanische Künste, transkultureller Tausch, ethnologische Sammlungen«. In: *Lettre international* 124, 12.

Küchler, Susanne/Carroll, Timothy (2021): *A Return to the Object. Alfred Gell, Art, and Social Theory*, Oxon, New York: Routledge.

Laely, Thomas/Meyer, Mark/Schwere, Raphael (2018): *Museum Cooperation between Africa and Europe: A New Field for Museum Studies*, Bielefeld: transcript.

Latour, Bruno (2005): *Reassembling the Social: An Introduction to Actor-Network Theory*, Oxford: Oxford University Press.

Leclerc, Gerard (1972): *Anthropologie et Colonialisme*, Paris: Fayard.

Leggasick, Martin/Rassool, Ciraj (2000): *Skeletons in the Cupboard: South African Museums and the Trade in Human Remains 1907–1917*, Cape Town: South African Museum.

Lehrer, Erica (2018): »From ›Heritage Communities‹ to ›Communities of Implication‹«. In: *Traces*, http://www.traces.polimi.it/2018/07/26/from-heritage-communities-to-communities-of-implication/ (23.07.2021).

Lehrer, Erica (2020): »Material Kin: ›Communities of Implication‹ in Post-Colonial, Post-Holocaust Polish Ethnographic Collections«. In: *Across Anthropology: Troubling Colonial Legacies, Museums, and the Curatorial*, ed. by Margareta von Oswald and Jonas Tinius, Leuven: Leuven University Press, 283–316.

MARKER, Chris/RESNAIS, Alain/CLOQUET, Ghislain (1953): *Les Statues Meurent Aussi*, Essay Movie, France.

MARRES, Noortje (2005): *Issues Spark a Public into Being: A Key but Often Forgotten Point of the Lippmann-Dewey Debate*. In: *Making Things Public: Atmospheres of Democracy*, ed. by Bruno Latour and Peter Weibel, Cambridge, MA: MIT Press, 208–217.

MBEMBE, Achille (2002): »African Modes of Self -Writing«. In: *Public Culture* 14:1, 239–273.

MBEMBE, Achille (2021): *Out of the Dark Night. Essays on Decolonization*, New York: Columbia University Press.

MODEST, Wayne/THOMAS, Nicholas/PRLIĆ, Doris/AUGUSTAT, Claudia (2019): *Matters of Belonging. Ethnographic Museums in a Changing Europe*, Leiden: Sidestone Press.

MIGNOLO, Walter (2002): »The Geopolitics of Knowledge and the Colonial Difference«, In: *South Atlantic Quarterly* 101 (1): 57–96.

MUDIMBE, Valentin-Yves (1991): *Parables and Fables. Exegesis, Textuality, and Politics in Central Africa*. Madison: The University of Wisconsin Press.

OFORIATTA-AYIM, Nana (2015ff.): »Mobile Museums-Projects«, https://www.anoghana.org/mobilemuseums (19.08.2021).

OWENS, David /CORBEIL, Jean Jacques (n.d.): »The Moto Moto Museum of White Father J.J. Corbeil«, https://www.youtube.com/watch?v=zdqnrfckd5o&t=569s, (23.06.2021).

OWUSU, Maxwell (1979): »Introduction«. In: *Colonialism and Change: Essays Presented to Lucy Mair*, ed. by Maxwell Owusu, Berlin: De Gruyter, 17–24.

PERALDI, Audrey (2017): »Oba Akenzua II's Restitution Requests«. In: *Kunst & Kontext* 1/2017, 23–33.

PHIRI CHITUNGU, Victoria (2021): »From the Cave Man to Craftsmanship; a Gendered Conversation: The Case of Ethnographic Displays in Zambian Museums«, https://boasblogs.org/dcntr/from-the-cave-man-to-craftsmanship-a-gendered-conversation/ (23.07.2021).

RABINOW, Paul (1977): *Reflections on Fieldwork in Morocco*, Chicago: Chicago University Press.

RASSOOL, Ciraj (2015): »Re-storing the Skeletons of Empire: Return, Reburial and Rehumanisation in Southern Africa«. In: *Journal of Southern African Studies* 41:3, 653–670.

RESTREPO, Eduardo/ESCOBAR, Arturo (2005): »›Other Anthropologies and Anthropology Otherwise‹. Steps to a World Anthropologies Framework«. In: *Critique of Anthropology* 25:2, 99–129.

ROGOFF, Irit (2002): »Hit and Run – Museums and Cultural Difference«. In: *Art Journal* 61:3, 63–73.

ROTHBERG, Michael (2009): *Multidirectional Memory. Remembering the Holocaust in the Age of Decolonization*, Stanford: Stanford University Press.

SARR, Felwine (2019): *Afrotopia*, trans. by Max Henninger, Berlin: Matthes & Seitz.

SARR, Felwine/SAVOY, Bénédicte (2018): *The Restitution of African Cultural Heritage: Toward a New Relational Ethics*, http://restitutionreport2018.com/sarr_savoy_en.pdf (19.08. 2021).

SAID, Edward W. (1978): *Orientalism*, London: Routledge.

SATTLER, Felix (2018): *The Dead, As Far As [] Can Remember*. Exhibition, Tieranatomisches Theater, Berlin.

SAVOY, Bénédicte (2021): *Afrikas Kampf um seine Kunst. Geschichte einer postkolonialen Niederlage*, Munich: Beck.

SCHÜTTPELZ, Erhard (2005): *Die Moderne im Spiegel des Primitiven: Weltliteratur und Ethnologie 1870–1960*, Munich: Fink.

SCHÜTTPELZ, Erhard (2017a): »Into the Whirpool. Part One: Soft Spots and Blind Spots«, https://boasblogs.org/dcntr/into-the-whirlpool/ (19.08.2021).

SCHÜTTPELZ, Erhard (2017b): »Into the Whirlpool. Part Two: Meanwhile, Back at the Ranch«, https://boasblogs.org/dcntr/into-the-whirlpool-2/ (19.08.2021).

SNOEP, Nanette J. (2020): »De la ConServation à la ConVersation. Le Pari de la Carte Blanche«. In: *Multitudes* 78, 198–202.

SNOEP, Nanette J. (2021): »It's Yours! 4 Autonomous Spaces«. In: *Resist! The Art of Resistance*, Exhibition, Rautenstrauch-Joest Museum, Cologne 2021/22, http://rjm-resist.de/en/its-yours-2/ (19.08.2021).

STRATHERN, Marilyn (2004): *Partial Connections* (Updated Edition), Oxford: Alta Mira Press.

VERRAN, Helen (2001): *Science and an African Logic*, Chicago, London: University of Chicago Press.

VERRAN, Helen (2019): *Joke: Papua New Guinea, 1998*, unpublished manuscript, n.p.

The Uganda Museum's Tribal Representation: Colonial Repositories and Community Reconciliation in Uganda

Nelson Adebo Abiti

Introduction

Colonial rule in Uganda introduced classifications of so-called ›tribal‹ groups to enforce British administrative units. The idea or imagination of the ›imperial‹ implemented by the British colonial government included exhibitions of ›tribal crafts‹ in the Uganda Museum. While such exhibitions and displays divided the population into ›tribes‹ for the convenience of the British, the protectorate government ordered its colonial officials to embark on the project of ›civilising society‹. The establishment of the Uganda Museum, therefore, should be understood as part of the process by which British protectorate rule was enforced; the museum was, in this sense, an institution of the colonial government structure (Peterson 2015: 5).

The imperial policy of indirect rule in Uganda was an instrument of dividing people into ›tribal‹ people (Mamdani 2018). Similarly, the foundation of the protectorate museum in Uganda from 1908 until the 1960s had served the problematic ethnographic project of the British colonial administration. It cannot be separated from the deliberative strategies to undermine the knowledge and the organization of native societies in Uganda. From my personal experience of encountering the ethnographic collections labelled as fetishes and charms on display in the Uganda National Museum, I was faced with the challenge of redressing colonial injustice.[1] But the underlying histories of protectorate rule at the Uganda Museum had infused the way the ethnographic artefacts were labelled with colonial classifications and the enactment of ›tribal‹ and ethnic differences.

The problematic task of displaying ethnic groups remained a challenge during the postcolonial period for the independent nation of Uganda. The idea of folkloric cultural competitiveness was promoted in the 1960s as Pan-Africanism. In 1983, Omare Konaré

1 I have been working as a conservator of ethnography at the Uganda Museum since 2008 and started my work by compiling inventories of ethnographic artefacts. This article is a result of reflections on my encounters with the hidden and unidentified information on the artefacts that were stored at the ethnographic store of the Uganda Museum during the colonial administration.

urn:nbn:de:hbz:6:3-zfk-2021-41926

noted that African ethnographic museums provided ratification for Western audiences to consume African exoticism (Konaré 1983: 146). This said, indigenous knowledge practices survived among the members of the various communities in independent Uganda, though the material cultural representation in, and through, the museum clung to a narrative disconnected from historical and contemporary social practice. As such, the reappearance of indigenous knowledge as a form of alternative cultural practice became a force of opposition against colonial epistemic violence.

In the recent report by Felwine Sarr and Bénédicte Savoy (2018), *Restitution of African Cultural Heritage. Towards a Relational Ethics*, the argument is made that the return of African Art objects to West African countries alone cannot fix the problems of colonial injustice. The scholarly debate on matters of restitution here focuses on rebuilding relations and engaging in rehumanizing them (Rassool 2015: 669; Sarr/Savoy 2018). Engaging with the knowledge practices that shape the museum (cf. Hicks 2020) would also entail putting the concept of the modern nation as an element of colonial ideology to the test, as it was established along the political, institutional and anthropological politics of representing ›tribal‹ people in Africa (Coombes 1994: 2). Therefore, restitution, decolonization and nation state formation must be addressed by re-evaluating violence against societies that have experienced land displacement, brutal killings and the looting of cultural objects, all of which have caused unresolved painful memories and injustice.

Yet, for too long, the representation of ›tribal‹ artefacts in the ethnographic galleries has remained immune to the disrupted intangible memories among young people in conflict situations. But it is precisely the loss of intangible memory that poses the risk of behavioural problems emerging from hopelessness and resulting in violence. Recently, indigenous knowledge has gained new grounds in memory practices of the community and has reawakened the need for reinterpreting and redefining the meaning of ethnographic artefacts. From the lessons learned during the encounter with ethnographic artefacts in the museum and from engaging with forms of social memory among the communities from which these artefacts originate, it has become apparent that it is precisely the question of restitution and decolonisation that has reconnected and reactivated the local knowledge of the artefacts and their immaterial significance and meaning.

Against this background, a collaborative community project in Northern Uganda was initiated to preserve the memorial landscape. It aimed at amplifying the elders' desire of restoring their cultural heritage in the aftermath of the civil war that had occurred between 1986 and 2006. After the cessation of hostilities between the Lord Resistance Army (LRA) and the government soldiers (Jahn/Wilhelm-Solomon 2015: 186f.), the community memorial practice was reviving the cultural practice initiated by the elders of the Acholi rituals processes of forgiveness and reburials. In a contested argument about the make-up of contemporary society, this project was geared towards a postcolonial reconstruction of social sensibility and aimed to help to reposition the moral authority of elders. The attempt to rethink the reconciliatory project of rebuilding society in Northern Uganda after the civil war entailed rethinking the ethnographic museum (Abiti 2018: 83). How could the colonially founded museum – with its ethnographic framing that has become the Uganda National Museum – reposition itself towards social healing in this post-conflict situation, while it continues to carry the burden of misinterpreting and misrepresenting cultural knowledge in Uganda? It is important to understand how the British colonial administration began to document ethnic societies and in doing so formed the nation of Uganda. Alongside the project of nation formation, the protectorate government promoted the colonial ›museum‹ project that emphasised and endorsed differences between communities in Uganda.

The Role of the British Protectorate in the Uganda Museum

The British government introduced an indirect rule policy to administer Uganda in 1894. Captain Frederick Lugard had coded the indirect rule policy in which the native societies were divided into ›tribes‹. Although Lugard did not govern Uganda for long, his approaches were incorporated as a form of effective imperial science in the East African protectorate of Uganda. The concept of ›tribal‹ structures was implemented administratively in Uganda by Henry Hamilton Johnston (also named Sir Harry Johnston) between 1899 and 1901.[2] When Hamilton Johnston was appointed as a special commissioner for the colonial protectorate government of the British in Uganda, he embarked on a survey and demarcated the country into ›tribal‹ provinces. Hamilton Johnston ensured that colonial rule administered the ›tribal‹ provinces as separated places and peoples. In the process of enforcing imperial rule, the formulation of the protectorate Museum was initiated to further the description of ›tribal‹ people as a basis of the modern nation state of Uganda. The colonial museum began as a project of collecting ethnographic artefacts (Uganda Protectorate 1939: 5, see Deming 1966: 2). The involvement of colonial administrators in the ethnographic work testifies to the discipline being designed in the nineteenth and early twentieth century to expand the imperial science of conquest.

The discipline of anthropology was developed in the nineteenth century. But it later became a category in its own right in terms of the way objects were collected and gathered as material culture in a modern museum. The anthropological museum was designated to implement and display the anthropological system of knowing the uncivilised society (Harris/O'Hanlon 2013: 8). When the discipline of anthropology became more pronounced in the early twentieth century, however, the ethnographic objectives of collecting, classifying and representing began to organize the work of anthropology as a field practice (Lidchi 1997: 161; cf. Clifford 1988: 25). Henrietta Lidchi (1997: 160) referred to ethnography as a discipline of human science that dealt with racism, primitiveness and exotic objects. Moreover, ethnography was considered a study of unknown societies by documenting their ways of life, behaviours, beliefs and artefacts from people's homes and places of worship as reference materials (Reeves/Kuper/Hodges 2008: 512). The language and the meaning of ethnography was designed in Europe. Ethnography was therefore a cultural practice of colonialism through which field activity, and the time spent for research, would qualify for working in a colonial state. Tony Bennett (1995: 4f.) pointed out that the beginning of the transformation of the modern public museum is part and parcel of

2 Racial descriptions of the people in the protectorate in Uganda were, according to Johnston (1902: 471), studied through natural history.

an ethnographic way of knowing ›uncivilised‹ societies in order to govern them. As such, the ethnographic museum is, in its origins, a colonial museum. If African museums were defined as ethnographic, it is important to lay bare the relationship of colonial structures on the one hand, and the use of the museum as an institution to train young colonial officers to have them administer effective processes of undermining native authorities on the other. In Eastern Africa, where the question of ethnography has been entangled with the ongoing politics of tribalizing, ethnicizing and traditionalizing this subject to colonial rule, the ongoing relevance of ethnographic museums has come under examination.

Consequently, the Uganda Museum was founded immediately under the British protectorate government in 1908 by Sir Henry Hesketh Bell (see Uganda Protectorate 1939: 5). The museum was also the oldest colonially established cultural institution in the East African region (Peterson 2015; Posnansky 1963). During the implementation of the 1900 Buganda agreement, the deputy commissioner of the British protectorate government Sir George William wrote in a letter:

> »I am directed to inform you that his excellency the Governor has made arrangements for the opening in Entebbe of a Protectorate Museum, for the collection of local curios of all descriptions, such as articles of interest and specimen of native weapons and manufactures, and local products, vegetable and mineral: in fact of all articles of historical, ethnological and local industries of interest« (Wilson 1908).[3]

Wilson was one of the colonial administrators employed to implement the policies of the protectorate government. He also coordinated a punitive expedition of the British military against the indigenous resistance in the territories of Buganda, Bunyoro, Ankole, as well as in Northern and eastern parts of Uganda (Wilson 1907: 118). The consolidation of colonial rule through the project of ethnological collections began in 1907. In his letter, George Wilson (1908) claimed he was instructed by his Governor Sir Hesketh Bell to begin the project of a protectorate museum, to collect several artefacts such as agricultural implements, cooking items, basketry, blacksmith tools, native weapons, fertility, religious and healing objects.[4] Wilson's letter further stated that the artefacts would first be stored at the Entebbe administrative offices of the scientific department of the protectorate government. He also indicated that a sum of money equivalent to £10 was made available to the collectors to purchase the artefacts (ibid.).

Following Wilson's letter, colonial officials acquired the artefacts and gathered them at Entebbe until 1908. However, there was no proper house for displaying the cultural objects to the public. In the absence of proper storage and space for public display, Hesketh Bell immediately allocated a sum of money equivalent to £200 for building the first Sikh

3 Wilson George's (1908) »Deputy Commissioner's Circular«, concerning the founding of the Uganda Museum, was issued to all collectors (See also Uganda Protectorate 1939: 5).

4 Wilson's (1908) circular tasked the District Commissioners to purchase a unique item, addressed to the Botanical, Forestry Scientific Department of the British colonial administration. He cautioned against duplication of the artefact(s) purchased or donated. The MEMO required a native name attached to the artefacts. Perhaps the scientific department took over the task on writing the rest of the information about the artefact.

Temple Museum of the protectorate at Kampala.[5] Bell sketched the design of the building and thereby approved the construction of the Protectorate Museum. When construction was completed at the Lugard's fort in Kampala, the artefacts were transferred there from the administrative offices in Entebbe in 1908 for public display at the protectorate building. Subsequently, the official Sikh Temple Museum of the British protectorate government of Uganda was built at Fort Lugard in Kampala to display the ethnographic materials to the public. The artefacts were crammed in a small space and tagged with paper labels.

During the process of collecting these ethnographic artefacts, punitive measures were routinely deployed. People were arrested, killed and their spears or tools were confiscated as relics of a primitive society. By way of example, the evidence suggests that Kibuuka regalia were coercively taken by Rev. John Roscoe during his visit to Uganda between 1899 and 1902. They were then shipped as »sacred items of the war god of the Bugunda people« (Thomas 2016: 340f.) to the Cambridge University Museum of Archaeology and Anthropology. As will be discussed in more detail below, the Kibuuka objects were returned to Uganda in 1962 and displayed at the Uganda Museum. Similarly, the collection of Mubende regalia (stored as E 53.83 to E 53.155) have become part of the Uganda museum holdings and were gathered within colonial rule and under violent measures of subjugation. Today displayed in the ethnography gallery of the Uganda Museum, they were objects of spiritual and medical activities at the Nakaima shrine. This shrine memorized the Chwezi-Dynasty (13–14th century) and continues to hold important community functions among the communities. Yet the present rivalry over the ownership of the shrine site and the holding of the objects at the Uganda Museum signify the presence of colonial injustice in postcolonial Uganda. The regalia were looted by the British colonial rule after the murder of Omukama (King) Kabalega of the Bunyoro Kitara kingdom who had resisted colonial rule in the Western part of Uganda from 1870s to 1898 (cf. Otunnu 2016: 91–93). When the British fought against him, they violently scorched the land and people, they arrested, humiliated and imprisoned the Omukama, exiling them to the island of Seychelles in the Indian ocean. After careful selection of the cultural artefacts, perhaps some of the objects were shipped as ethnographic artefacts to western Europe while other objects – considered damaged or of negligible value – were crammed into the colonial administrative offices.

Interpretation and Presentation of Artefacts in Protectorate Museum-Uganda

The colonial government decided to relocate the ethnological artefacts from the administrative and scientific offices at Entebbe to the site of Lugard's fort. The site was selected on the hill of Kampala where the Imperial British East African Company (IBEAC) under Captain Lugard had established his military fort in 1891 (Otunnu 2016: 82f.). During this period of relocating the ethnographic artefacts, the objects so violently gathered were stored at the Sikh temple where they contributed to governing the society ›in a tribal

5 The Sikh Temple Museum was derived from the Sikh religious naming from India (See Uganda Protectorate 1939: 5).

mode‹. While the Sikh Temple Museum had been built and established by the special commissioner Hesketh Bell in 1908 to popularize the protectorate administration, it soon proved too small for the colonial propaganda of civilizing the indigenous society (Trowell 1957: 71, see Uganda Protectorate 1939: 6). In any case, the description of the artefacts in the protectorate museum revealed how the colonial masters reinterpreted the objects. Most of the artefacts were piled up in a small space having a wooden and glass case cabinet to both store and present ethnographic material to the public. As such, the interpretation and meanings of ethnographic artefacts corresponded to different meanings ascribed to the collection and the museum. To the local population, the presentation of the first museum was called *enyumba ya amayembe* (house of spirit). The keeper of the museum was *omukulu ya amayembe* (the head of spirit). The local communities had no interest in the museum collections because the colonial administration intentionally relabelled the artefacts (Deming 1966: 2; Trowell 1957: 72). The indigenous audience was unhappy with the presentation of the objects because the colonial administrators misinterpreted the cultural objects with negative attitudes as witchcraft or fetishes.

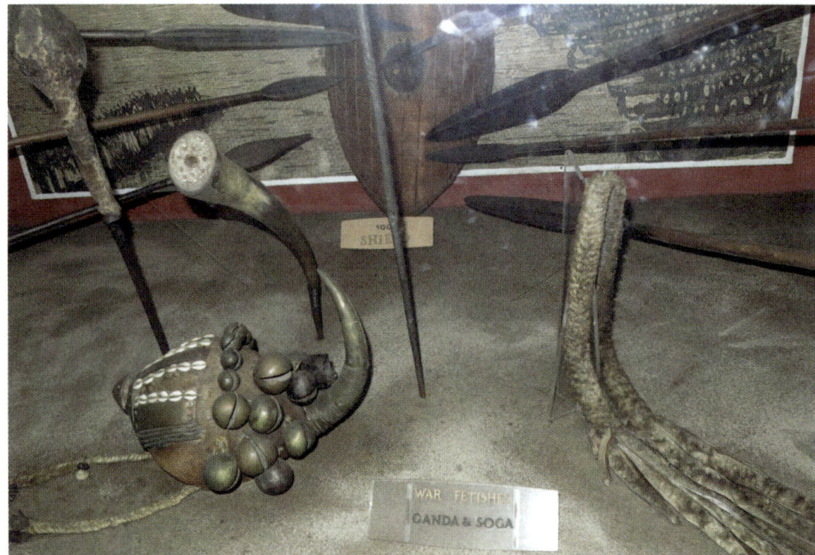

Fig. 1: Object label: Ganda Fetish, Ethnography Gallery No. E25. Uganda Museum. Photo: Nelson Adebo Abiti.

Towards the period of World War II, the colonial administration was faced with the challenge of a financial crisis, which also led to the neglect of the ethnological objects collected by colonial agents. Hence, most of the collection suffered damage. As a consequence, Margaret Trowell, an art teacher at the School of Art of Makerere College, opted to relocate the ethnological artefacts from the Protectorate Museum to the newly formed Art school at Makerere college in 1942. Trowell also transformed the art studio to create space for the incorporation of ethnographic material just until 1953, when the Uganda Museum building was completed (Trowell 1957). After the transfer of the artefacts, a catalogue listing the ethnological material was published as *Tribal Crafts of Uganda* (Trowell/Wachsmann 1953). The catalogue was developed from the descriptive work of the colonial administrative officers, the police and the judiciary services. The young police recruits were known to provide information used for the labels of the individual artefacts. They also helped in the illustration of the artefacts by providing indigenous knowledge (Trowell 1957). The catalogue was also significant in structuring the layout for the classification and arrangement for the exhibitions of an African gallery at the Uganda Museum. The name of the gallery was slightly modified in 1961 to the ›Ethnography Gallery‹. Yet the mode, style of display, and labels for the artefacts remained unchanged, apart from occasional restoration. This showed that the colonial enterprise of cultural orientation had established the Protectorate Museum as an instrument of power to implement violent and coercive domination. Colonialism was also presented as part of both a supposed benevolent social uplifting, as well as a form of governance along the concept of ›tribe‹. Although the museum project was aimed at civilizing the native people in the enlightenment framework of ethnographic practice, it undermined pivotal indigenous knowledge and thus deprived communities in Uganda of the root for cultural rejuvenation and the survival of their society.

The first phase of museum development as a Protectorate Museum was, however, entirely an ethnographic project. As of 1954 in particular, the Uganda Museum was developed as a modern cultural institution in Uganda to expand the ethnographic project. The museum was opened on 30th June 1954 by Uganda's Governor, Sir Andrew Cohen. During the enforcement of the last stages of colonial rule, the official opening of the Uganda Museum was deemed a failure in terms of its exhibition displays (Wachsmann 1954: 3). There were encounters from farmers' groups and trade union boycotts against the colonial regime (Kibanja et al. 2012: 412). Many of the artefacts in the wooden cabinets remained in the basement storage. The visitors were directed toward the basement storage area and the objects in it were labelled ›ethnographic‹ (Wachsmann 1954: 4). In addition to displaying ethnographic objects from the museum's storeroom, the museum curators also created an installation in the newly-finished exhibition gallery to illustrate a certain category of ›tribal‹ people as Nilo-Hamite ›tribes‹. This exhibition was also interactive, offering a sound installation of ›tribal‹ music played from upstairs (ibid.). Hence, in this first exhibition of what was crafted as a modern museum in Uganda, the society was divided into ›tribes‹.

As the transformation of the Protectorate Museum took effect, the incorporation of the ethnographic artefacts paved the way for the process of civilizing the society. The project that the colonial masters embarked on was to train young people in missionary schools to adopt Western ways of life against the purportedly primitive life of the natives. The indigenous life and the material culture were deemed to be of low quality and were termed a primitive technology (Bennett 1995: 6). The young Ugandan people were told to stay away from this primitive life. Hence, the perspective of the colonial civilization aimed to antagonize Ugandan cultural knowledge. The missionary training then depicted young people from the ›savage‹ culture with fetish objects of a past primitive life. Within the museum framing, the idea of fetishized objects was carefully reorganised into the ethnographic displays. The modern Uganda Museum and its curatorial practice took a hold of its ethnography as a discipline and exhibitionary architecture of ›tribal‹ people. Inside the museum, this was illustrated by a diorama map of the people and landscape of Uganda, distinctively identifying separated people, fixed in a constant location.

The Uganda Museum and Nation Formation

Following Uganda's independence from colonial rule in 1962, the management of the museum and the ethnographic collections became state policy. This national state was a project of ethnography through the colonial framework of policies and regulations that were aimed at governing the society. When the ›tribal‹ ethnographic objects were assembled at the Uganda Museum, they were arranged into agricultural tools, homestead utensils, leisure, adornment and clothing, hunting, local industries of blacksmithing, salt mining, leather works and barkcloth making (Trowell 1957: 74). There was also an introduction of scientific and industrial ›development‹ exhibition models and a presentation of modern photography in Uganda. Alongside the ethnographic displays and the modern industrial shows at the Uganda Museum, Kibuuka objects were considered of national significance in the ethnographic collections in 1962. These were a set of ritual objects belonging to Kibuuka who was chief of the god of war in the Buganda kingdom. Kibuuka was a contemporary of King Nakibenge of the Buganda kingdom. Kibuuka's remains had been preserved in a barkcloth. The jawbone, umbilical cord and other objects were kept by priestess Muzingu in a shrine for worship in Mpigi within the Buganda area (Roscoe 1911: 301; Welbourn 1962: 16). However, before Uganda's independence, the Buganda minister of education Abubakar Kakyama Mayanja campaigned for the return of the Kibuuka objects in 1961 (Mayanja 1961; Bennett 2018: 217). After the Kibuuka objects were returned to Uganda in July 1962, they were first remade into historical objects and subsequently national treasures. They were then integrated into the ethno-history gallery of the Uganda Museum (Peterson 2015: 15). The Kibuuka objects were returned on long-term loan by the Museum of Archaeology and Anthropology at the University of Cambridge to the Uganda Museum. The assemblage of the Kibuuka objects on display coincided with the opening of the Science Gallery at Uganda Museum by the Prime Minister Milton Obote on the eve of independence on 8th October 1962. They were thus integrated into attempts to reintroduce ethnically defined cultural artefacts into the modern nation state.

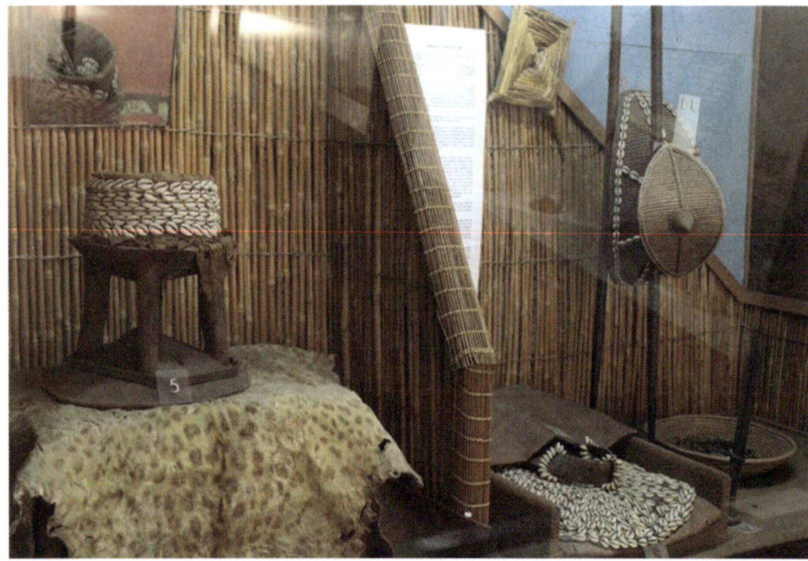

Fig. 2: Kibuuka Objects redisplayed in 1962 after they were returned from the Cambridge University Museum of Archaeology and Anthropology. Ethnohistory Gallery, Uganda Museum. Photo: Nelson Adebo Abiti.

Politically, Mayanja was celebrated for having repatriated the Kibuuka artefacts, as Nicholas Thomas puts it: »Kibuuka relics were returned to Kampala« (Thomas 2016: 340f.). The process of repatriation was also supported by the Uganda Museum curators. Nonetheless, at the time of the returning Kibuuka Mayanja's involvement was viewed with caution by the new government since the ethnic divisions were rampant and had escalated to physical violence by the time the British protectorate government began to enforce colonial conquest. Mayanja's political demand for the return of Kibuuka in 1961 was partially achieved through the Cambridge University deciding on the Kibuuka objects to be repatriated and displayed at the Uganda Museum in Kampala. Since 1961, the continued holding of the Kibuuka objects in Uganda had been contentious. As Nicholas noted, in November 2007, the Kibuuka's followers had stormed the Uganda Museum, intending to seize the relics but were prevented by the police guards of the Uganda Museum (Thomas 2016). Hence the British colonial power had much influence on the Uganda Museum concerning the conservation and presenting the cultural objects that belonged to indigenous communities.

However, the politics of national identity and museum practice in the post-independence period led to abolishing the functions of a royal system of governance that later caused the attack on the Buganda palace in 1966 and the subsequent confiscation of royal regalia by President Milton Obote in 1967. The confiscation of the royal artefacts was part of the militarization of the nation (Peterson 2015). National policies also led to changes in the state's approach to governing the collection of objects. This suggests that the militarization of the nation and the violence in Uganda had, and continue to have, implications for the ways through which 21st century museum practices are thought, and through which they change the meanings of ethnographic objects.

In contrast to the above, however, the Uganda National Museum also began to engage in documenting, collecting and exhibiting experiences of violence. This is pertinent given that the museum has aimed to recover the memory of violence and trauma experienced between 1986 and 2006 through its more recent work. Particularly in the Northern part of Uganda, a civil war had occurred for a period of two decades between 1986 and 2006 which had a devastating and traumatic impact on women and children. The hostilities, spanning two decades, saw the government soldiers of Uganda on the one side and the Lord Resistance Army (LRA) rebels led by Joseph Kony on the other. The prolonged civil war in Northern Uganda caused death, displacement, and the abduction of children. More than two million people were forced to seek refuge in congested Internally Displaced People (IDPs) camps (Mwenda 2010). About twenty-five thousand children were abducted. This culminated in the phenomenon of night commuters in Uganda – children walking into Gulu at night seeking protection in the urban area and in camps for internally displaced people (Annan/Blattmann/Horton 2006). The issue in the post-conflict situation was to understand the memory of traumatic experiences, consciously appropriated as spirit beliefs and Acholi culture in the region.

The conflict had changed the landscape in Northern Uganda as well as people's mind-set, it required a process of resettlement in addition to reconstruction programs that could take the communities' cultural memory into account. In post-conflict reconstruction efforts, it is crucial that communities acknowledge the suffering caused to the survivors of the wars and the victims' experience of bodily harm suffered in the course of the violence and injustice enacted against the indigenous community. The recognition of the elders by the Uganda National Museum as key stakeholders in the reconstruction of cultural heritage was a positive step for documenting the difficult heritage of war. Indeed, the elders of Northern Uganda had foreseen the need to document cultural sites with significant memories and to preserve traditional dances, songs, and rituals as a way of rebuilding society with a dignified identity. This insight was a result of their long-standing experience in peace mediation, conciliatory effort, and uniting community.

Community Reconciliations

In Northern Uganda, the community memorialization was a form of bottom-up approach in a process of remembering the pains of war in a post-conflict situation. This community memorialization was a result of the aftermath of what happened when the civil war between the Lord's Resistance Army (LRA) in Northern Uganda and National government soldiers broke out. The project on *A Memorial Landscape in a Post-Conflict Situation* and a mobile exhibition was implemented as *The Road to Reconciliation*. The team from the Uganda Museum collaborated with the communities and also continued to engage with civil society, religious leaders, the elders and the survivors. The beginning of a dialogue on memorial practices enabled the Uganda Museum to start rethinking its strategy towards community memorialization. In my involvement with the project, the idea of an alternative model of learning with divergent views in a contested space of violence came to the fore (Abiti 2018). The experiences and knowledge gained from continuous interactions with people living in and around the four sites in Northern Uganda provided the project with an outcome for the exhibition on reconciliation and forgiveness.

The transition from war to peace required the re-introduction of *Mato oput*. This traditional ritual of healing and reconciliation was a form of reintegrating offending individuals – including former members of the LRA rebels – into their communities. The complexity of working with communities who knew their members as perpetrators, victims and bystanders was resolved by the communities themselves. The Ugandan writer Okot P'Bitek (1971: 155) pointed out that »the blood-feud, *kwor,* must be settled and if it is not settled the ghost of the deceased will bring much trouble to his kinsmen« (see also Onyango-Ku-Odongo/Webster 1976: 61–65). In addition to *Mato oput*, the Northern Uganda Transition Initiative (NUTI) was also founded in order to undertake reburials and reintegrate former abductees into the communities by stepping on eggs, or *wong tong* – a purification ritual in Acholi. In this context, reburials were »efforts to remake homes and reorder lives«, in a continued climate of uncertainty, by relocating the dead or materialities associated with them »from sites of displacement to former homesteads« (Jahn/Wilhelm-Solomon 2015: 182). These ritual ceremonies were performed because of post-war, psycho-social traumas that occurred when communities lost their relatives in the wars. At the site of my own participation, the implementation of the program demonstrated that the Uganda National Museum's work not only documented the reburials, it also helped to shed light on the problems that the continuous existence of unburied dead and missing persons – having neither graves nor representation – posed to the survivors and communities. The unresolved questions created a demand for curatorial practices at the museum as a forum of dialogue. By 2010, the Uganda National Museum had, as such, sought to change its curatorial practice by enabling processes of mediation. The conversations with the survivors of war became meaningful when the communities began opening up by talking and providing ideas as to what is meant by knowledge of the past. The question, for example, of how we can make such knowledge useful to young people was posed. To which the answer emerged that it was the respect we gave them, and our deep listening that provided a platform for us to create a fruitful network of working with post-conflict survivors. Women and men were equal, each of them taking responsibility. We ate food together and we shared moments of joy. Yet the question remains: How do you maintain a network of diverse needs and how do you continue working with people that have narratives contrary to the official stories of national and state policies?

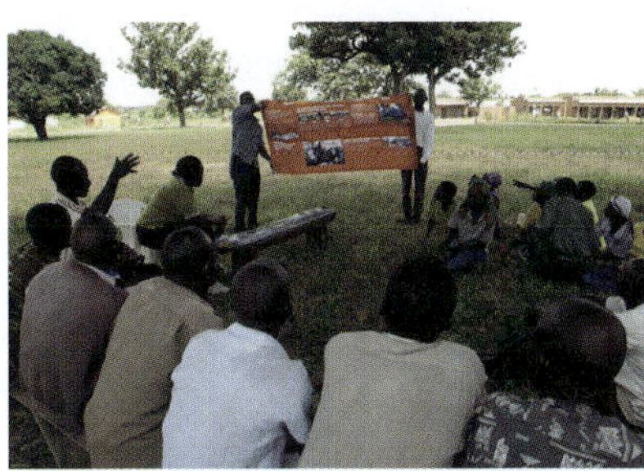

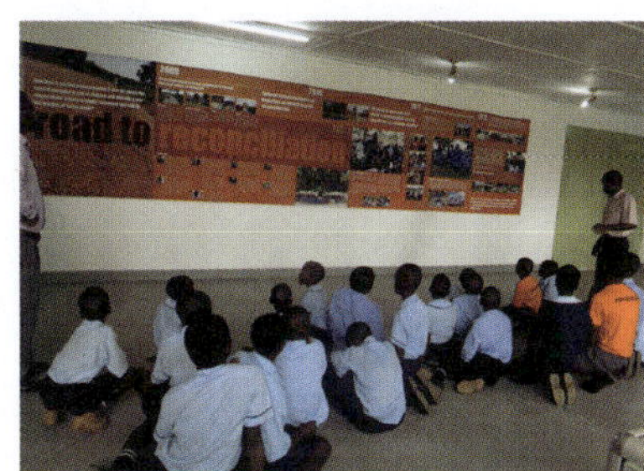

Fig. 3 and 4: Dialogue on the community-led exhibition »road to reconciliation«: with survivors of a massacre at the IDP camp Barlonyo, and with a young audience. Photo: Nelson Adebo Abiti.

Artefact Reactivation

Certain cultural objects, such as spears, were central in the mediation work. The Uganda museum began to collaborate with the community in reinvigorating the *Mato oput* ritual practice. Why is it that the idea of new forums and community collaborations became significant to the society? The *Mato oput* ritual is an indigenous mode of a certain traditional justice mechanism, which was used to reconcile families from the angers and pains of violence that had occurred in the recent civil wars. The Uganda Museum, therefore, also used its space to create a forum of creating community exhibitions on reconciliation. The collection of spears in the museum provided an important means to ritually integrate the communities into rituals of reconciliation. Originally collected by the colonialists as artefacts of warriors, they had been mainly displayed to show ›tribal‹ wars. In contrast, when the Uganda Museum decided to take the objects from storage and to offer them to the community for rituals, it reactivated their lives. Important artefacts such as spears also inherited the injustice and cruelty that had been enacted against communities. Originally, the spears had been serially classified on the basis of ethnic identity. Dialogical efforts made by the Uganda Museum to reunite artefacts with communities would begin a process of addressing structures, which have been in place since the foundation of colonialism. Beyond the violence that has burdened and caused traumas to communities, the Uganda Museum is attempting to remake the personhood of artefacts into a new form of knowledge that enables communities to perform certain rituals and ceremonies.

Documenting memories of violence is not a question of obsessively collecting objects, it is about enabling voices of communities and amplifying their ritual practices.

The concept sought out and collected traces of material culture that would enable community memorials to take place rather than simply collecting everything into museum storage. The spears in Northern Uganda became important cultural objects for performing rituals of forgiveness during the reburial of the dead, the enthronement of cultural leaders and for mediating peaceful resolution in events of clan conflicts. Beyond their use as weaponry, they perform a healing process. The presence of oral histories and local knowledge systems embodied in artefacts challenges the colonial idea of transforming cultural materials into tangible museum objects in displays. Although colonial structures disrupted the orality of heritage, it is certainly the case that feasts, which are of importance to the society, as well as stories and touch have now been re-enacted to renew the life of artefacts. The physical materiality is remade in intangible practices.

My argument here is that orality is important in expressing the utility of tangible cultural material. The ›spear‹, which was once reduced to a serialised artefact of fighting amongst the warriors, regains its capacity to resolve conflict in the post war reconciliation process of Northern Uganda. Notably, memorial spaces of the communities in Northern Uganda have remade the material objects such as drums, spears, beads, and musical instruments as important tools for reconciliation and peace-building initiatives. Indeed, some fundamental questions emerge in addressing the community practices of memorialization in Northern Uganda; first, why are the communities using the spears in dances or *Mato oput* rituals for reconciliation when, in a very real sense, spears are meant as tools for hunting or fighting in war?

The spear has been the most important object embodied in the ritual process of reconciliation. In the account of these, the spear manifests itself as a symbol of authority, dancing ephemera and bending into performing reconciliation ceremonies. In mythical tales, the spear belonged to the eldest son whose father would hand over his power of authority through the spear. In contrast, certain situations reveal that the inheritors of the spear are not necessarily the eldest heirs. Colonial anthropologists have documented certain intangible beliefs whereby the function of the spear is to perform the ceremony of the *Jok* spirit in the Patiko chiefdom (Girling 1960). However, the original meaning of such intangible practices is not so readily comprehensible in the written records. When I asked the current chiefs in Northern Uganda whether they had such important royal spears in their possession, they were able to identify the objects but they did not own any of the typical double-head spears in the regalia. There are possible reasons why spears were lost during the war or why there are no specialised blacksmiths making such spears in this particular society. It is clear that the double-headed spears are not easily seen within the communities; they possess secret functions among the indigenous communities. But although the intangible knowledge of reactivating the power of spears was threatened by colonial violence it survived in the transmission of oral expressions amongst the elderly population. Moreover, accessing important cultural objects remained often difficult for the elderly and thus the challenge remained to demonstrate the intangible knowledge practices such as the *Mato oput* and reburials at all. Therefore, the community collaborations with the museum are a form of sharing the artefacts and the immaterial knowledge. While the Uganda Museum once held the artefacts, they now become useful to the communities in order to facilitate solutions to their problems. The museum is being redefined to work outside of its structural wall through the activity of engaging with the communities.

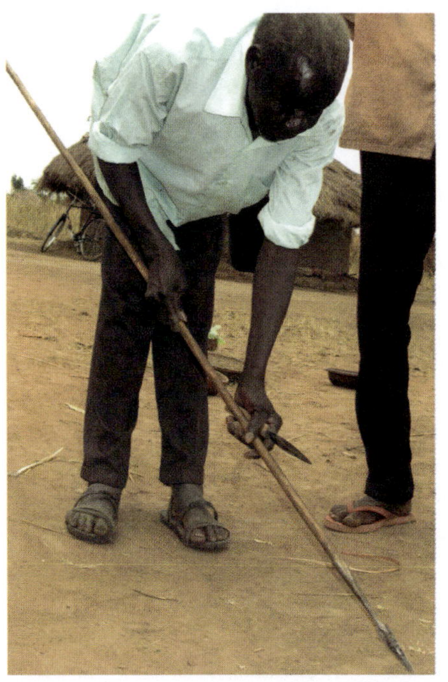
Fig. 5: Elder demonstrating ritual use of spear for Mato Oput, in Okoro village, Gulu district, Northern Uganda. 2014. Photo: Nelson Adebo Abiti.

Following the above discussion, spears are clearly significant objects in ritual performance as well as symbols of authority. In most cases the spears animate spirits during the annual feasts of *Jok* presided over by the priest or *Ajwaka* (p'Bitek 1971). When the spears are transformed from an artefact into a spirit, they acquire a power, by which they embody the new life of ancestors (Ocholla-Ayayo 1980: 101). In contrast, the ethnographic practices of collecting artefacts were violent. By displaying ethnographic objects without providing an historical analysis, we continue to ignore colonial violence, and we continue to promote colonialism and the acts of injustice. Yet the style of the museum, with its ethnographic gallery display, is old and it raises the question of visualising exotic representation. Unfortunately, Ugandans are faced with the question of mirroring themselves in the foreign narratives enacted in the museum. What kind of stories do we want to tell contemporary Ugandans? How does a young audience interact with the exhibitions linked to violence? Will the Ugandan Museum's old exhibitions be reorganized? And if so, how and who will be involved? Will the process of reimagining the practice of a new museology become institutionalized in management practice? What will finally happen to the concept of ethnography in museums? Should it be a dialogue, a rethinking, a reconciliation and a questioning of the old gallery?

A focus on investigating the ideas on colonialism suggests that the problems encountered within the ethnographic museum were constituted by discriminatory policies of divide and conquer as well as the creation of ethnic or ›tribal‹ cultures. Yet these museums accumulated the cultural property of colonial injustices, which enabled the imperial powers to subdue human beings in an evolutionary scheme. In the language of imperialism, the clue to the native society was to use the materiality of their cultural objects to understand and control local systems of power. Hence, the ›tribe‹ in Uganda is linked to the colonial marker of managing people into ›tribal peoples‹ as seen in the present ethnographic diorama display at the Uganda Museum.

Therefore, the community memorial practice – proffered in the new form of museum practice – is an attempt to enable a museum community to work on restitution, decolonization and healing from violence in the form of a community project. Yet bridging the gap of colonial injustices and rebuilding the society require, in my view, a public discourse of listening to, and working with, the relevant societies. The example of the communities in Northern Uganda, who embarked on social ceremonies as form of healing, are significant insofar as they highlight cultural ways of transmitting knowledge. It has shown how the reactivation of intangible memories can help to manage conflicts and rebuild societies, using objects to express reconciliation in Northern Uganda (Abiti 2018). The process of community memorial also points to a debate on understanding the processes of memory-making in a local community, including how people's participation in a museum project might define its future outcome.

This article has undergone a double-blind peer-review.

Literature

Abiti, Nelson Adebo (2018): »The Road to Reconciliation. Museum Practice, Community Memorials and Collaborations in Uganda«. In: *Museum Cooperation between Africa and Europe: A New Field for Museum Studies*, ed. by Thomas Laely/Marc Meyer/Raphael Schwere, Bielefeld: transcript Verlag, 83–96.

Annan, Jeanie/Blattman, Christopher/Horton, Roger (2006): *The State of Youth and Youth Protection in Northern Uganda. Findings from the Survey for War Affected Youth*. Kampala: UNICEF, https://chrisblattman.com/documents/policy/sway/SWAY.Phase1.FinalReport.pdf (30.06.2021).

Allen, Tim/Vlassenroot, Koen (Eds.) (2010): *The Lord's Resistance Army: Myth and Reality*, London: Zed Books.

Assmann, Jan (2013): »Communicative and Cultural Memory«. In: *Cultural Memories. The Geographical Point of View*, ed. by Peter Meusberger/Michael Heffernan/Edgar Wunder, Dordrecht: Springer, 15–27.

Bennett, Alison (2018): »Diplomatic Gifts: Rethinking Colonial Politics in Uganda through Objects«. In: *History in Africa* 45, 193–220.

Bennett, Tony (1995): *The Birth of the Museum: History, Theory, Politics*, London, New York: Routledge.

Clifford, James (1988): *The Predicament of Culture: Twentieth-Century Ethnography, Literature, and Art*, Harvard: Harvard University Press.

Coombes, Annie E. (1994): *Reinventing Africa: Museums, Material Culture, and Popular Imagination in Late Victorian and Edwardian England*, New Haven, London: Yale University Press.

Deming, L. M. (1966): *The History of the Uganda Museum*. Kampala: Uganda Museum.

Girling Frank K. (1960): *The Acholi of Uganda*, London: Her Majesty's Stationery Office.

Harris, Clare/O'Hanlon, Michael (2013): »The Future of Ethnographic Museums«. In: *Anthropology Today* 29(1), 8–12.

Hicks, Dan (2020). *The Brutish Museums. The Benin Bronzes, Colonial Violence, and Cultural Restitution*, London: Pluto Press.

Jahn, Ina Rehema/Wilhelm-Solomon, Matthew (2015): »›Bones in the Wrong Soil‹: Reburial, Belonging and Cosmologies Exhumed in Post-Conflict Northern Uganda«. In: *Critical African Studies*, 7(2), 182–201.

Johnston, Harry Hamilton (1902): The Uganda Protectorate. *An Attempt to Give Some Description of the Physical Geography, Botany, Zoology, Anthropology, Languages and History of the Territories Under British Protection in East Central Africa, Between the Congo Free State and the Rift Valley and Between the First Degree of South Latitude and the Fifth Degree of North Latitude*, Vol. 2, London: Hutchinson and Co.

Kibanja, Grace/Kajumba, Mayanja/Johnson, Laura (2012): »Ethnocultural Conflict in Uganda: Politics Based on Ethnic Divisions Inflame Tensions Across the Country«. In: *Handbook of Ethnic Conflict*, Boston: Springer, 403–435.

Konaré, Alpha Oumar (1983): »Towards A New Type of ›Ethnographic‹ Museum in Africa«. In: *Museum International* 35(3), 146–151.

Lidchi, Henrietta (1997): *The Poetics and Politics of Exhibiting Other Cultures*, London: Sage/Open University Press.

Mamdani, Mahmood (1996): *Citizen and subject: Contemporary Africa and the Legacy of Late Colonialism*, Princeton: Princeton University Press.

Mayanja, Abubakar (1961): *Letter to the Vice Chancellor of the Cambridge University*, Museum of Archaeology and Anthropology at the University of Cambridge, file AA4/5/15.

Mwenda, Andrew (2010): »Uganda's Politics of Foreign Aid and Violent Conflict: The Political Uses of the LRA Rebellion«. In: *The Lord's Resistance Army: Myth and Reality*, ed. by Tim Allen/Koen Vlassenroot, London: Zed Books, 45–58.

Ocholla-Ayayo, A. B. C. (1980): *The Luo culture: A Reconstruction of the Material Culture Patterns of a Traditional African Society*, Wiesbaden: Steiner.

Otunnu, Ogenga. (2016): *Crisis of Legitimacy and Political Violence in Uganda, 1890 to 1979*, Cham: Palgrave.

P'Bitek, Okot. (1971): *Religion of the Central Luo*, Nairobi: East African Literature Bureau.

Onyango-Ku-Odongo, Jamal Mikla/ Webster, James Bertin (1976): *The Central Lwo During the Aconya*, Nairobi: East African Literature Bureau.

Peterson, Derek (2015): *Politics of Heritage in Africa*, Cambridge: Cambridge University Press.

Posnansky, Merrick (1963): »The Uganda Museum, Kampala: The Programme and the Organization«. In: *Museum International* 16(3), 149–162.

Rassool, Ciraj (2015): »Re-storing the Skeletons of Empire: Return, Reburial and Rehumanisation in Southern Africa«. In: *Journal of Southern African Studies* 41(3), 653–670.

Reeves, Scott/Kuper, Ayelet/Hodges (2008): »Qualitative Research Methodologies: Ethnography«. In: *Bmj* 337, https://doi.org/10.1136/bmj.a1020 (30.06.2021).

Reis, Ria (2013): »Children Enacting Idioms of Witchcraft and Spirit Possession as a Response to Trauma: Therapeutically Beneficial, and for Whom«. In: *Transcultural Psychiatry* 50(5), 622–643.

Roscoe, John (1911): *The Baganda: An Account of Their Native Customs and Beliefs*, London: Macmillan.

Sarr, Felwine/Savoy, Bénédicte (2018): *The Restitution of African Cultural Heritage: Toward a New Relational Ethics*, http://restitutionreport2018.com/sarr_savoy_en.pdf (30.06.19).

Thomas, Nicholas (2016): »The Inhabited Collection«. In: *The Antioch Review* 74(2), 333–342.

Trowell, Margaret (1957): *The African Tapestry*, London: Faber and Faber.

Trowell, Margaret/Wachsmann, Klaus P. (1953): *Tribal Crafts of Uganda*, London: Oxford University Press.

Uganda Protectorate (1931): *The Report of the Protectorate Museum, Kampala:* Uganda Museum Archive.

Uganda Protectorate (1939): *Report of the Uganda Museum Committee*, Entebbe: Uganda.

Wachsmann, Klaus (1954): »Curators Report«. In: *Uganda Museum Occasional Paper*, 3–4.

Welbourn, Fred B. (1962): »Kibuuka Comes Home«. In: *Transition* 5, 15–20.

Wilson, George (1907): »The Progress of Uganda«. In: *Journal of the Royal African Society*, 6(22): 113–35.

Wilson, George (1908): *Deputy Commissioner's Circular of January 15, 1908*, Uganda National Museum Archive, Courtesy of the Uganda National Museum.

Table of figures

Challenges of Re-Writing the Iziko Ethnographic Collections Archives: Some Lessons from the Khomani San/Bushmen Engagement

Paul Tichmann and Lynn Abrahams

The authors of this article are both museum professionals within the Iziko Museums and as such have come to inherit the ›skeletons in the cupboard‹. We would prefer to believe that, having been active participants in the struggle against apartheid and wrestling with issues of identity in post-apartheid South Africa, we have a critical approach in our museum practice. However, as insiders of an institution that has roots in the colonial and apartheid eras and which continues to wrestle with transforming its structures, practices, and content, we cannot avoid complicity. The dilemma we face, then, is how to be agents of transformation while, at the same time, being part of an institution that has its foundations in colonialism and apartheid.

Achille Mbembe argues »Archiving is a kind of internment, laying something in a coffin, if not to rest, then at least to consign elements of that life which could not be destroyed purely and simply« (Mbembe 2002: 22). He further argues that the process of assigning materials to archives gives such materials an unquestionable authority that neutralises the violence and cruelty of the ›remains‹ (cf. ibid.: 22). This certainly holds true for much of the ethnographic collections in South African museums. While several museums in South Africa grapple with the reburial of human remains in their collections, a spectre from the colonial past, the equally important task of interrogating the museum archives, linked to ethnographic collections, is yet to be adequately addressed.

Laura Gibson contends that South African museums have failed to interrogate the ›rules of practice‹ for constructing knowledge, pointing out that »cataloguing, classifying and collecting processes are the foundational level at which museums produce knowledge« (Gibson 2019: 25). Similarly, Leslie Witz et al. argue that in South Africa the museum has failed »to critically examine its own history of collecting« and museums, therefore, remained trapped in their »classificatory system in which the exhibitionary and ethnographic work« (Witz et al. 1999: 13) remains separate from notions of history. There is often a tendency to separate museum collections from the idea of archives, and museums have neither confronted their collecting practices nor systematically interrogated the museum documentation or archives. Witz criticizes that museums, instead of interrogating their classificatory formations, opted to become inclusive by simply

urn:nbn:de:hbz:6:3-zfk-2021-41930

adding more »voices, objects and explanations to give them the authority of a factual past« (Witz 2012: 13). Contributing to this argument, Steven Dubin argues that museums were »playing catch up, striving to fill in what they recognize as wide gaps in their holdings« (Dubin 2009: 5). In attempting to enact transformation in democratic South Africa, the tendency has been for museums to adopt an add-on approach that seeks to ›fill the gap‹ by bringing in some new narratives and interpretations rather than critically engaging with the flawed narratives that are part of their legacy of colonialism and apartheid. These add-ons, according to Witz et al., allowed museums to insert themselves into the discourse on »South Africa's public history and the heritage of all citizens« (Witz et al. 1999: 12). Rogoff, furthermore, argues that the add-on effect is carried forward by the »belief that we can simply insert other histories into a grand narrative of Modernism and ignore the conflict between hegemonic and marginally-located cultures« (2002: 5).

As Gibson states, »we need to understand not only the types of narratives that are told by the museum's collections and documentation but also why and how others are (still) excluded« (Gibson 2019: 236). If museums want to meaningfully engage with cultural diversity and decolonize their collections, classificatory and exhibitionary practices, and processes, they have to »recognize the shift from the compensatory projects of atoning for absences and replacing voids, to a performative one in which loss is not only enacted, but is made manifest from within the culture that has remained a seemingly invulnerable dominant« (Rogoff 2002: 3).

A focus on the ethnographic archive at the Iziko Museums cannot avoid acknowledging the complexities of the human remains, which form part of these collections. Ciraj Rassool (2015: 654) has pointed out that the collecting of artefacts relating to the San, now located in our museum, was carried out alongside the ›plunder of graves‹. Legassick and Rassool (2000) have demonstrated the involvement of museums in South Africa in the trade in human remains for purposes of racial science during the colonial period. They also suggest »it might be the case that the entry of such remains into museums and such racial research at the beginning of the twentieth century were at the centre of the transformation of the museum in South Africa as an institution of order, knowledge and classification« (Legassick/Rassool 2000 1f.). To what extent are we still bound by these systems of »order, knowledge, and classification«?

An innovative attempt to raise critique concerning museum classification and knowledge production came in the form of the exhibition *Miscast: Negotiating the Presence of the Bushmen*, curated by Pippa Skotnes and installed at the South African National Gallery in 1996. The exhibition attempted, through a strong visual display that included body casts, photographs, anthropological field notes and museums accession notes, to critique the misrepresentation and dehumanisation of the Bushmen in museums in South Africa. Thus the curator intended to make Western scientific practices inherited by museums visible and bring into question museum practices related to human remains and the representation of ›other‹ cultures. In a review on the exhibition, Michael Morris argued that the exhibition would »invigorate difficult debates in cultural museum circles on displaying human remains to illustrate and explain the identity, nature and culture of people« (Morris 1996). Though the exhibition was met with ambivalence, it provoked substantial debate and dialogue on the representation of San material culture and human remains. In its *Sunday Culture* column, the Sunday Independent of 26 May 1996 pointed out that the exhibition provoked »animated and heated debate in the media and in university seminars and staff tearooms. In addition, a plethora of local groups had emerged claiming to be descendants of the Khoisan and the legitimate representatives and custodians of Khoisan past« (Sunday Independent 1996: 23). In many of the reviews on the exhibition, Skotnes was severely criticised and her motives questioned. She was accused of ›self-promotion‹, of being ›insensitive‹, and of ›appropriation‹ and ›recolonization‹ of history. On the other hand, there were some who »wholeheartedly endorsed and praised« the *Miscast* exhibition (ibid.: 26). Some critics classified the exhibition as thought-provoking, raising both genuine praises and concerns (ibid.). Irrespective of its reception, the exhibition's success can be measured in the dialogue on transformation and identity it brought into the public domain. It forced people to rethink how they were classified as well as how knowledge concerning their history and culture is produced, interpreted and narrated.

The Iziko Museums have come to inherit these human remains, procured by the South African Museums, and the challenge is to restore dignity and humanity to these remains as well as to the descendants, including Khoi, San and Nguni communities.[1] Objects of San[2] material culture, human remains, and photographs were collected from the early formation of the South African Museum (now the Iziko South African Museum), which was established in 1825. Ciraj Rassool points out that »these collections and records were assembled in the attempt to study pasts without memory that were active and effective in the present« (Rassool 2015: 654). Human remains and grave goods were collected and incorporated into the ethnographic collections of museums as objects, either for display or in pursuit of ›racial science‹. These indigenous San objects, human remains, and grave goods were framed through the scientific lens of anthropology and archaeology, and were incorporated into museums as ethnographic collections. In South African museums indigenous objects and remains were collected and »exhibited in natural history museums, as opposed to cultural history museums or art museums« (Coombes 2003: 209). This was to »illustrate the progress made by European civilization and the white race, compared to primitive cultures« (Gore 2004: 33). It is this agency of power and authority over the production and dissemination of knowledge that has to be interrogated, investigated and re-interpreted in the post-apartheid museum. Indigenous communities started demanding representation in museum narratives but also wanted to become active participants in the rewriting of the colonial archive, represented through museums as well as government archives, which had ›locked them in time‹. These demands created tension between the colonial archive represented through museums as well as state archives, and the post-apartheid mandate of an inclusive archive which purports representation of the nation's diverse history. In addition, these demands are linked to

1 The human remains collection at the Iziko Museums also includes remains from Namibia, Botswana and Australia.

2 Some indigenous communities prefer to be identified as ›Bushman‹ rather than ›San‹. A number of researchers have commented on the fact that both of these terms are problematic, having been thrust on communities, and that some indigenous communities prefer to ›self-identify‹.

reclaiming identity, language, culture, and the restoration of dignity, as well as to the need for an alternative voice to the narratives of colonialism and apartheid.

The Iziko Museums hold 195 unethically-collected human remains, including a number of body casts and moulds. The human remains and casts are not available for exhibition, research or viewing. The Iziko Museums developed a human remains policy in 2002 in an attempt to chart a way forward for the reburial and repatriation of human remains. However, the process of restitution and repatriation has been hampered by, amongst other challenges, the lack of a national policy and legislation for restitution and repatriation, incomplete documentation on the remains collected, and lack of a budget to cover the costs of consultation and reburial ceremonies. A positive step towards reburials was recently taken through a collaborative project involving the Iziko Museums, the Department of Sport, Arts and Culture (DSAC), the South African Heritage Resources Agency (SAHRA), the Khoi-Boesman, and the Nguni Coalition, all in relation to the so-called Colesberg 52. At the time of the *Miscast* exhibition, a Griquas group lobbied the government in an effort to focus attention on their ancestral burial graves and called for the reburial of the »Colesberg remains« (Maykuth 1996). The Colesberg 52, victims of a smallpox epidemic in 1866, were exhumed from a grave outside Colesberg in the Northern Cape and incorporated into the South African Museum collections for purposes of ›race-based science‹. According to Tanya Peckmann »these individuals were probably an indigenous Khoe community who lived on the outskirts of town but provided the rural and urban population with a cheap source of labour« (Peckmann 2003: 290). The Covid-19 pandemic and subsequent lockdown unfortunately thwarted plans to hold a consultation meeting with the community of Colesberg planned for 22 March 2020.

In considering how to rewrite the colonial archives linked to our social history collections at the Iziko Museums, we have to acknowledge and interrogate the violence and racism that is, in a sense, a stain on the Khomani San collections in our museums. We also have to acknowledge the power of museums in creating ›knowledge‹ and ›truths‹ through the selections we make in exhibiting objects of material culture. Patricia Davison points out that »museums give material form to authorized versions of the past, which in time became institutionalized as public memory« (Davison 1998: 145).

After many years of discussion and deliberation, the controversial Ethnographic Gallery at Iziko South African Museum was finally de-installed on 15 September 2017. The decision elicited a range of interesting and conflicting responses. While a number of Khoisan chiefs and descendants asserted that the closure of the gallery was overdue, several members of the public, including some Khoisan descendants, complained about the closure. A retired historian from the University of Cape Town argued that it was a »grave mistake« to close the diorama as it could be used »to show the history of what colonialism did to the hunters and herders of the Cape« (Smith 2017: 9). One group of doctoral students staged an intervention, closing the Ethnographic Gallery space off with tape declaring the space to be »A colonial crime scene« and holding a performance; *Ndabamnye neenkumbulo nemiphefumlo enxaniweyo* (I became one with memories and thirsty souls). The curators of the intervention argued that »the objects in the gallery are in fact evidence of colonial crimes and require decolonial investigation« (Art Africa 2018).

One of the stakeholders we consulted about the closure of the Ethnographic Gallery was the Khoi-Boesman-Nguni Coalition, which was critical of the ethnographic display and proposed a cleansing ceremony in the space. They then performed the ceremony on 7 August 2017, in order to pray for forgiveness, demonstrate repentance for the way in which the history and culture of black peoples had been portrayed, and to sanctify the space. The Khoi-Boesman-Nguni Coalition was formed around March 2017 to campaign for the return of human remains. »Led by Chief Melvin Arendse of the Kei Korana, the Coalition brought together Khoi-, San- and Xhosa-speaking groups. Chief Arendse asserted that the ›Nguni and Khoi‹ had a long history and formed the first alliances against colonialism« (Evans 2017).

One of the questions we face as museum practitioners is how to acknowledge the violence, dislocation and pain that haunts collections such as those of the Khomani San in a way that contributes to healing and social justice. Anne Wanless has indicated that a set of manacles, used on Bushmen prisoners, was amongst the collections donated to the South African Museum by the collector Dr Louis Fourie, Medical Officer for the Protectorate of South West Africa and amateur anthropologist (cf. Wanless 2007: 20). These manacles are not part of the San collections. Instead, they have been grouped with artefacts associated with slavery as opposed to falling within the narrative of San oppression and dislocation. This kind of *unremembering* of history testifies to the ways in which colonial archives were twisted, falsified, and or marginalized. If we wish to decolonize the colonial archive, we need to interrogate processes and practices that lead to such *unremembering*, while beginning a process of correcting such historical falsifications.

There have been shifts within the museums in South Africa. These have variously occurred as both a result and interplay of reflections on particular practices and their relevance, as well as external pressure from the government and relevant stakeholders. During the colonial and apartheid period, collections relating to the Bantu-speaking groups, Khoi and San, were housed at the South African Museum alongside natural history collections, while collections relating to Europe and European descendants, as well as to Asia and Asian descendants, were housed in the South African Cultural History Museum. Ironically, the South African History Museum, occupying a site that was formerly that of the Dutch East India Company's Slave Lodge, made virtually no reference to the history of slavery at the Cape. In an often-quoted speech given during a Heritage Day address at Robben Island Museum in September 1997, Nelson Mandela called for the transformation of South African museums, stating that

> »when our museums and monuments preserve the whole of our diverse heritage, when they are inviting to the public and interact with the changes all around them, then they will strengthen our attachment to human rights, mutual respect and democracy, and help prevent these ever again being violated« (Mandela 1997).

On 4 December 1998 the Cultural Institutions Act was promulgated, providing for the amalgamation of some of the national museums to form two flagship institutions: the Northern Flagship (now Ditsong Museums) in Pretoria and the Southern Flagship (now Iziko Museums) in Cape Town.

The Iziko Museums decided, in an attempt to transform the way in which collections were classified, to break down the divisions of the colonial and apartheid past and build diversity in museum representation, to integrate the European, Asian and ethnographic collections as social history collections. However, it has become clear that in order to bring about real integration, museum archives needed to be rewritten. Documentation accompanying the archive continues to reflect the conditions of colonialism and apartheid under which these collections were acquired. Various researchers have analysed and published on aspects of these collections. For example, Vibeke Viestad has examined San costume in depth, rejecting the myth of the ›naked Bushman‹ and demonstrating that »far from being naked, or nearly naked, Bushmen of colonial southern Africa had a complex and meaningful practice of dress that was intimately related to subsistence, identity and their perception of how to live life in the world as they knew it« (Viestad 2014: 21).

The Iziko Museums were approached by representatives of the Khomani San in November 2017 with a proposal to hold an exhibition titled *Light in the Darkness* in the space that had formerly served as the Ethnographic Gallery. The Khomani San were in the process of setting up a creative collective and in their motivation for the exhibition they stated that it was »a narrative that zooms in on the contemporary relevance of traditional Bushmen world views, unifying Bushmen communities on the one hand, but also the wider global audience that is currently looking to indigenous culture for ways of reconnecting to the natural world and to each other« (Bodenham 2017: 1). The Iziko Museums management pointed out to the Khomani San representatives that a decision had been taken not to exhibit on the Khoi and San in the gallery space until the question of exhibiting on human history alongside natural history had been resolved. The response by the Khomani was that the dichotomy between natural history and human history was a Western construct and that, in the San worldview, humans and nature are one. The proposal was turned down, much to the disappointment of the Khomani San representatives. The Collections and Digitisation department saw an opportunity to engage with the Khomani San around the collections and to bring in community narratives to Khomani collections.

Arrangements were made to transport and accommodate four leading members of the Khomani Communal Property Association – Chief Petrus Vaalbooi, traditional leader of the Khomani San, Itzak Kruiper, Lydia Kruiper and Annamarie Vaalbooi. The idea was, that the four would spend some time engaging with the collections and in discussion with the staff for the Iziko collections. We requested permission to record the proceedings via video recorder, which was granted, and a Memorandum of Agreement was concluded around the project. Interestingly, the first hurdle we ran into with the project was a challenge from the Khoi-Boesman-Nguni Coalition, who accused us of separating out the cultural history of the Khoisan, in a colonial fashion, arguing that the Khoi and San had always had an interlinked history. We acknowledged that their histories were interlinked but pointed out that we were looking at collections from a particular geographical area. This challenge left an uncomfortable feeling, however, as it raised the question of whether our approach was not ›ethnicising‹ the analysis of the history of indigenous communities. In addition, the inadequate and/or falsified recording of information in the colonial archive posed additional challenges in reconfiguring the archive. However, we also needed to acknowledge that the Khomani San were a scattered people who had been brought together for the purposes of a 1999 Land Claim. The South African apartheid government had forcibly removed the Khomani San from their ancestral lands in 1971 and the clan had become widely scattered across the Northern Cape.

The Iziko Collections and Digitisation department held a preliminary meeting with the Khomani San representatives in December 2018 to discuss the aims and objectives of the workshop around the collections and to agree on logistics and a preliminary programme. The workshop ran from the 4th to the 8th of February 2019 and was conducted in Afrikaans as the delegates did not feel confident in their English. On the first day we revisited the aims and objectives and provided an overview of the social history collections. During the discussions, Petrus Vaalbooi expressed concern over the »dying of the Nxu language«, arguing that more attention was paid to the preservation of Nama while Nxu speakers were gradually dying out. There was a sense of frustration in that several government departments had been approached but to no avail. As a collections department, we unfortunately could not be of much help in this regard. Another issue raised was the identity of the San, with Vaalbooi stating that the Bushmen had been subjected to a range of identities that had been imposed on them, from Bushman, to coloured, to San, and that his earliest recollections were of his elders using the term Saa for their self-identity. The first day of the workshop also saw the group examine the various objects in the collections, discuss the memories evoked by the collections, and also examine and comment on the information generated by the museum on the objects. Their comments on the objects of spiritual significance, such as a whisk that was used during the trance dance, and the rattles that were tied around the ankles of the dancers, made from cocoons and containing tiny stones, were of particular interest. They explained how the shaman would use the whisk to sprinkle a medicine over each dancer to give them protection and strength to access the spirit world and bring healing. They also commented on the use of tortoise shells to store buchu[3] and other medicinal herbs and the potency of the tortoise shell. In addition, they commented on the bows and arrows used during a hunt. They also mentioned the blunt arrows used in courtship. A suitor would shoot the arrow at his intended partner and if she picked it up and broke it this meant she was not interested in him. If, however, she held it against her heart, this meant she accepted his overtures.

On the second day we began with a reflection of the first day's activities. We then resumed our interaction with the object collections and the catalogue cards linked to the objects. The third day was spent on an examination of, and discussion on, the photographic collections relating to the Khomani San. During the examination of the photographs, the group, in a moment of excitement, began to communicate with each other in Nxu and we had to request that they translate the interaction in Afrikaans. In the Bleek and Lloyd photographic collection, the group were able to identify relatives and community members they had known. Lydia Kruiper identified her father, brothers and other community members, who had been photographed during a healing ceremony, as well as during hunts. She was able to provide background information on her family and other community members. Petrus Vaalbooi identified his mother, Elsie Vaalbooi, who had been a fluent Nxu speaker and a member of the Khomani San Council of Elders. She passed away in 2002. Petrus and his mother had been involved in an initiative to trace surviving Nxu speakers in the Northern Cape. Curiously, Petrus Vaalbooi commented

3 Buchu is an aromatic fynbos herb with healing properties. It was used for centuries by the indigenous peoples of the Cape in various rituals and as a medicine.

that, contrary to the images projected of the San, his grandfather rode a horse, hunted with a gun, and was a sheep farmer.

The fourth day was dedicated to a visit to the Iziko South African Museum where the group did a walk-through of the Rock Art Gallery and reflected on the messages associated with the different rock art paintings. They also visited the Mammal Gallery and the Discovery Room. As Petrus Vaalbooi had expressed an interest in assisting the Iziko Museums with resolving the question of the restitution of human remains, we held a meeting with the Executive Director of Core Functions to discuss possible areas of collaboration. The group offered to speak to other groups, including the Khoi-Boesman-Nguni-Coalition, to encourage everyone to come to the table in the interest of reburying the human remains as they found it deeply disturbing to think of their ancestors lying in boxes in museums. They also suggested that the San Council be involved in deliberations as they are, ostensibly, tasked with representing the interests of all San groups in South Africa.

The final day was spent on an oral history interview with the group, followed by a discussion on how to proceed. We had been considering how we could broaden such an exercise to include other San groups, as well as Khoi groups. Interestingly, this was also an issue that was raised by the Khomani San group. We considered how the issues discussed during the workshop could be taken back to the broader community in the Kalahari, given the challenges of distance – one thousand and seventy-nine kilometres to the Kgalagadi Transfrontier Park to Cape Town. We provided the group with images of the object collections and copies of the photographic collections and also wrote up a report, which was sent to the San Council so that the community could receive some feedback from the museum. Other factors to consider were the lack of electricity and the high rate of illiteracy within the community.

We are hoping to build on this exploratory project and, together with the Khomani group, reach out to other Khoisan groups so as to open the museum collections to communities and bring community narratives to these collections. One of our concerns is that while museums focus on the past history of the Khoi and San, there is little focus on the resurgence of San and Khoi identity and on how the past speaks to the present. There is a sense of frustration amongst the indigenous communities, as museums are perceived to have neglected their histories. There is little or no contemporary collecting taking place around the material culture of the San and Khoi descendants. There is also a need for a dynamic oral history project that can trace the narratives that have been handed down through the generations.

In attempting to rewrite the museum archives we must consider not only the language and content of the archives but also the collections that raise ethical questions. For example, we know of at least one artefact, a skin bag, that was in the ownership of one of the San prisoners used in the Ethnographic Gallery casting project. Given the violence and racism that were an integral part of the making of the San casts in the exhibition diorama, how should such artefact be treated? This also raises the question of how much research has been conducted into how the collections were acquired. We need to research all collectors who sold or donated collections to the museums in order to try and understand how these items may have been acquired. Vibeke Viestad's study makes mention of »photographs of naked people taken by Dorothea Bleek« in the South African Museum collections, though she adds that »these have of course never been published online unlike her other field photographs« (Viestad 2014: 40). What are the rights of descendant communities when faced with photographs that violate their ancestors? As a collections department tasked with the digitizing and care of the collections, we realise that the rewriting of the museum archives is an enormous task, which calls for partnerships that can provide valuable research assistance. In order to truly integrate the social history collections, we need to rewrite the documentation on the objects while also acknowledging the flawed interpretations stemming from the periods of colonialism and apartheid. We should be working towards an inclusive museums archive, which recognizes the multiplicity of voices and histories of people as they crossed paths with history, and which also critically addresses the violence and racism underlying the narratives linked to our ›ethnographic collections‹. The lesson from the *Miscast* exhibition is that if we do not involve communities in these endeavours, our knowledge production systems will remain flawed.

This article has undergone a double-blind peer-review.

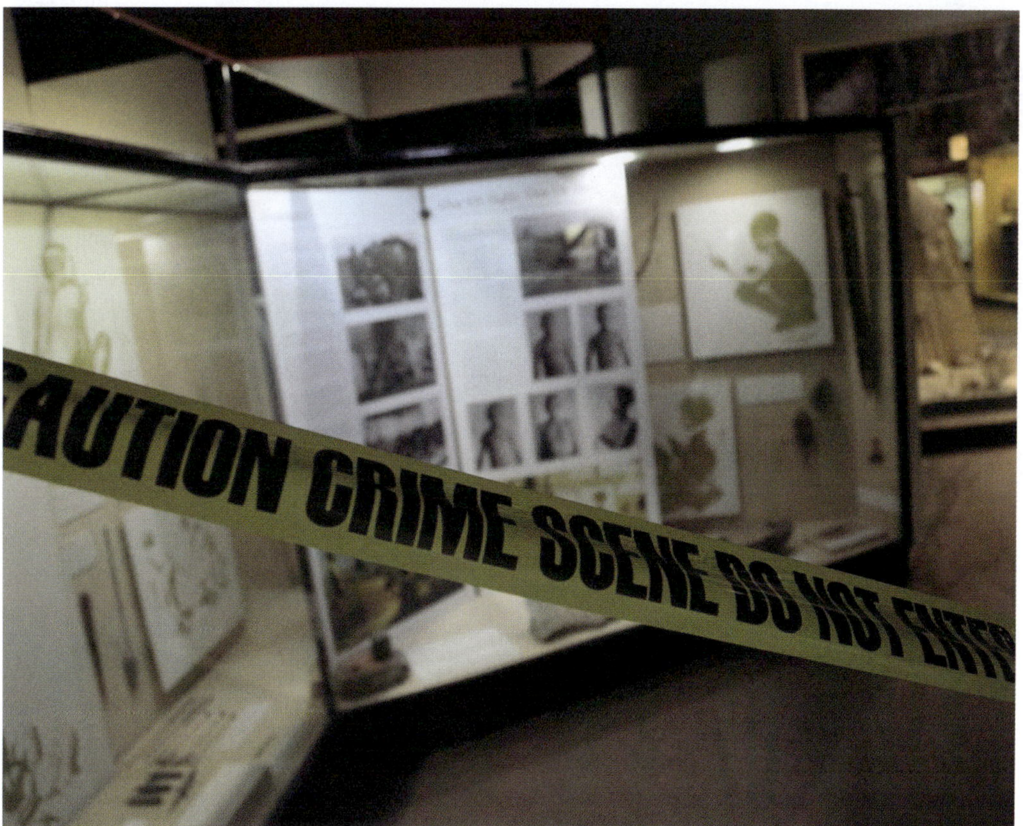

Fig. 1: The Ethnographic Gallery at the Iziko South African Museum declared a ›colonial crime scene‹. Photo: Wandile Kasibe, Iziko Museums.

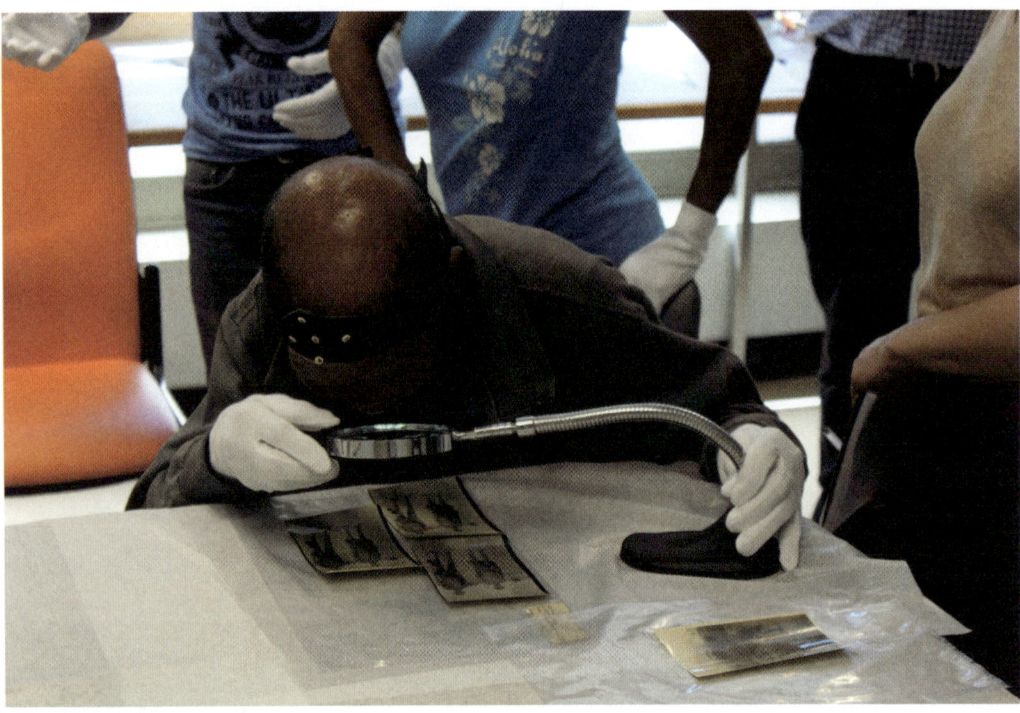

Fig. 2: Petrus Vaalbooi, Traditional Leader of the Khomani Bushman/San examines photographs at the Iziko Social History Centre. Photo: Janene van Wyk, Iziko Museums.

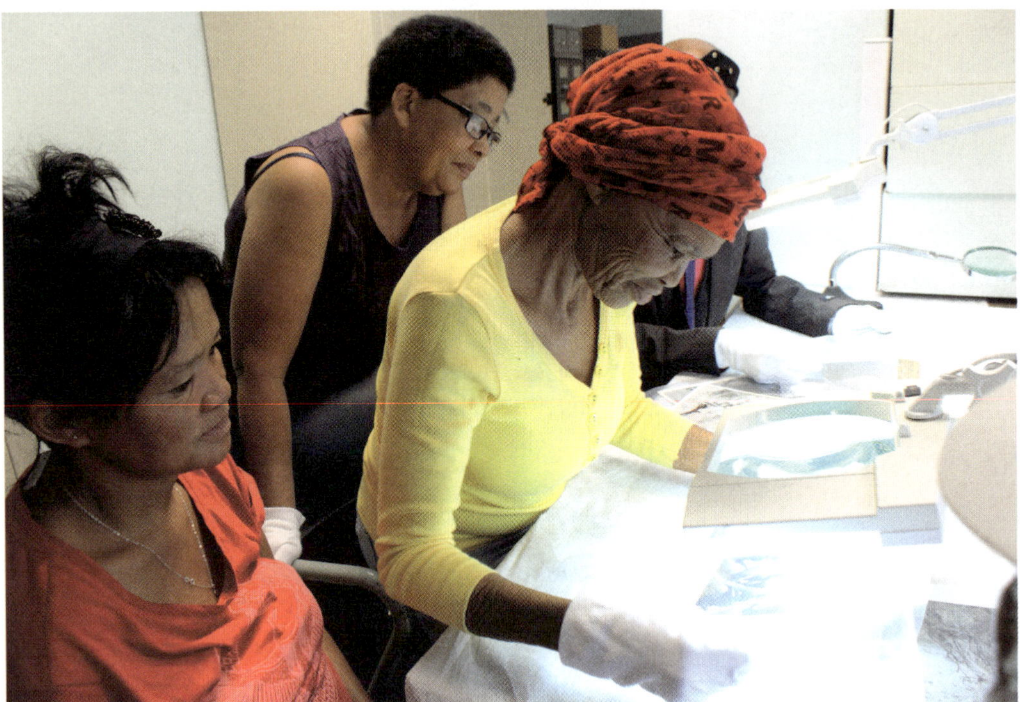

Fig. 3: From left to right: Anna Marie Vallbooi, Lydia Kruiper and Iziko staff member, Marie Scheepers, examining photographs from the Bushman/San collection at the Iziko Social History Centre. Photo: Janene van Wyk, Iziko Museums.

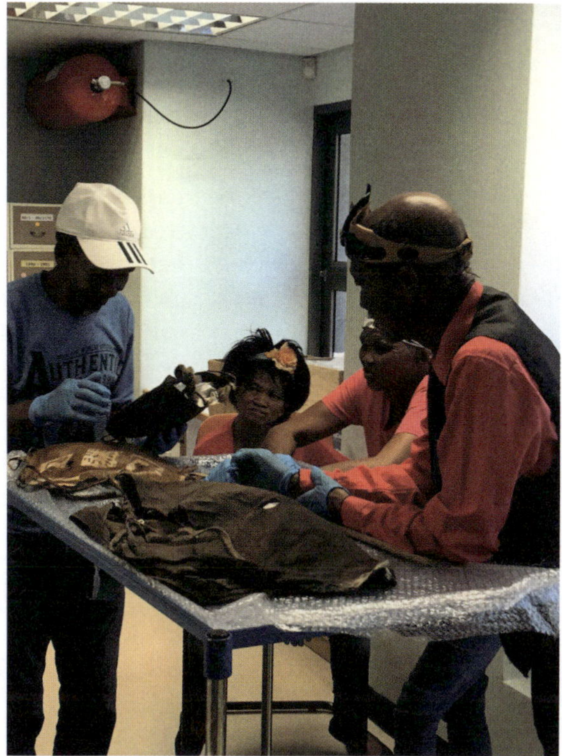

Fig. 4: Isak Kruiper (in white cap), Anna Marie vaalbooi, Lydia Kruiper and Petrus Vaalbooi examining bags and a coat fashioned from animal skin, Iziko Social History Centre. Photo: Janene van Wyk, Iziko Museums.

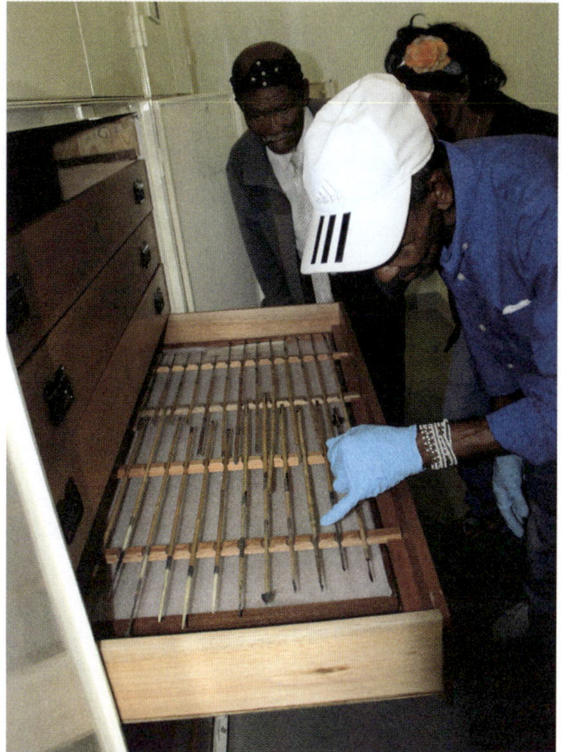

Fig. 5: Isak Kruiper and Petrus Vaalbooi inspecting Bushman/San arrows at the Iziko Social History Centre. Photo: Janene van Wyk, Iziko Museums.

Literature

ART AFRICA (2018): »Curating the Colonial Crime Scene: Heritage & Violence of Ethnographic Racism«, https://artafricamagazine.org/curating-colonial-crime-scene/ (30.06.2021).

BODENHAM, Hugo (2017): »Light in the Darkness«. In: *Exhibition proposal submitted to Iziko*, 3 November 2017.

SMITH, Andrew (2017): »It was a Grave Mistake to Have Got Rid of the Diorama at the SA Museum«, *Cape Times*, 16. August 2017, 9.

COOMBES, Annie (2003): *History after Apartheid: Visual Culture and Public Memory in a Democratic South Africa*, Durham: Duke University Press.

DAVISON, Patricia (1998): »Museums and the Reshaping of Memory«. In: *Negotiating the Past: The Making of Memory in South Africa*, ed. by Sarah Nuttall/Carli Coetzee, Cape Town: Oxford University Press, 113–160.

DUBIN, Steven (2009): *Mounting Queen Victoria: Curating Cultural Change*, Auckland Park: Jacana Media.

GIBSON, Laura (2019): *Decolonising South African Museums in a Digital Age: Re-Imagining the Iziko Museum's Natal Nguni Catalogue and Collection*, PhD Thesis: Department of Digital Humanities, London: King's College.

GORE, J.M. (2004): »A Lack of Nation? The Evolution of History in South African Museums c.1825–1945«. In: *South African Historical Journal* 51, 24–46.

LEGGASICK, Martin/RASSOOL, Ciraj (2000): *Skeletons in the Cupboard: South African Museums and the Trade in Human Remains 1907–1917*, Cape Town: South African Museum.

MANDELA, Nelson (1997): *Address by President Mandela on Heritage Day*, 24 September 1997, http://www.mandela.gov.za/mandela_speeches/1997/970924_heritage.htm (30.06.2021).

MAYKUTH (1996): »Colsberg Remains«. In: *Philadelphia Inquirer*, 5 June 1996.

MBEMBE, Achille (2002): »The power of the archive and its limits«. In: *Refiguring the Archive*, ed. by. Carolyn Hamilton/Verne Harris/Jane Taylor et al., Dordrecht/Boston/London: Kluwer Academic Publishers, 19–26.

MORRIS, Michael (1996): »Baring the True Culture of Bushmen: The National Gallery Exhibition Offers a Fresh Approach to History«. In: *Miscast – Centre for Curating the Archive – University of Cape Town*, http://www.cca.uct.ac.za/cca/projects/miscast-archive (30.06.2021):

PECKMANN, Tanya (2003): »Possible Relationship between Porotic Hyperostosis and Smallpox Infections in Nineteenth Century Populations in the Northern Frontier, South Africa«. In: *World Archaeology* 35: 2, 289–305.

EVANS, Jenny (2017): »We Want Bones of Our Ancestors Back from Europe, says Khoi Chief«, *news24*, 10. March 2017, https://www.news24.com/news24/SouthAfrica/News/we-want-bones-of-our-ancestors-back-from-europe-says-khoi-chief-20170310 (01.07.21).

RASSOOL, Ciraj (2015): »Re-Storing the Skeletons of Empire: Return, Reburial and Rehumanisation in South Africa«. In: *Journal of Southern African Studies* 41: 3, 653–670.

ROGOFF, Irit (2002): »Hit and Run – Museums and Cultural Difference«. In: *Art Journal* 61: 3, 63–73.

Sunday Independent (1996): »As Museumgoers Literally Walk all Over the Brutal Fate of the Bushmen, They Seem to Miss the Point«. In: *The Sunday Culture/Sunday Independent*, 26. May 1996.

Viestad, Vibeke M. (2018): *Dress as Social Relations: An Interpretation of Bushmen Dress*, Johannesburg: Wits University Press.

Wanless, Ann (2007): *The Silence of Colonial Melancholy*. PhD Thesis, Johannesburg: University of the Witwatersrand, http://wiredspace.wits.ac.za/handle/10539/5710 (12.04.2021).

Witz, Leslie (2012): »Making Museums as Heritage in Post-Apartheid South Africa«. Göteborg: International Journal of Heritage Studies/Heritage Seminar at University of Gothenburg.

Witz, Leslie/Minkley, Gary/Rassool, Ciraj (1999): *The Castle, the Gallery and the Sanatorium: Curating a South African Nation in the Museum*, Kimberley: McGregor Museum.

Table of figures

Fig. 1: The Ethnographic Gallery at the Iziko South African Museum declared a ›colonial crime scene‹. Photo: Wandile Kasibe, Iziko Museums.

Fig. 2: Petrus Vaalbooi, Traditional Leader of the Khomani Bushman/San examines photographs at the Iziko Social History Centre. Photo: Janene van Wyk, Iziko Museums.

Fig. 3: From left to right: Anna Marie Vallbooi, Lydia Kruiper and Iziko staff member, Marie Scheepers, examining photographs from the Bushman/San collection at the Iziko Social History Centre. Photo: Janene van Wyk, Iziko Museums.

Fig. 4: Isak Kruiper (in white cap), Anna Marie vaalbooi, Lydia Kruiper and Petrus Vaalbooi examining bags and a coat fashioned from animal skin, Iziko Social History Centre. Photo: Janene van Wyk, Iziko Museums.

Fig. 5: Isak Kruiper and Petrus Vaalbooi inspecting Bushman/San arrows at the Iziko Social History Centre. Photo: Janene van Wyk, Iziko Museums.

Problematic Museum Heritage in a Postcolonial Context: The Case of the Moto Moto Museum *Chisungu* Collection

Mary Mbewe

Introduction

Chisungu is a female puberty initiation ceremony practiced by most ethnic groups in Zambia, but predominantly by the Bemba of Northern Zambia. While these rites are still practiced in some form today, their nature and conduct is significantly different from which was observed and recorded by anthropologists and missionaries during the colonial period.[1] During that time, *chisungu* dealt with the transition from girlhood to womanhood in society, and involved public and secret rites that formalised the entry of girls who had come of age into womanhood, and solemnizing their right to marriage and reproduction. Unlike similar ceremonies in other parts of Africa, *chisungu* did not involve circumcision or virginity testing. In a month-long secluded ceremony, elderly specialised women called *banacimbusa* used songs, dances, performances, floor and wall paintings, and most importantly, moulded pottery emblems – collectively called *mbusa* – to impart esoteric knowledge to the initiates. This knowledge embraced a range

1 Contemporary *chisungu* rituals are devoid of many aspects of the rituals that were practiced in the colonial period, such as the intricate rituals that took place in the forests as described by Audrey Richards and Jean Jacques Corbeil. During the colonial period, when formal education for girls was not widespread, women married a few years after puberty. Consequently, *chisungu* was associated with preparing girls for marriage and motherhood. *Chisungu*, as observed at puberty, is no longer associated with marriage or marital relations; hence teachings on marital relations are no longer part of the puberty rites, although *chisungu* is still stereotyped as a place of sexual education. The widespread adoption of Christianity during the colonial period and its continued growth in the post-colonial period also led to changes in *chisungu* and other cultural practices, resulting in Christianised versions of these practices. Today, there is great variety of ways in which *chisungu* is conducted, based on socio-economic status, beliefs and so on. Many families no longer practice *chisungu* rites at puberty. These are included in traditional teachings just before a woman marries in what has become generally known as kitchen practices, a formal bridal shower in which a bride is also taught traditional marital lessons and given gifts to start her new home. Where some form of *chisungu* is held at puberty, it is significantly shorter and less elaborate. For details, see Rasing (2001).

urn:nbn:de:hbz:6:3-zfk-2021-41941

of practices and beliefs including religion, sexuality, sex education and marital relations, childbirth and childrearing, as well as family and social obligations. Women, exclusively, held the authority in this important rite, the ramifications of which embraced the health and well-being not only of the individual but also of the lineage and the entire social body. Consequently, the significance of *chisungu* went beyond ensuring the transition from girlhood to womanhood. Indeed, it was at the heart of ensuring the health and progress of society, and defining differences between different generations of women, between men and women, and between initiated and uninitiated women. The British anthropologist Audrey Richards observed this ceremony in June 1933, and in 1956 she produced one of her most outstanding works describing and analysing this ceremony based on this participant-observation (Richards 1956). Jean Jacques Corbeil, a priest of the Catholic Church belonging to the order of the Missionaries of Africa, also studied the *chisungu* after Richards. Although not well known in scholarly circles, perhaps owing to the fact that he was an amateur ethnographer as opposed to a professional one, Corbeil's work was significant because it led to the collection of hundreds of objects and texts on *chisungu*. These included more than 200 clay objects (*mbusa*), wall and floor emblems and songs and other oral texts. Corbeil collected these objects as a result of five decades of ethnographic work among the people of northern Zambia, with whom he worked as a Catholic priest from 1943 to 1989. These *chisungu* objects, together with thousands of other objects, came to make up the Moto Moto Museum, which is today one of Zambia's five national museums. Corbeil's work also led to the publication of a book on the ceremony (Corbeil 1982).

In this paper, I focus on the body of *chisungu* objects that Corbeil collected, and pose questions around the status of the objects during a) the colonial period when Corbeil started the collection and constituted the Moto Moto Museum, and b) in the postcolonial period, discussing what has become of the objects now. I demonstrate that the collection of the *chisungu* objects by Corbeil was done within a broader context of epistemic violence and cultural appropriation. Through processes such as enculturation, missionaries prohibited and changed cultural practices in order to make the work of Christianization of indigenous communities possible. These processes of cultural appropriation corresponded with ethnographic studies conducted on indigenous societies by the missionaries. One result of these studies was the collection of cultural objects and the establishment of the Moto Moto Museum. These collections and their representation in the museum's permanent exhibition and storage rooms remain problematic, in terms of the static and primitivised ways in which they represent people and practices. Despite this, the Moto Moto Museum, through its public programs, has formed partnerships with members of the community. These involve revisiting the *chisungu* collection, reinvesting it with new meanings and using the collection for public programs and education in which contemporary problems such as HIV/AIDS, gender-based violence, and child sexual abuse and early marriages are addressed. The dynamic and innovative ways in which this collection is used demonstrates how collections with problematic histories can begin to transcend such problematic legacies in so far as they are used productively by communities.

Missionaries, Ethnography, and the History of the Moto Moto Museum

»Ignorance of African customs and beliefs on the part of the missionary could certainly result in a lack of understanding of his flock and their manner of reasoning with the consequent stifling of his apostolic work.«[2]

The history of the Moto Moto Museum and the foundation of the *chisungu* collection is encapsulated in the history of the establishment of the Catholic Church in Northern Zambia by an order of mostly French priests called the Missionaries of Africa, popularly known as the White Fathers.[3] The White Fathers' missionary work was hinged on the appropriation of local customs and practices with the result that ethnography and evangelisation were parallel processes. The formation of the museum was part of a long history of the production of indigenous ethnographic texts and heritage by the White Fathers. Because of the centrality of this background to understanding Corbeil's work and the nature of the foundations of the Moto Moto Museum, I will focus on this background in more detail in the foregoing sections.

The White Fathers arrived in Northern Zambia in 1886. Although their work of conversion focused on different groups of people in Northern Zambia such as the Mambwe, Lungu, Namwanga and Bisa, their main interest was in the Bemba, who were the most dominant group, and whom Indian (Arab) Slave traders and early colonial administrators depicted as superstitious and heathen. In 1889, with the help of Bishop Joseph Dupont, the British South African Company occupied Bembaland, paving the way not only for formal colonisation by the company on behalf of Britain, but also for the Catholic church to declare this portion of Northern Zambia as its »sphere of influence« (Roberts 1976: 3; Rotberg 1965; Hinferlaar 2004: 49).

From the beginning, the production of the ethnographic heritage of the Bemba and other groups was a core part of the White Fathers' proselytising work and was done to make the work of Christian evangelism possible. Missionaries needed to understand African languages and customs to translate the Christian message in order to make converts. Missionary work and converting Africans to Christianity was premised on prohibiting competing African religious practices and customs. Despite this prohibition of certain indigenous practices, the missionaries took a strong stance of salvaging such practices and cultures. The intention was to legitimise their ethnographic work and eventually position themselves as the protectors of, and experts on, African culture.

As early as 1910, priests such as Frs. Jan Van Sambeek, Eugene Welfele, François Tanguy, Louis Guillerme and Eduard Labreque wrote extensively on the religious practices and

2 White Fathers Archive (hereafter WFA), Lusaka, I-M-C 66, Tanguy Francois, his notes in view of a booklet for students at the Language Centre.

3 The museum was named after Bishop Joseph Dupont, a French pioneer missionary of the White Fathers. His biography and role in the Catholicization of Northern Zambia are central to the construction of Catholic heritage in the region. He was nicknamed *Bwana Moto Moto*, which can be translated as fire fire, allegedly because of his fiery temper and his habit of pipe smoking for which he habitually demanded an open flame.

customs of the Bemba and surrounding peoples such as the Bisa, Mambwe, Lungu, Shila and others.[4] The range of themes covered was vast and included the whole spectrum of Bemba life, religious, social, political, and economic systems. Notable themes were the religious practices and beliefs, female initiation and marriage systems, natural environment, clan systems, witchcraft and sorcery, death rituals and rituals related to sexuality and reproduction, as well as political systems. Eduard Labreque for example studied and wrote on the *chisungu* ceremonies from as early as 1912. In the 1930s, he published several accounts in international journals such as *Anthropos* and *Africa* (Labreque 1931).

Between 1920 and 1960, the White Fathers introduced a series of readers on the Bemba for use in schools for literacy classes. One of the most famous of these were the *Ifya Bukaya* (of familiar things) readers, which were, in essence, ethnographic texts (Oger 1994: 127). These readers were also evangelical tools, as the sections on customs commented on customs that were considered negative and unchristian, such as ancestral worship.[5] In 1947, the General Chapter of the White Fathers had appealed to older missionaries to edit everything that had been compiled and written on African history and customs. It also expressly asked the bishops and heads of missions to organise a methodical study of African customs and ways of life, following a pre-established ethnological plan of enquiry.[6] White Father publications such as *Imyendele Isuma* (rightful living) were also used to arbitrate behaviour, customs, and lifestyle. They dispensed instructions on rightful living in terms of family life, and proper behaviours for husbands and wives in different situations (Hinfelaar 2015: 66). The White Fathers' ethnographies and Bemba-readers crystallised centuries-old, but dynamic, oral histories in ways that were fixed and bounded. Derek Peterson notes: »through these and other documentary practices the routines of human life were lifted out of the dynamic real world, placed outside the reach of change and innovation, and rendered anachronistic at the moment of publication« (Petersen 2015: 1f.).

Policy of Inculturation

Beginning around the late 1940s, the Roman Catholic Church adopted a new set of policies concerning the Church's relationship with non-Western cultures. This was the Church's response to challenges that resulted from the social, political, cultural and technological developments of the post-war period which were characterised by liberalism, the increasing recognition of the autonomy of formerly subjugated societies and the growth of nationalism globally. Both as a response to these changes and as a result thereof, the church convened the Second Vatican Council (1962–1965), which sought to usher the Roman Catholic Church into the modern era. An important part of this post-war reformation was the opening of dialogue with the contemporary world and other cultures and religions. In Africa, this led to what has generally been perceived as a

4 WFA, Various documents (Oger 1991: 127).

5 WFA, 3-P-Sc16, White Fathers Chilubula, Ifya Bukaya (second Bemba Reader 1931: 16).

6 WFA, circular letter Durrieu, 1948, Chapters decisions, 48 (referenced in Oger 1991: 128).

more accepting attitude to African cultural practices, through processes that have broadly become known as inculturation.[7]

The key position of inculturation was cultural adaptation in which non-Western and non-Christian cultures and their customs were allowed to practice Catholicism within the boundaries of their culture. What this meant in practice, especially for the church in Africa, is that African customs were subjected to scrutiny and sieved of elements that were deemed negative and intolerable. These were given a Christian facelift, adopted and re-codified as African customs. These processes bear significant similarities with the new modes of colonial governance through the policy of indirect rule that Mamdani describes insofar as the Church claimed not just to acknowledge difference but also to shape it (Mamdani 2012: 2). As with the language of indirect rule, the language of inculturation was benign. Inculturation was presented as »partnership«, »mutual exchange«, and »dialogue of cultures« (Ott 2006: 25).

Significantly, the language of inculturation and the ethnographic work and collection of cultural objects that made it possible was posited as benevolent. It was a language of protection and preservation of indigenous custom, which missionaries saw as increasingly defiled by modernity and undesirable Western influences, and which were prone to extinction. It is this stance of salvation that Corbeil used as a justification for his *chisungu* collection (Corbeil 1982). The paradigm of salvation generally legitimated racist representations of indigenous communities and the conversion of indigenous practices, even sacred ones such as *chisungu*, into an object of spectacle.

Inculturation worked in several ways. One example is a process which Steven Kaplan terms assimilation, in which Christian missionaries incorporated aspects from a non-Christian setting into an already existing Christian ritual (Kaplan 1994: 19). Another was Christianization, in which missionaries sought to »create Christian versions of traditional African rites and practices« (ibid.: 16). These processes had begun even before the Second Vatican Council. In 1957, the General Chapter of the White Fathers decided upon the opening of centres for the study of African languages and customs. In Northern Rhodesia's Chinsali District, the Ilondola Language and Culture Study Centre was opened in 1958.[8] In Northern Rhodesia, the White Fathers began adapting Christian practices to local customs beginning in the late 1940s, a period which correspondingly witnessed more deliberate approaches to the study and collection of Bemba customs and what has generally being presented as tolerant attitudes to these customs. This was also an enhanced ordering of knowledge on indigenous people. In this later period, the White

7 Although couched as a more liberal and accommodating attitude towards African cultural practice than the earlier labelling of African culture as pagan, inculturation was a more pervasive and repressive form of cultural control and appropriation. This enabled the Catholic missionaries – usually male and white – to become adjudicators of African culture. This is most clear in how the Catholic Church created a Christianised version of the female initiation ceremony and replaced other cultural practices that they deemed unchristian and pagan with what was perceived to be more Christian and thus a more acceptable form of the practice.

8 WFA, Circular Letter Volker (1958: 78).

Fathers' headquarters in Rome requested their missionaries posted in different territories to send detailed ethnographies of indigenous people.[9]

The Moto Moto Museum

The Moto Moto is located in a rural district called Mbala, at the northernmost tip of Northern Zambia, 1000 miles from the capital Lusaka. It was officially opened as a National Museum on 17th April 1974, joining the Copperbelt Museum and the Livingstone Museum as national museums in the sense of being owned and managed by the state. Until then, the collection was managed by the Diocese of Mbala and owned by Jean Jacques Corbeil.

The museum has its beginnings in 1956, when Corbeil, a French-Canadian priest, began collecting cultural artefacts from among the people of Northern Zambia.[10] His first posting later that year was in Northern Rhodesia, at Mulilansolo Mission in Chinsali District, in the heart of Bemba territory. He spent six months at the Language and Customs Study Centre there, before being posted to Katibunga Mission where he was to spend ten years as parish priest. Remote and far-removed from other European settlements, Katibunga mission would have given Corbeil further opportunity to immerse himself in the learning of the local languages and culture.

In 1954, after a year's home leave in Canada, Corbeil was transferred back to Mulinlansolo mission. As part of the processes of inculturation described earlier, Corbeil, together with another priest, was entrusted with the adaptation to Bemba of Catholic liturgy, which until then had been conducted in Latin. By 1956, this enhanced engagement with African culture led Corbeil to start collecting artefacts. The structure of Catholic evangelism helped him in this regard. Bemba territory was vast but sparsely populated. This, coupled with an inadequate number of priests, made the church adopt a system whereby one priest used a rota to visit his congregants, camping at one location for approximately two weeks. Living among the local people, away from conventions of mission stations and white settlements, helped him to participate in the local ways of life and cultural practices. With the help of mostly male mission-educated catechists, Corbeil collected artefacts that he stored in the respective mission stations.[11]

The early history of the collection reflects Corbeil's missionary career – it was a collection in motion. The collection moved from place to place as Corbeil was moved from one mission station to another. He carried several objects with him and would make additions wherever he went. The collection was at Chinsali, Isoka, then Kayambi missions between 1956 to 1964, and then Serenje from 1964 to 1970 when Corbeil transferred, along with the

9 WFA, I-M-C 07 Etienne Louis: Answer in the name of the Vicariate of Kasama to »enquetes sur les costumes indigenes: Tribu des Babemba (N. Rhodesia)«, asked by the generalate of the White Fathers in Rome, in the 1950s. 63 pages. French.; I-M-C 10 »Table d'enquete sur les moeurs et coutumes africaines, par le generalat des w.f. responses par le P. Tanguy«.

10 Corbeil had recently been ordained in Montreal under the Missionaries of Africa in 1943.

11 A documentary on the Moto Moto Museum and Corbeil gives a picture of his collection work. See Owens 2014 and https://www.youtube.com/watch?v=zdqnrfckd5o.

collection, back to Isoka and ultimately to Mbala in 1973. The Bishop of Mbala donated a former carpentry workshop to house the collection, a huge building which was part of a complex of Catholic institutions located in the Catholic settlements of St Paul's and St Mary's villages. It included a primary school, a chapel, the Bishop's house, the Catholic cemetery and a skills training centre. The carpentry workshop was fitted with shelves on which the hundreds of objects that Corbeil had collected were assembled, thematically displayed and hand-captioned. This former carpentry workshop has been the museum's main gallery ever since, and is today the ethnography gallery.[12]

Collecting Female Initiation Secrets and Objects

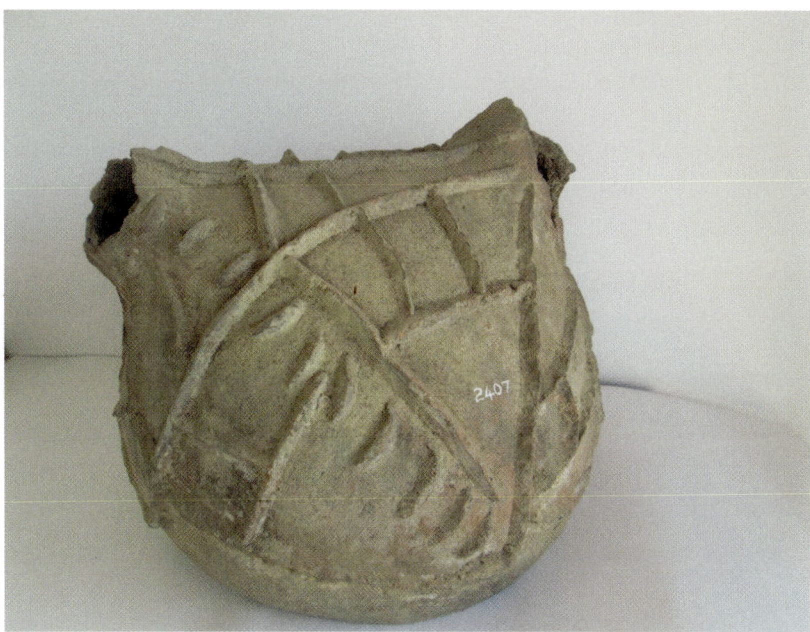

Fig. 1: Example of *chisungu* object collected by Corbeil. Photo: Moto Moto Museum.

Until 1960, Corbeil had been unable to observe and collect *chisungu* initiation objects due to their sensitive nature and due to the secrecy with which the ceremony was conducted. In 1960, Helena Mubanga, a Bemba royal princess of Mubanga village in Chinsali District (the same district where Audrey Richards had conducted her *chisungu* research in 1933) left the Catholic Church to join the Lumpa Church, a flourishing Africanist church that was one of the most significant challenges to Catholicism and colonial rule at the time. Perhaps as a result of the success of the Catholic Church's attempts to win back the thousands of converts that they had lost to the Lumpa church and fearing punishment from the Catholic priests, Helena requested to be readmitted to the Catholic Church at Mulilansolo Mission. Corbeil, who at that time was stationed at the Mission, ascended to this request on the condition that Helena be punished for leaving the Catholic Church by revealing

12 For a video documentary on the exhibitions see Owens 2014.

to Corbeil the secrets of the *chisungu* ceremony. Alarmed at this unusual request, Helena refused to divulge the details of the ceremony. Not only was Corbeil male and white and therefore prohibited from knowing the details of the ceremony as an uninitiated person and outsider, the Catholic Church was known for its negative attitude towards African practices such as *chisungu*. Corbeil, however, went on to convince her: »If it is a bad ceremony, I should know about it as a priest who is responsible for souls. If it is a good ceremony, why not reveal it to me?«[13] After much hesitation, Helena agreed to secretly sing some of the initiation ceremony songs to Corbeil and his clerk who recorded them under the cover of night. When the community members realised what was happening, they forbade further revelation of the secret knowledge of the ceremony. Using the same argument, namely that missionaries had the right to knowledge about these practices, Corbeil convinced the elderly women who were in charge of the ceremony to reveal further details (Carey 2002: 1–7). In time, Corbeil was given access to all aspects of the ceremony. The midwives re-enacted the ceremony for Corbeil at the missionaries' house, while another priest, Charles Van Rijhoven, operated the tape recorder and two male African catechists/teachers acted as interpreters. Corbeil observed the actual ceremonies in the community, including the secret aspects that took place in enclosed spaces in the village and in the bush. These and subsequent encounters led to the collection of more than 100 songs and, as of 1968, more than 200 sacred objects used during the secret rituals, which included clay models and floor as well as wall models and paintings.[14] It is clear from this instance of collection of such sensitive cultural objects that missionaries such as Corbeil abused their positions of authority and thus collected from positions of power.

The collection of *chisungu* objects became the biggest curiosity and attraction in Corbeil's collection of African artefacts. Helena Mubanga remained one of Corbeil's chief informants at the ceremony. Accession registers held in the Moto Moto Museum show that she continued supplying Corbeil with objects and information on the ceremony as late as 1976.[15] In 1982, Corbeil published *Mbusa: Sacred Emblems of the Bemba,* detailing the conduct of the ceremony and the teachings and songs of the objects. The interpretation of the *chisungu* teaching in this book was sanitised of the deeper cultural meanings and especially the teachings regarding intimacy and sexual matters. The book was instead modelled on the Catholic Church's teachings on marriage, sexuality and family life. One reviewer of the book bemoaned the fact that through the book and the *chisungu* displays at Corbeil's museum, practices whose significance lay in their secret and symbolic nature were exposed and diminished through such processes of ethnographic study, collecting and public display (Musambacime 1983). These processes of studying and controlling female initiation are part of the broader discourses on how the colonial and even postcolonial governments attempted to control black women's bodies and sexuality, and undermined women's authority in very significant ways (Thomas 2003; Hayes 2006).

13 Roan Selection Trust 1969: 8–12; Corbeil 1982.

14 This story is narrated by Corbeil in many unpublished and some published texts. See for example Roan Selection Trust (1969: 8–12).

15 Mbala, Moto Moto Museum collection and accession registers 1960 to 1976.

The Christianised interpretation of *chisungu* in the book mirrors the processes by which the Catholic Church introduced Christian versions of the initiation rites. Their teachings were codified by appointed lay organisations within the church who were tasked with conducting these Christian versions, in many cases attended by the missionaries. Specifically, aspects that were removed included some forms of ancestral veneration or ancestral worship which were significant to the rituals; teachings on sex, the use of indigenous medicines and charms purposed to make the initiates sexually attractive; dances and songs that were perceived to be sexualised, like beer brewing and drinking etc.[16] These processes of sanitisation of meaning are also reflected by the way in which Corbeil presented the *chisungu* objects in the museum. The implications of these racialized discourses have been commented on by numerous scholars. Central to the practice of colonial ethnography/social anthropology and related fields, these racialized notions enabled a temporalisation and spatialisation of time, a »denial of coevalness« to other people which Johannes Fabian defines as »a persistent and systematic tendency to place the referent(s) of anthropology in a time other than the present of the producer of anthropological discourse« (Fabian 1982: 31). The result was hierarchical classification of societies, with non-Western societies at the bottom of the ladder. With these processes, the epistemic agency of the owners of the practices and knowledge was compromised. It is the legacy of epistemic violence, in collections such as this, with which we need to contend.

The *chisungu* Permanent Exhibitions in Recent Years

Between 2007 and 2016, the Moto Moto Museum embarked on a project of refurbishing the old exhibition, which had not significantly changed since Corbeil's times. A detailed discussion of this permanent exhibition is beyond the scope of this current paper. Suffice to say, it perpetuates the problematic representations in ways that signify why so many ethnographic collections with colonial foundations continue to be sites of debate and contestation. In summary, about 30 *chisungu* objects that were collected by Corbeil and some models made from his original collections, as well as ten photographs from Richards' 1931 study of the ceremony, were enlarged and displayed on the boards behind, and on the sides, to compliment the object display. The exhibits and photographs are accompanied by texts, which mirror those from Richards' and Corbeil's publications. This representation perpetuates a construction of the *chisungu* ceremony as an ›authentic‹ and ›timeless traditional‹, thereby sustaining the problematic epistemic conditions of its creation. Consequently, the museum's current *chisungu* permanent exhibition presents a static representation of the ceremony, the knowledge of which was produced within specific historical contexts and practices. These representations are also ahistorical, devoid of a historicised narrative, which would locate the ritual, related issues of womanhood and the collection within a broader historic frame of social and political changes and contexts.

16 A well-known example of the introduction of Christianized versions of *chisungu* was done by the famous missionary to Central Africa Mable Shaw (Morroe 1986). See General Missionary Conference of Northern Rhodesia (1939).

The Museum as a Place of Knowledge Transitions – The *Chisungu* Collection and Community Engagement

Despite these limitations, the museum, through its public programs run by the education department, has developed engaging and productive ways in which, through partnerships with community members, the *chisungu* collection is used to address issues affecting society, such as HIV/AIDS, gender-based violence, reproductive health and so on. Karp and Kratz develop the idea of museum friction in recognition of the museum as a »varied and often changing set of practices, processes and interactions« (Karp/Kratz 2006: 2). Drawing on experiences from the District Six Museum in Cape Town, Rassool also suggests that the museum should not be seen as a place or a collection, but should be viewed as a »space for conversation and debate«, and as a place for »knowledge transactions« involving different actors and their respective agency (Rassool 2006: 296). This idea engages the ways in which different actors mediate the processes of meaning-making and knowledge production and its representation at different stages of museum processes. I want to apply this notion of the museum as a »space of knowledge transactions« to the ways in which the *chisungu* collection at the Moto Moto Museum has been reconstituted through the contributions and relationships between different actors like the ethnographers, museum curators, exhibition experts and *chisungu* traditional experts drawn from the community.

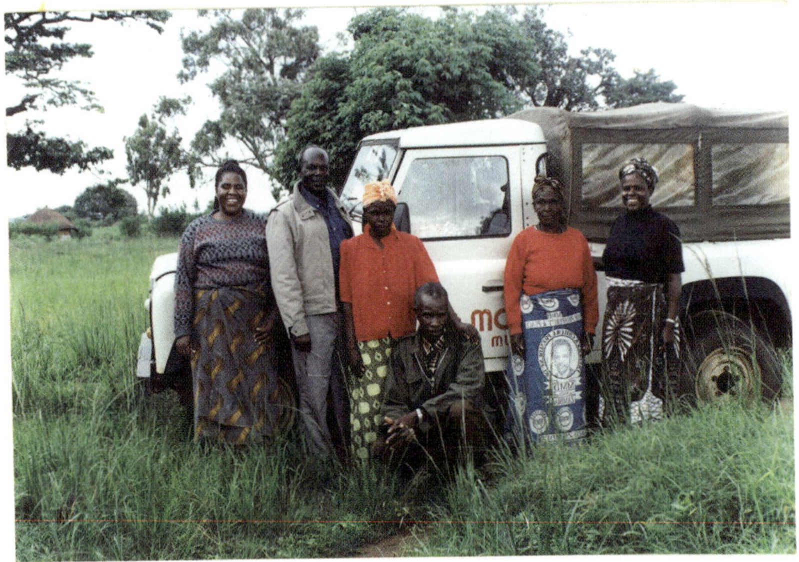

Fig. 2: *Chisungu* counsellors from the community carrying out museum programs. Photo: Moto Moto Museum.

In 1996, the museum constituted the *mbusa* group, which was composed of and driven by members of the community who were considered experts in *chisungu* initiation rites. The *mbusa* group members were part of the Museum's Education Department and could come up with their own programs. One collaborative success between the museum and the community members has been that of documenting and interpreting the *chisungu* objects. Corbeil did not adequately document individual objects, and when he did, the interpretations were sanitised as alluded to earlier. By collaborating between the museum professionals and local experts in knowledge production, a form of co-authoring in interpreting the indigenous knowledge embedded in the *chisungu* objects is enabled. When I joined the museum in 2006, I had a basic idea of the meanings of the different *chisungu* objects and the significance of the *chisungu* rites. Through years of interacting with the *chisungu* experts I acquired a significant understanding of the workings of *chisungu* and a renewed appreciation of their significance. The community members have also been integrated into museum processes such as exhibition-making and interpretations, with their guidance, allowing for a culturally sensitive way of engaging with the objects. In this way, the spiritual and cultural values that the community attaches to the objects and related practices are respected through museum-community collaborations.

Significantly, the collaboration between the museum curators and community members led to processes through which the *chisungu* objects were reinvested with new meanings and interpretations in the service of addressing contemporary problems faced by society. As the *chisungu* female initiation rites deal with issues of reproductive health, these practices have long since been seen to be important sites through which reproductive health issues and education could be addressed. In the initial stages of the HIV/AIDS pandemic, practices like *chisungu* were seen to be negative and were generally thought to contribute to the spread of the disease as it was thought that they encouraged unsafe behaviours such as early marriages, unsafe sexual practices and a subservient role of women which negatively affected their reproductive health. While some of this was true, it has since been recognised that indigenous practices like *chisungu* have knowledge that is relevant and useful in addressing problems of sexual, gender and reproductive health.

The partnership between the museum and the community members led to the successful implementation of programs in which traditional *chisungu* experts from communities carry on a dialogue on how the female initiations are done and how they could be used as tools for education. Through the museum-community partnership, various local and international agencies like the Ministry of Health of the Republic of Zambia, Irish Aid, and the United States President's Emergency Plan for AIDS Relief (PEPFAR) funded different projects in which *chisungu* traditional experts were engaged to include education on HIV/AIDS, gender-based violence and reproductive health in their cultural practices. The museum was used as a forum through which community experts and museum staff received formal training in these areas via workshops and other formats. Dialogues over practices of *chisungu* and the implications of the different teachings over reproductive health and gender relations were part of these conversations. The museum education team and the *chisungu* experts then went into the communities, especially in the rural areas, to engage other *chisungu* counsellors on how *chisungu* teachings could be an intervention and educational platform for issues related to HIV/AIDS, gender relations and reproductive health. Programs were developed targeting different demographic groups, where culturally appropriate conversations occurred. In typical *chisungu* teachings, women were taught to be subservient to men, to the extent that women were expected to tolerate male infidelity, while male infidelity and having multiple sexual partners was usually considered a sign of virility. The *chisungu* experts are encouraged to tackle such attitudes during premarital and marriage counselling. For younger audiences, dialogues involved issues appropriate to them. For example, early marriage remains a problem in many communities today. The *chisungu* experts were encouraged to include these issues in their teachings and to enter into dialogues with traditional leaders, guardians and young people on the laws and organisations that protect young people from child marriages. The range of themes to which the *chisungu* practices could be used is wide. As a result of these collaborations, the museum and the *chisungu* experts produced two booklets that exemplify how selected *chisungu* objects have been reinvested with new meanings. One, written in ChiBemba is *Imbusa Sha CiBemba Ishafwa Ukusalanga Ubulwele Bwa HIV/AIDS* (»*chisungu* teachings that help to spread HIV/AIDS«) was produced by the *chisungu* experts in 2007. Another, specifically targeting young people was produced in 2013 (Phiri/Mateke 2013).

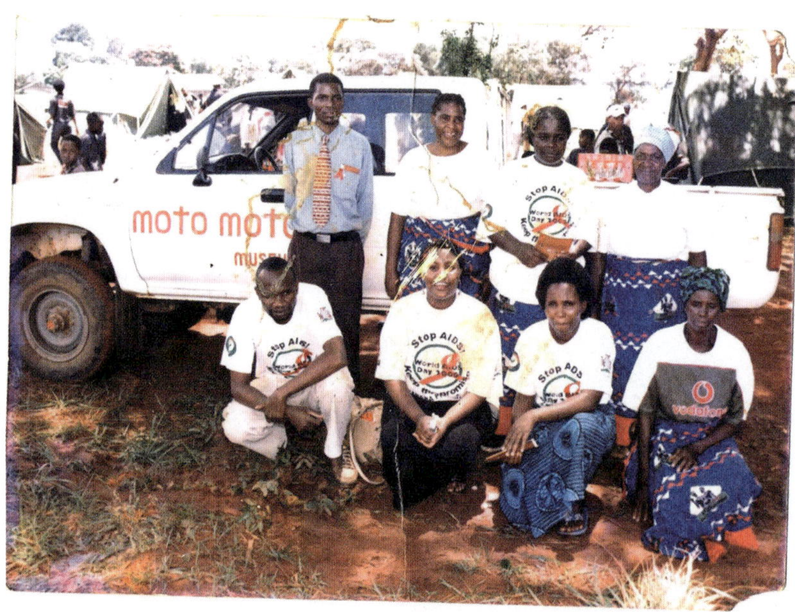

Fig. 3: Museum staff (the two gentlemen, and author in black skirt) with the Mbusa club members during a museum outreach program for the commemoration of World AIDS day, December 2006. Photo: Mary Mbewe.

This validation, however, is not without its problems. The museum-community collaboration works by encouraging the inclusion of these and other positive social teachings in *chisungu* practice while discouraging *chisungu* teachings that are thought to be negative. This perpetuates notions that indigenous practices – especially those dealing with women and their sexuality – are seen as sites of potentially negative practices and need to be ordered, normalised and validated by formal institutions such as the museum, the NGOs involved in the processes, and the Ministry of Health. When I interviewed the former Education Officer of the Moto Moto Museum, I wondered why the title of the *chisungu* book that the Mbusa Club and the museum education department produced, implicitly posited the *chisungu* teachings as helping in spreading HIV/AIDS. He explained that the initial concept for the book was to emphasise the positive aspects of *chisungu* teachings but that the concept of the book had to change because the NGO that funded its production was at that point focusing on dissuading indigenous practices that were thought to be contributing to the spread of HIV/AIDS. Hence, the theme of the book had to conform to the objectives of the funding project.[17] My raising this critique is not intended to undermine the efforts of the collaborations the museum has made and the meaningful ways that the *chisungu* is used, but to point to some of the problems that have been brought about by such collaborations.

Conclusion

Collections that have their foundations in colonial knowledge projects remain sites of contestations and debate today. These collections, such as the Moto Moto Museum collection, were results of cultural appropriation and epistemic violence on indigenous communities. And yet, these collections retain indigenous knowledge that is still relevant and useful to the indigenous communities. Despite its troubled history, the *chisungu* collection at Moto Moto Museum has been reinvested with new meanings through collaborative work between the museum and members of the community. Through these initiatives, the *chisungu* collection has been used to address contemporary issues such as HIV/AIDS. This case study demonstrates that collections like the *chisungu* collection, which have their foundations in problematic histories of cultural appropriation, can be reinvested with new meanings and used to serve the community. Despite some of the problems involved with this particular collaboration, this example of a postcolonial museum practice, within these specific contexts highlights the potential of collections with problematic legacies.

This article has undergone a double-blind peer-review.

Literature

CAREY, Margret (2003): »Missionaries in Zambia«. In: *Journal of Museum Ethnography* 15, 1–7.

CORBEIL, Jean Jacques (1982): *Mbusa: Sacred Emblems of the Bemba,* Mbala, London: Moto Moto Museum, Ethnographica Publishers.

FABIAN, Johannes (1982): *Time and Other: How Anthropology Makes its Object*, New York: Columbia University Press.

GENERAL MISSIONARY CONFERENCE OF NORTHERN RHODESIA (1939): *Report of Proceedings of the Eighth Conference held at Lusaka, August 5th to August 8th 1939*, Lovedale Press, http://www.historicalpapers.wits.ac.za/inventories/inv_pdfo/AD1715/AD1715-15-8-8-001-jpeg.pdf (01.11.2020).

HAYES, Patricia (2006): »Efundula and History: Female Initiation in Pre-colonial and Colonial Northern Namibia«. In: *Towards New Perspectives of African History: Women, Gender and Feminism*, ed. by Tominaga Chizuka/Nagahra, Yoko/Osaka: National Museum of Ethnology Japan, 27–48.

HINFELAAR, Hugo (2015): *History of the Catholic Church in Zambia: 1885–1995*, Lusaka: Fenza Publications.

17 Interview with Mr. Chanda Mutale, Mbala, December 2019.

Kaplan, Steven (ed.) (1994): *Indigenous Resposes to Western Christianity*, New York: New York University Press.

Kratz, Corrine A./Karp, Ivan (2006): »Introduction: Museum Frictions: Public Cultures/Global Transformations«. In: *Museum Frictions: Public Cultures/Global Transformations*, ed. by Ivan Karp/Corinne A. Kratz/Lyn Szwaja/Thomas Ybarra-Frausto, Durham, London: Duke University Press, 1–34.

Labreque, Eduard (1931): »Le mariage chez les Babemba«. In: *Africa* 4: 2, 209–221.

Mamdani, Mohmood (2012): *Define and Rule: Native as Political Identity*, Cambridge: Harvard University Press.

Morroe, Sean (1986): »No Girl Leaves the School Unmarried: Mabel Shaw and the Education of Girls at Mbereshi, Northern Rhodesia, 1915–1940«. In: *The International Journal of African Historical Studies* 19: 4, 601–635.

Musambacime, Mwelwa (1983): *Review of Mbusa Sacred Emblems of the Bemba*, Zambia Museums Journal.

Oger, Louis (1991): *Where a Scattered Flock Gathered Ilondola 1934–1984: A Catholic Mission in a Protestant Area*, Lusaka: Missionaries of Africa.

Ott, Martin (2006): *African Theology in Images*, Lilongwe: Kachere Series.

Owens, David (2014): *Moto Moto Museum*, documentary, https://www.youtube.com/watch?v=zdqnrfckd5o&t=569s (20.11.2020).

Petersen, Derek (2015): »Introduction: Heritage Management in Colonial and Contemporary Africa«. In: *Politics of Heritage in Africa: Economies, Histories, and Infrastractures*, ed. by Derek Petersen/Kodzo Gavua/Ciraj Rassool, Cambridge: Cambridge University Press, 1–36.

Phiri, Victoria/Mateke, Clare (2013): *Vilengo and Mbusa: Towards an HIV/AIDS Free Youth in Zambia*, https://www.academia.edu/38969309/ Vilengo_and_Mbusa_Towards_an_Hiv_Aids_Free_Youth_in_Zambia (02.07.21).

Rasing, Thera (2001): *The Bush Burnt, the Stones Remain: Female Initiation Rites in Urban Zambia*, Leiden: African Studies Centre.

Rassool, Ciraj (2006): »Community Museums, Memory Politics, and Social Transformations in South Africa: Histories, Possibilities, and Limits«. In: *Museum Frictions: Public Cultures/Global Transformations*, ed. by Ivan Karp/Corinne A. Kratz/Lyn Szwaja /Thomas Ybarra-Frausto, Durham, London: Duke University Press, 286–321.

Roan Selection Trust (1969): *Horizon January 1969.*

Richards, Audrey Isabel (1956): *Chisungu: A Girls' Initiation Ceremony among the Bemba of Northern Rhodesia,* London: Faber and Faber.

Roberts, Andrew (1976): *A History of Zambia*, London: Heinemann.

Rotberg, Robert Irwin (1965): *Christian Missionaries and the Creation of Northern Rhodesia*, Princeton: Princeton University Press.

Thomas, Lynn (2003): *The Politics of the Womb: Women, Reproduction and the State in Kenya*, Berkeley: University of California Press.

Table of figures

Eugen Zintgraff's Diary as a Document of Theft and Destruction of Art Treasures in the Colonial Context

Richard Tsogang Fossi

Introduction

Eugen Zintgraff (1858/Düsseldorf – 1897/Tenerife) was a ›prominent‹ explorer in the early years of German colonization of Cameroon (Nkui Nchoji 1989), whose name is deeply rooted in the local collective or grassroots memory (Tsogang Fossi 2019). It is also linked to many cultural or zoological objects as well as human remains, namely skulls, currently in German museums, like in Berlin, Braunschweig, Detmold, Hildesheim, Leipzig, Oldenburg or Stuttgart. Though not himself a military man, he was in charge of several ›exploratory trips‹ between 1886 and 1892, which he misleadingly referred to as ›punitive expedition‹ and ›pacification warfare‹. These partly very violent exploratory were specifically to the coastal forest area (Wouri, Bodiman, Yabassi, Bakundu, Anyang and Banyang), the Grassland region (Bali, Bafut, Mankon, etc.) and the north of the colony (Adamaua, Banyo, Tibati, Sokoto and Yola). Despite the enthusiastic support of Baron Julius von Soden,[1] the first governor of German Cameroon (1885–1891), the ›excursions‹ were in violation of the 1884 Protectorate Treaty, which forbade the Germans access to the hinterlands. Zintgraff not only met and harassed people during these ›trips‹, he also came across many art assets of the forest areas and the Grasslands. These included large drums, wall paintings, carved statues and door frames, sacralized rocks for worshiping, jewelry, and so on. In his diary, *Nord-Kamerun* (1895), Zintgraff describes his attitudes, i.e. his behavior, feelings, and (inter)actions, with African art and cultural objects. As such, the diary appears to provide reliable testimony concerning the loss of these objects. Interestingly, these attitudes showcase different mechanisms of violent destruction or appropriation of cultural objects during colonial times.

1 In recognition of his ›loyal‹ services to the German Nation, a street still carries his name in Düsseldorf-Urdenbach (Soden-Straße), an urban quarter whose streets have been especially devoted to former ›prominent‹ colonial actors (Adolf Woermann, Lüderitz, Julius von Soden, Carl Peters, etc.). Julius von Soden, who also supported one of the first putsches in an early African kingdom (Bimbia), harassed local rulers and embezzled some lands of the Duala for colonial and personal purposes, is another such example. He is, however, surprisingly recast in the city narrative of Düsseldorf as a »harmless colonialist«. See Michels (2017); Linden-Museum (2021).

urn:nbn:de:hbz:6:3-zfk-2021-41955

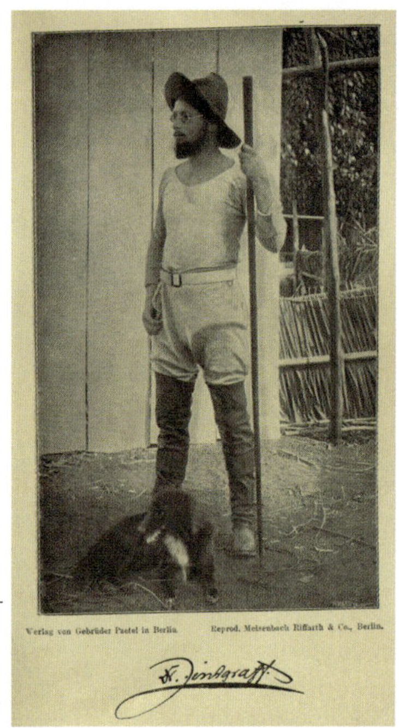

Fig. 1: Eugen Zintgraff. Photo from his diary Nord-Kamerun (Zintgraff 1895: IX).

Focusing on the art treasures of the Banyang and the Grasslands of Cameroon, the descriptions and narratives to be found in his diaries, and which concern his encounters with such objects, are enriching for at least four reasons. First, they help the different communities he confronted in rediscovering parts of their bygone traditions. Second, they enrich existing insights into the types of encounters that European travelers, colonial officers, traders, scientists, missionaries, administrators, colonial doctors and teachers had with local artistic and cultural treasures. Third, they testify to the importance of diaries for research on the provenance of existing art treasures and, analogously, help to shed more light on lost art objects, which had been destroyed by Europeans simply because the objects were too unwieldy to be transported. Finally, they could help establish a network of (inter)connections to people from the same period, context or location with whom he was in contact, and who shared the same ethnographical or anthropological views. These connections are of great importance for research on the provenance of objects that were collected either without the use of force and constraint, or alternatively in problematic contexts and under questionable circumstances (Grimme 2017).

Four main attitudes towards these artifacts are immediately identifiable in Zintgraff's diary: admiration, the desire for looting, followed by destruction, and finally awareness. I have structured the present article in accordance with these four prevalent attitudes, which I identified as giving a discernible pattern to his actions and strategies.

Admiration

As Zintgraff and his men travelled through the Bakundu region in 1886–87, just two years after the official start of German colonization of Cameroon, they made certain ›discoveries‹. Apart from colorful butterflies and other insects in assorted sizes, which his assistant,

2 Zintgraff's rather masculine and narcissistic stance in this portrait from his diary is somewhat reminiscent of the Colossus of Cecil Rhodes striding from Cape Town to Cairo, and is symptomatic for the colonial gaze of the man. Zintgraff considered himself superior to the colonized, whose sole right was to bow to his ultimate authority and to be at his mercy. As a result, he frequently sentenced people to fifty strokes with the colonial cane (*shambock* or *kimboko*), thus going beyond the limit of corporal punishment by flogging permitted at that time (twenty-five strokes). He even sentenced some local people to death, such as one of his translators, Soppo Bell. Moreover, Zintgraff went as far as signing a contract with the Bali ruler, Fon Galega, taking entirely into his own hands »the power of life and death« over any Bali native. See Zintgraff (1895); Tsogang (2019).

lieutenant Zeuner, and later on the entomologist Paul Preuss, collected[3] (Zintgraff 1895: 63-64), they also found in N'Djanga, in the neighborhood of Kumba, in the South-West region of today's Cameroon, very tall columns of rocks, some of them as high as 75 meters. Borrowing his words from European mythology, Zintgraff compares them to »cyclops«, observing them from above: »Most striking were some strange, towering basalt formations in the middle of the forest, which, some 50 to 75 metres high, looked down upon us like giant cyclop's fortresses« (ibid.: 35).[4] How it was that these basalt rocks, 50 or 70 meters in height, came in this special and somewhat spectacular shape is not mentioned in the diary. Nonetheless, their uncommon shape also gave them a special significance in the culture and beliefs of the region. Hence, they were sacralized and appeared as such in many cults in association with many other accessories (skulls, carvings, calabashes, hats, etc.). This rendered them valuable ethnological finding in the eyes of European ›visitors‹. Depending on which populations were using them, some of these smaller rocks – though still as tall as human beings – were placed in particular positions alongside various accessories at the entrances of assembly halls. In this position, they were given names in accordance with their designated purpose:

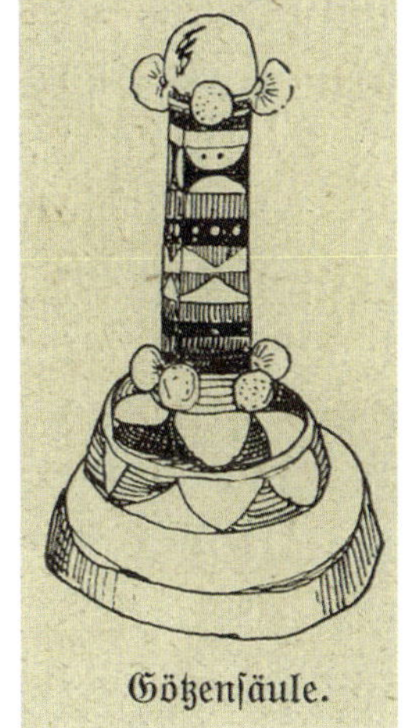

Fig. 2: A *Dikoki* drawn later by Ernst Vollbehr (Vollbehr 1912: 150).

»Each of these assembly houses in the middle, right at the entry, has a man-sized upright stone, called *Dikoki*[5], which, together with the small area in front of it, is considered ›taboo‹. This stone is a basalt that at great pains has been dragged over from the western parts of the protectorate that I already had the occasion to mention. It is painted with brown, white and black squares, a cap decorates its uppermost part while the rest is adorned with many amulets, with sacred objects lying at its feet«.[6]

3 Paul Preuss became the director of the Botanical Garden in Victoria (today Limbe), founded under the support of the then governor Baron Julius von Soden around 1890–1891. Initially, it functioned as a center for the collection of a wide variety of objects of zoological and botanical interest until the surge in German plantations, when it came to serve more as a laboratory for analyzing crops diseases or for experiencing new varieties of plants. See Notizblatt des Königl. Botanischen Gartens und Museums zu Berlin, No. 21, (1900); Michel (1970).

4 »Auffallend waren mitten in dem Walde seltsame, hohe Basaltformationen, die an 50 bis 75 Meter hoch wie ungeheure cyklopische Burgen auf uns herabschauen.«

5 The name *Dikoti* certainly refers to a deity for the *Losango* cults and practices (*Losango* also stood for different local cult societies, sing.: *Isango*) that were widespread in this region and even to people alongside of the Wuri- and Cross-Rivers. See Bureau (1962).

6 »Jedes dieser Versammlungshäuser hat in der Mitte gleich am Eingange einen aufrecht stehenden Stein von Manneshöhe stehen, *Dikoki* genannt, der mit einem kleinen Platz davor als ›tabu‹ gilt. Dieser Stein ist Basalt, der oft mit vieler Mühe aus den westlichen Gegenden des Schutzgebietes, die ich bereits im ersten Kapitel zu erwähnen Gelegenheit hatte, herangeschleppt wird. Er ist mit braunen, weißen und schwarzen Vierecken bemalt, eine Mütze ziert sein oberes Ende, während ihn im Übrigen zahlreiche Amulette schmücken oder geweihte Gegenstände zu seinen Füssen liegen« (Zintgraff 1985: 46). On these rocks as symbolic representations of the royal ancestors, see Brain (1981: 357); on the culture and belief systems of the region, see also Mansfeld (1908: 212, 218f.).

Zintgraff expressed enormous admiration for artifacts and cult objects when he reached the Banyangland, where he discovered many wall paintings, high quality tools and, in his own words, very large, ethnologically valuable drums. In all his travels throughout the colony, he had never seen wall paintings executed nor homes decorated to such a standard.[7] He writes:

> »There is one thing that the Banyang have the advantage over all negro tribes from Cameroon to the Benue: their dwellings are extraordinarily neatly built and even furnished to a certain comfort. The clay walls and the sofas with arm rests, also made of clay, are meticulously polished, painted in black, frequently also adorned with beautiful ornaments in black, white, red and blue color« (Zintgraff 1895: 121).[8]

The high artistic quality of the objects soon gave rise in Zintgraff to an increased desire for looting, a longing to acquire them for his own anthropological research.

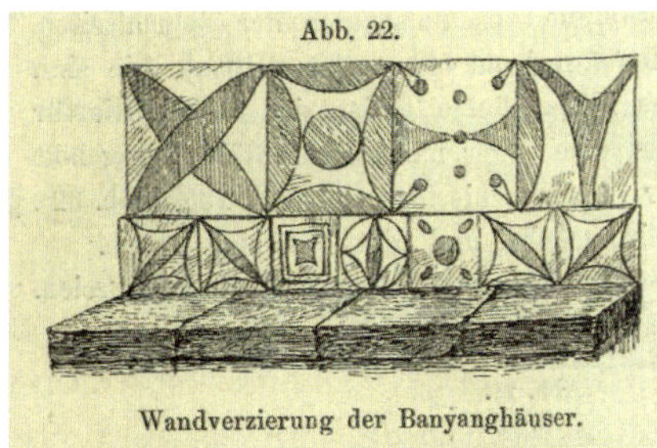

Fig. 3: Wall paintings in Banyangland (Hutter 1902: 278).

Fig. 4: Carved stools of the Banyangland (Hutter 1902: 280).

Desire to Loot Artifacts and Skulls

If Zintgraff had been relatively indifferent to possessing the ›ethnological rocks‹ to this point, this was no longer the case for the other objects he found in Baduma. Based on his personal account, it was the first time he saw such skillfully carved and highly valuable »idols«. Just as Max Buchner (1914: 269) had secretly wondered how he could obtain the marvelous artifacts from the hut in the Bakundu area, which had been offered him as a sleeping area in 1884–1885, Zintgraff's own desire to acquire objects grew stronger and stronger. At first, he tried in vain to purchase them. Since the villagers were not at all willing to sell their ›gods‹, Zintgraff devised a plan to »mistakenly« (so he claims) kidnap at least

7 Some wall paintings were also reported for the Yabassi region, where Zintgraff had sojourned during his first trips into the interior of »Cameroon« in the outgoing 1886/7. See Ziemann (1907: 135).

8 »Eines haben die Banyang sämmtlichen [sic!] Negerstämmen von Kamerun bis zum Benue voraus: ihre außerordentlich sauber gebauten und mit einer gewissen Bequemlichkeit eingerichteten Wohnhäuser. Die Lehmwände sowie die gleichfalls aus Lehm gefertigten Sophas [sic!] mit Armlehnen sind tadellos glatt poliert, mit schwarzer Farbe bemalt, oft auch mit schönen Verzierungen in schwarz, weiß, roth [sic!] und blau ausgestattet« (Zintgraff 1895: 121). Editors' note: The terms n****/N**** are highly discriminatory and are therefore generally avoided today. But to delete them from colonial sources would obscure the violence and racism of colonial regimes.

one of them while leaving in the early morning. Yet, a further obstacle impeded him from realizing his plan, namely the size of the cult objects. Just as with previous »idols« in the Bakundu-land, these were also all as tall as a human being, the carvings however were even more attractive. Zintgraff shamelessly describes his desire to steal the »idols«: »In Baduma I also for the first time saw excellently carved idols, which, however, no money could gain; also their man-sized height did not allow to reap one of them ›mistakenly‹ at the crack of dawn« (Zintgraff 1895: 83).[9] Did Zintgraff revisit this place during his stay in the colony? It is not mentioned. Yet one such ›idol‹, *Dikoi*, would eventually turn up in Switzerland some ten years later in 1898, brought by a missionary of the Basler Mission named Nathanael Lauffer.[10] At the 1909 Basler Mission exhibition, the ›idol‹ was proudly presented as »Beutestück des Stärkeren« (»looted piece of the strongest«) (Ratschiller 2013), the strongest here referring to the courageous messengers of a Christian God (priests), who considered the religion and beliefs of the local populations as those of pagans or heathens. Such practices were to be destroyed by all means, of which one of the most frequently utilized was destruction by fire (Opoku 2015).

Zintgraff's expression »no money could gain« clearly indicates that he did his utmost to buy them, and that he must surely have tried to bribe some of the locals. Once arrived in the Kombone village, whose inhabitants were said to be ›cannibals‹, Zintgraff made no attempt to conceal his intention to take human skulls home for scientific analysis. He tried to retrieve skulls from the ashes in a forest where it was rumored that secret ceremonies took place (Zintgraff 1895: 85f.). At that time, the act of collecting cult or art treasures and human remains of the so-called ›inferior‹, ›savage‹ and ›barbaric‹ races was considered part of heroic and patriotic actions destined, so the claim goes, to advance scientific, medical and anthropological research; all of which were to become significant tools of colonialism. Skulls, in particular, were both useful and sought after as according to anthropological convictions at the time they, more than other parts of the human body, could demonstrate through biological anthropology/craniometry the supposed inferiority of the colonized, specifically by comparing the sizes of the brain cavit for instance. Furthermore, colonial collections were generally intended to raise one's prestige, status and income or that of the domestic institution (Tsogang Fossi 2020). Yet no matter the extent to which resisting peoples were crushed, particularly large artifacts would simply never be looted, and were thus destined to be destroyed.

Zintgraff's Destruction of Art Treasures by Burning and ›Recycling‹

In the colonial history of Cameroon, the Tange was, of course, the first notable object to have escaped destruction by fire. The Tange was a beautiful and colorful ship bow that served as an emblem for the King of Hickory Town (today Bonaberi), Lock Priso. It continues

9 »In Baduma sah ich auch zum erstenmale [sic!] ausgezeichnet geschnitzte Götzenbilder, die indessen für kein Geld zu erhalten waren; auch gestattete es ihre mannshohe Größe nicht, eins etwa morgens in aller Frühe beim Aufbruch ›aus Versehen‹ mit einzupacken« (Zintgraff 1895: 83).

10 A photograph of the *Dikoti* can be found on the website of the Basler Mission Archives (International Mission Photography Archive, n.d.), or in Gardi 1994.

to be a bone of contention between the Bele Bele community (led mostly by Kum'a Ndumbe III) in Duala and the Bavarian State (Splettstösser 2019) up to this day. In July 1884, Lock Priso had already refused the German flag to be hoisted on his territory and to submit himself to the German colonial power. In December 1884, following an attack of the Lock Priso's men and Joss people against King Bell, an ally of the Germans, on the grounds that King Bell had sold the land to the Germans for his sole interest, the German navy waged war against Lock Priso and the Joss people. Priso's palace was then set ablaze and heavily shelled and bombarded under the orders of German admiral, Knorr, who sought thereby to »enhance psychological effects« as he put it at that time. Max Buchner, acting as representative of the German civil administration, searched the palace before it was burnt down. He discovered the Tange, which he described as his most prominent find and sent it to his homeland Bavaria (Buchner 1914: 194). Terming it a most prominent find suggests that he did indeed find other objects, but that the remnants were consumed in the fire. It is difficult for me to qualify and quantify them as Buchner kept no inventory. Thus, Buchner's book title – *Aurora Colonialis* – entailed also indescribably difficult times for peoples, art and cult treasures in Cameroon and throughout the colonies.

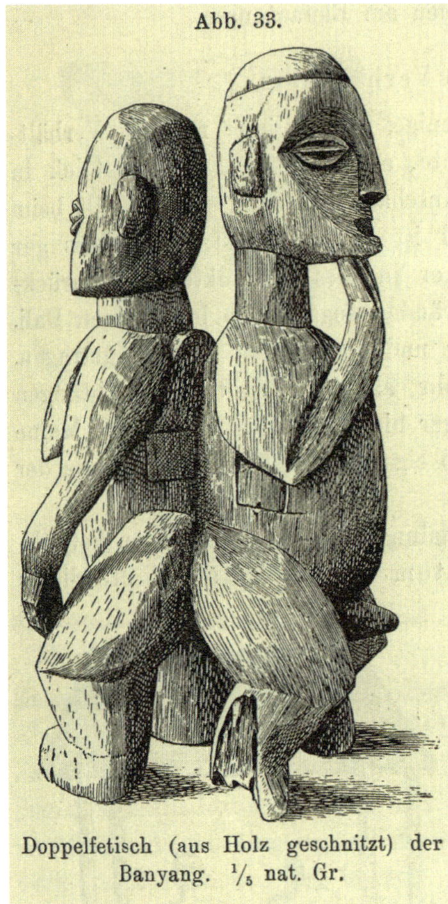

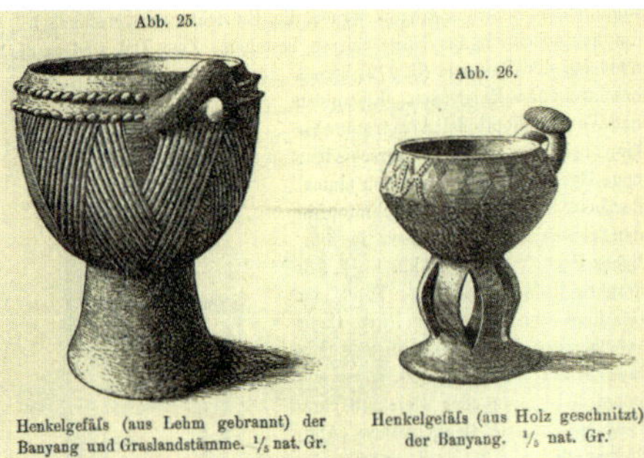

Fig. 5 and 6: Double ›idol‹ figures of the Banyang (Hutter 1902: 296) and tools of the Banyang (Hutter 1902: 280).

Zintgraff's decision to reduce the compounds of Banyang paramount chief N'Tok Difang to ashes (»levelled to the ground«), – following N'Tok Difang's obstruction of Zintgraff's path inland – draws a similar pattern. The wall paintings he had earlier admired, as well as the drums and other artifacts that were fated to disappear in the fire, including the compounds 10 km around, encompassed nearly the whole Banyang land. This was a difficult spectacle for Zintgraff, above all because, as he himself laments, he could not transport the treasures he was destroying.[11] Ten people were killed on N'Tok Difang's property, as well as a further seventy people in Bahuang, another Banyang settlement. What became of the art treasures? Zintgraff, his own words, watched »the very valuable ethnological objects disappear in the fire«. Again owing to their great size, he was unable to transport them. As he relates in his own personal account:

»The number of people killed was later given as 70 by themselves whilst about 25 hamlets within a radius of 10 kilometres were levelled to the ground. *Many remarkable objects, precious for anthropology, like big drums draped with human skulls with jaws rattling when beaten, had to be destroyed since, to my greatest distress, it was not feasible to drag them along*« (Zintgraff 1895: 152; my emphasis).[12]

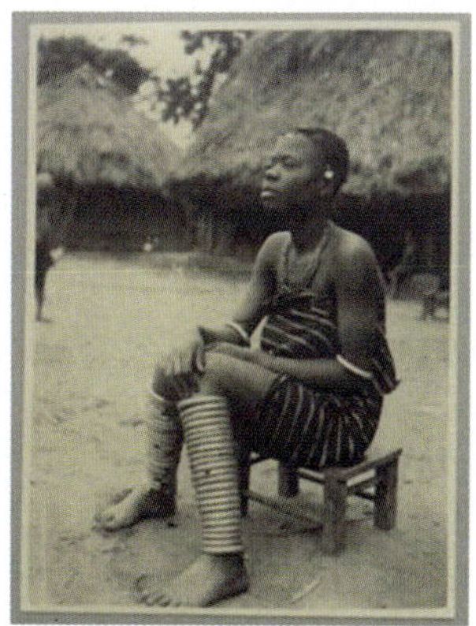

Fig. 7: A bride from the Cross River area in the 1920s. This gives an idea of the quantity of brass jewel that a queen, according to Zintgraff's account, could be wearing at the time he took them hostage (MARKK Hamburg, Photo: Tsogang Fossi).

Yet, fire was not the only employed by Zintgraff in his dealing with the art and artifacts of the region. His attitude toward women's jewelry should also be highlighted. During the war against N'Tok Difang, 20 of his richly adorned wives were taken hostage. As queens, they wore many brass jewels. Brass figured significantly in weddings, while the jewels from them also served to indicate status, as is the case with ivory bracelets in the coastal Duala community. As a matter of fact, women of noble descent, as well as queens, could be adorned with more than eight kilograms of such jewels at a given

11 The destruction of villages was both a human and an artistic catastrophe. With significant insight, Oskar Nuoffer (1926) later described the art of the grassland region. This art equally suits the case of the Banyang, as is attested to in the following citation: »Comprehensive palaces were created with domed roofs and galleries of pillars, the portals flanked by posts richly embellished with figures, the walls with ornamental friezes; in the chambers there were thrones, majestic beds and sedan chairs, portable stretchers with human and animal sculptures both in the round and pierced; big drums with lavish ornaments, not to think of the numerous wooden dance masks. The whole people takes a vivid delight in beautifully carved house ornaments, in stools, dishes, bowls, drinking horns and other fine household goods, especially pipes« (»Umfangreiche Paläste erstanden mit Kuppeldächern und Säulengallerien, die Tore von figurenreichen Pfosten flankiert, die Wände mit Ornamentfriesen; in den Gemächern Throne, Paradebetten und Sänften, Tragbahren mit Menschen und Tieren in Rundplastik und durchbrochener Arbeit; große Trommeln mit reichem Ausschmuck, der zahlreichen hölzernen Tanzmasken nicht zu gedenken. Im ganzen Volke lebt die Freude an schöngeschnitzten Hausverzierungen, an Hockern, Schüsseln, Schalen, Trinkhörnern und anderen feinen Hausrat, besonders der Pfeife«; Nuoffer 1926: 32).

12 »Die Gefallenen wurden später von ihnen selber auf 70 angegeben, während etwa 25 Weiler im Umkreise von 10 Kilometer dem Erdboden gleichgemacht waren. *Viele merkwürdige, für die Völkerkunde werthvolle [sic!] Gegenstände, darunter große Trommeln mit Menschenschädeln behangen, die beim Trommeln mit den Kinnladen klapperten, mussten vernichtet werden, da deren Mitschleppen zu meinem größten Kummer nicht angängig war*« (Zintgraff 1895: 152; my emphasis).

time (Skolaster 1910: 49–50). We can therefore surmise, at no risk of exaggerating, that the twenty queens may well have been wearing more than 160 kg of brass jewels!

Yet Zintgraff was lacking in ammunition; he took the unprecedented and incredible decision of harshly and ungentlemanly seizing the jewels, which he then recycled by transforming them into bullets. Very cynically, he goes so far as to hope that the families of these queens would soon regret their generosity to them because the jewels were to become bullets for the extermination of the generous donors:

»To remedy this sensitive need of ammunition we had to use the serpentine rings of the captured womenfolk that were made of strong brass wire and worn as jewellery around their arms and legs. We ungallantly pulled them from their limbs and had them smashed with a chisel into buckshot size pieces by the carpenter who used his axe as an anvil. In this shape they were fired, as lethal greetings, towards their fathers, husbands and brothers, who in view of this unexpected and fatal use we made of their former generosity, may have bitterly regretted it« (Zintgraff 1895: 151–152).[13]

Such destruction of African artifacts and art would occur both during and after the German colonial period. It was equally enacted by different missionaries, who understood the practice as a sign of conversion from ›paganism‹ to Christianity. The new convert would passionately take part in such apostasy as proof that he had changed life and was newly born in Christ. Paul Steiner reports cases around the Muyuka, Balong and Bombe areas, where new converts either developed an interested in selling their former carved ›gods‹ as »curiosities« to the Europeans, or where they simply allowed the objects to perish in missionary fires:

»Bit by bit idol worship also began to lose its reputation and the national heathendom received a heavy blow. People started to sell their carved or clay baked Losango (human and animal figures) as curiosities or had them burned. Notably the downfall of an important Balong chief, who, as a dreaded Losango-man, had exerted great pressure on the people by means of his magic, lead to idol burning fires flaring up in almost all Balong and Bakundu villages« (Steiner 1909: 77).[14]

13 »Um nun dieser empfindlichen Geschoßnoth [sic!] abzuhelfen, mussten die aus starkem Messingdraht gewundenen Ringe der gefangenen Weiber herhalten, die sie als Schmuck um Arme und Beine trugen. Wir zogen ihnen die Reifen sehr ungalanterweise von den Gliedern und ließen sie dann durch den Zimmermann auf einer als Ambos dienenden Axt mit einem Meißel in rehpostendicke Stücke zerschlagen. In solcher Gestalt flogen sie als todtbringende [sic!] Grüße ihren Vätern, Männern und Brüdern entgegen, die wohl Angesichts dieses unerwarteten und verhängnisvollen Gebrauchs von ihrer einstigen Freigebigkeit solche bitter bereuen mochten« (Zintgraff 1895: 151–152).

14 »Allgemach verlor auch der Götzendienst an Ansehen, und das nationale Heidentum erlitt einen starken Stoss. Die Leute fingen an, ihre geschnitzten oder aus Lehm gebrannten Losango (Menschen- und Tierfiguren) als Kuriositäten zu verkaufen oder sie verbrennen zu lassen. Besonders der Fall eines bedeutenden Balong-Häuptlings, der als gefürchteter Losangomann durch seine Zaubermittel einen großen Druck auf das Volk ausgeübt hatte, führte dazu, dass fast in allen Balong- und Bakundudörfern die Götzenfeuer emporloderten« (Steiner 1909: 77).

Jakob Keller, a missionary who dwelled in the Bakossi lands from the 1890s, also witnessed and actively encouraged public apostasy as accompanied by the destruction of objects belonging to local cults. The objects in question were either cast into flames or thrown into rivers. Through this ›trick‹ however, he was also able to save certain objects that he later took to Basel. He reports:

»As it was, the Bakosi tribe had bidden farewell in *corpore* to heathendom. At a large public gathering they officially bade farewell to heathendom. Mountains of skulls, bones etc. were burned and thrown into the river Mongo. Few things could I save and bring to Basel« (in Gardi 1994: 56).[15]

However, it is obvious in these instances that the iconoclastic attitude of the population is a result of their recent inclusion in the new church and is, as such, not precisely forced, though not totally entirely voluntary or free from the manipulation and intimidation of the colonial and missionary administration. In some cases, certain rituals and cults were even banned, while in the same stroke missionaries insisted that Sundays be institutionalized as a holy day (see Steiner 1909: 116; Wurm 1904: 27f.). In such cases, no other cult or religious practice was allowed, and the complaints of missionaries against offenders would lead to punitive police or military interventions, whereby the offenders were imprisoned and their cult objects seized. Some leaders of the secret society were also hanged. This exemplifies another aspect of the collaboration and mutual help that coexisted between the missionary societies and the colonial administration (see Berger 1978: 81). Seizing cult objects in such instances also became a means for administrators and European missionaries to provide collectors with so-called curiosities, in cases where they were not themselves interested in the objects.

The fourth attitude of Zintgraff towards art treasures of the regions he »visited«, may be termed »awareness«.

›Egoistic‹ Awareness

Upon arrival in the Western Grasland of Cameroon, Zintgraff was warmly welcomed by one of the great rulers of the area; Fon Galega of Bali. Fon Galega dreamed of expanding his domination over the neighboring kingdoms Bafut and Mankon, and decided to protect Zintgraff from his notables and other rulers, who were urging him to kill the stranger. He saw in the modern technology that the visitor displayed (weapons) a solid chance to achieve his plans for hegemony in the region. Zintgraff, for his part, viewed the ruler, who had an unlimited power over his subjects, as an ideal partner for his colonial projects. Both men would eventually sign a blood pact by mixing their blood and drinking it, swearing mutual and infallible assistance. Zintgraff would later seek out and sign a

15 »Der Bakosistamm hatte nämlich in *corpore* dem Heidentum den Abschied gegeben. An einer großen Volksversammlung wurde offiziell dem Heidentum Abschied gegeben. Ganze Berge von Schädeln, Knochen etc. wurden verbrannt und in den Fluss Mongo geworfen. Wenige Sachen konnte ich retten und nach Basel bringen« (in Gardi 1994: 56).

formalized contract with Galega, thus rendering the local ruler harmless for colonial power (Tsogang Fossi 2019).

Zintgraff's view was that the artistic practices of the people inland were undergoing a constant, yet dramatic change due to contact with the European world. As a result, he claimed, a visible loss of originality or authenticity in African art was occurring. We can thus summarize: ›Culture‹ (›Kultur‹) seemed to be destroying ›nature‹ (›Natur‹ or ›die primitive Kunst der Naturvölker‹), i.e. the art of the African ›savage‹. One way or the other, the position is paradoxical, given that the colonizers, and thus Zintgraff himself, arrived with the assumption that they had been assigned a sort of divine mission to civilize the ›savage‹. His position, however, conflicts with an assumption known as ›the white Man's burden‹ insofar as he claims to be the ›apostle‹ of civilization, while at the same hoping that the ›savage‹ remain authentic, that is, consistently ›savage‹. He did not want European ways of life to be imitated, giving way to what were derogatively referred to at the time as »Hosennigger«, that is, those who were; »too civilized to be authentic but not able to do more than mimic true civilization« (Aitken/Rosenhaft 2013: 14). Despite this underlying contradiction, Zintgraff rather accurately articulates – as one of the first colonizers – the start of a form art trafficking in the early years of European colonialism. Though the African's ›authenticity‹ appeared to be waning, certain European art dealers were keenly aware of the increasing value of African art and artifacts in Europe. They were unscrupulous and rather a little too eager to engage in producing the ›exotic‹ at/from home (Europe) in order to lure unsuspecting African art collectors:

> »Like with all tribes in inner Africa, who have been touched by culture, here too there is a gradual transformation of indigenous customs and craftsmanship taking place. The Bali already have started to digress from their old patterns and to imitate European ones, and the time, when a sword forged from indigenous iron will be a rarity, is probably not far away, since they can get better things equally cheap by way of trade from the coast. The weapons of the Haussa and Mandingo in West Africa as well as Massai spears from East Africa even now are already partly counterfeited in Europe and sold to inexperienced collectors as genuine« (Zintgraff 1895: 218).[16]

Yet it should be emphasized that Zingraff's concern here is not the fate of the African, but that of the poor European collector, who would probably become the victim of this trick. In this sense, Zintgraff, in his capacity as an eager collector of African artifacts, was acting in defiance of what could well have become his own fate.

16 »Wie aber bei allen Stämmen im Inneren Afrikas, die von der Kultur berührt werden, so vollzieht sich auch hier eine allmähliche Umwandlung der einheimischen Gebräuche und Kunstfertigkeiten. Bereits fangen die Bali an, von ihren alten Mustern abzugehen und europäische nachzuahmen, und die Zeit ist wohl nicht mehr fern, wo ein aus einheimischem Eisen geschmiedetes Schwert eine Seltenheit sein wird, da sie bessere und ebenso billige Sachen auf dem Wege des Handels von der Küste erhalten. Die Waffen der Haussa und Mandingo in Westafrika, sowie in Ostafrika die Speere der Massai werden zum Theil [sic!] schon jetzt in Europa nachgeahmt und an unerfahrene Sammler als echte verkauft« (Zintgraff 1895: 218).

Conclusive Remarks

The above-described attitudes of Zintgraff toward Cameroonian cultural assets demonstrate the fate of African art and cult objects from the early years of European colonialism until today. Debates on the restitution of art treasures from colonial contexts, which presently appear to some, erroneously, as new motives (Savoy 2020) continue in the absence of any meaningful action or result.[17] Despite measures and resolutions taken by UNESCO and ICOM (Le Courrier de l'UNESCO 2020) to protect cultural heritage and discourage art trafficking, art dealers prove to be very inventive. These attitudes also unveil some challenges that await researchers of the provenance of art and cult treasures from questionable contexts. Apart from the insects which Zintgraff openly admits to collecting, he does not, at any point in his diary, clearly state whether or not he collected artifacts or not, admitting only to their destruction. His silence on these activities as a collector is certainly misleading, until one considers the diary in relation to other sources, either from the same author or those who accompanied him, such as Franz Hutter (letters and reports to the colonial administration, letters with museum institutions). In point of fact, there is no more room for doubt: not only did he collect artifacts and insects – to be found in Braunschweig, Detmold, Berlin, Oldenburg, Leipzig, Stuttgart, and Hildesheim – but human remains as well, namely skulls.[18] Although no word of this appears in the diary, the first contingent of artifacts collected, received or looted by Zintgraff arrived Europe as early as 1887, that is, from the very beginning of his ›trips‹ in Cameroon. Is there any specificity to the ›objects‹ he collected? When, where and how did he collect these art assets? Is there any identifiable network of collectors, or links to specific museums? These are some of the questions in the next steps to gain greater insight into the collection history of this ›explorer‹.

Seeking to determine the provenance of art treasures that were simply transported, taken forcibly, or looted as booty from their original owners helps us understand the asymmetrical relations of power of colonial times. Furthermore, the failure to consider objects that had been voluntarily destroyed by the conquerors may contribute to erasing collective memory and the cultural heritage of a given population. Future discussions should be extended to various forms of destroyed artifacts, which need comparative studies of different historical materials and records. Reconstruction of a bygone artistic know-how appears to be a symbolic reparation of the wrongs endured by source communities. It also helps in nation-building narratives as a counter-discourse to the colonial assumptions that legitimated colonial ideology and practices as a humanitarian enterprise, casting colonialism as a ›divine‹ mission of the ›civilized‹ Europe to the benefit of the ›uncivilized‹ local African.

17 Only recently did Germany promise to restitute looted Benin bronzes to Nigeria. See Monks (2021).

18 Enough skulls were harvested in the Grasslands during campaigns against resisting villages. As Franz Hutter launched a punitive expedition against the Bamigni, the Bangoa, the Bafortchu in October 1891, more than 200 human skulls were collected (»looted« in his own words) and carried back to Bali where Zintgraff dwelled. See Hutter (1901: 22). Some of these skulls likely ended up at the Charité in Berlin where they have preoccupied a team of researchers investigating human remains in Berlin's institutions with links to the colonial period (Holger Stoecker, Sarah Fründt and Thomas Schnalke).

Literature

AITKEN, Robbie/ROSENHAFT, Eve (2013): *Black Germany. The Making and Unmaking of a Diaspora Community, 1884–1960*, Cambridge: Cambridge University Press.

BERGER, Heinrich (1978): *Mission und Kolonialpolitik. Die Katholische Mission in Kamerun während der deutschen Kolonialzeit*, Immensee: Neue Zeitschrift für Missionswissenschaft.

BRAIN, Robert (1981): »The Fontem-Bangwa: A Western Bamileke Group«. In: *Contribution de la Recherche Ethnologique à l'Histoire des Civilisations du Cameroun/The Contribution of Ethnological Research to the History of Cameroon Cultures*, ed. by. Claude Tardits. Paris: Editions du Centre National de la Recherche Scientifique, 355–360.

BUCHNER, Max (1914): *Aurora Colonialis. Bruchstücke eines Tagebuchs aus dem ersten Beginn unserer Kolonialpolitik*, München: Verlag Piloty & Loehle.

BUREAU, René (1962): *Ethno-Sociologie Religieuse des Duala et Apparentés*, Yaoundé: Institut des Recherches Scientifiques du Cameroun.

CHILVER, E. M. (1966): *Zintgraffs Explorations in Bamenda, Adamawa and the Benue Lands 1889–1892*, Victoria: Basel Missions Press.

INTERNATIONAL MISSION PHOTOGRAPHY ARCHIVE (n.d.): *The Idol Dikoki (?); Masks and Staffs for Losango Worship. Cameroon*, http://digitallibrary.usc.edu/cdm/ref/collection/p15799coll123/id/18302 (12.05.2021).

GARDI, Bernhard (1994): *Kunst in Kamerun. Waldland und Grassland – Ausgewählte Stücke aus den Sammlungen des Museums für Völkerkunde Basel und der Basler Mission*, Basel/Muttenz: Schwabe & Co. AG.

GRIMME, Gesa (2017): »Annährungen an ein ›Schwieriges Erbe‹ – Provenienzforschung in Linden-Museum Stuttgart«. In: *Provenienzforschung zu ethnographischen Sammlungen der Kolonialzeit. Positionen in der aktuellen Debatte*, ed. by. Larissa Förster/Iris Edenheiser/Sarah Fründt/Heike Hartmann, Berlin: Arbeitsgruppe Museum der Deutschen Gesellschaft für Sozial- und Kulturanthropologie, 157–170, https://doi.org/10.18452/19029 (01.07.21).

HUTTER, Franz (1902): *Wanderungen und Forschungen im Nord-Hinterland von Kamerun*, Braunschweig: Friedrich Vieweg und Sohn.

OPOKU, Kwame (2015): *Price of Kota Sold in Paris is Interesting but what about Loss to Creators and Original Users?*, http://www.africavenir.org/de/newsdetails/archive/2015/july/article/kwame-opoku-price-of-kota-sold-in-paris-is-interesting-but-what-about-loss-to-creators-and-original.html?tx_ttnews%5Bday%5D=13&cHash=522bbeb-5f776951545f05d129d26e9f1 (05.07.2019).

LE COURRIER DE L'UNESCO (2020): *Trafic Illicite des Biens Bulturels, 50 ans de Lutte*. No 3. https://fr.unesco.org/courier/2020-4 (01.07.21).

MANSFELD, Alfred (1908): *Urwald-Dokumente: Vier Jahre unter den Crossflussnegern Kameruns*, Berlin: Dietrich Reimer.

MICHEL, Marc (1970): »Les Plantations allemandes du Mont Cameroun (1885–1914)«. In *Revue Française d'Histoire d'Outre-Mer*. Tome 57: 207, 183–213.

MICHELS, Stefanie (2017): »Julius von Soden«, in *Koloniale Verbindungen*, http://deutschland-postkolonial.de/portfolio/soden/ (22.06.2021).

MONKS, Kieron (2021): »Germany to return looted Benin Bronzes to Nigeria«, *CNN online*, https://edition.cnn.com/style/article/benin-bronzes-germany-restitution/index.html (22.06.2021).

Nkui Nchoji, Paul (1989): *The German Presence in the Western Grassfields 1891–1913. A German Colonial Account*, Leiden: African Studies Centre/Yaoundé: Computer Services of Scientific Research.

Notizblatt des Königl. Botanischen Gartens und Museums zu Berlin (1900): No. 21.

Nuoffer, Oskar (1926): *Afrikanische Plastik in der Gestaltung von Mutter und Kind*, Dresden: Carl Reissner Verlag.

Ratschiller, Anna (2013): »›Die Zauberei spielt in Kamerun eine böse Rolle‹. Die ethnographischen Ausstellungen der Basler Mission (1908–1912)«. In: *Mission Global. Eine Verflechtungsgeschichte seit dem 19. Jahrhundert*, ed. by Rebekka Habermas/Richard Hölzl, Wien/Köln/Weimar: Böhlau Verlag, 241–264.

Savoy, Bénédicte (2021): *Afrikas Kampf um seine Kunst. Geschichte einer postkolonialen Niederlage*, München: C.H. Beck.

Linden-Museum (ed.) (2021): *Schwieriges Erbe. Linden-Museum und Württemberg im Kolonialismus. Eine Werkstattausstellung*, booklet about the eponymous exhibition, Stuttgart.

Skolaster, Hermann (1910): *Kulturbilder aus Kamerun*, Limburg/Lahn: Druck und Verlag der Kongregation der Pallottiner.

Splettstösser, Anne (2019): *Umstrittene Sammlungen. Vom Umgang mit kolonialem Erbe aus Kamerun in ethnologischen Museen. Die Fälle Tange/Schiffschnabel und Ngonnso'/* Schalenträger in Deutschland und Kamerun, Göttingen: Universitätsverlag.

Steiner, Paul (1909): *Kamerun als Kolonie und Missionsfeld*, Basel: Verlag der Missionsbuchhandlung.

Sydov, Eckart von (1930): *Handbuch der westafrikanischen Plastik*, Berlin: Dietrich Reimar und Ernst Vohsen.

Tsogang Fossi, Richard (2020): »Itinerary of a Cameroon Cross River Collection in Art Market Networks. An Analysis of Transaction Correspondence between Hamburg-Berlin-Leipzig«. In: *Journal for Art Market Studies* 4:1, https://doi.org/10.23690/jams.v4i.101 (10.05.2021).

Tsogang Fossi, Richard (2019): »›Du bist wie ein Küchlein in mein Haus gekommen, Weißer…‹. Intermediale Erinnerung an eine Männerfreundschaft des deutschen Kolonialismus in Kamerun«. In: *Koloniale Verbindungen – Transkulturelle Erinnerungstopografien. Das Rheinland in Deutschland und das Grasland in Kamerun*, ed. by Albert Gouaffo/Stefanie Michels, Bielefeld: transcript, 111–130.

Wurm, Paul (1904): *Die Religion der Küstenstämme in Kamerun*, Basel: Verlag der Missionsbuchhandlung.

Vollbehr, Ernst (1912): *Mit Pinsel und Palette durch Kamerun. Tagebuchaufzeichnungen und Bilder*, Leipzig: List und von Bressensdorf.

Ziemann, Greta (1907): *›Mola Koko‹! Grüsse aus Kamerun*, Berlin: Wilhelm Süsseroth.

Zintgraff, Eugen (1895): *Nord-Kamerun. Schilderung der im Auftrage des Auswärtigen Amtes zur Erschliessung des nördlichen Hinterlandes von Kamerun während der Jahre 1886–1892 unternommenen Reisen*, Berlin: Verlag der Gebrüder Paetel.

Table of figures

The ›Mystery‹ of the Konkomba's Severed Thumbs: Historical Fact, Colonial Rumour or Legend of the Defeated?

Bernard Müller

»Forgetting and remembering are equally inventive.«
Jorge Luis Borges (1970)

The former ethnographic museum could reinvent itself by exhibiting not only objects but also stories. It is important to allow for anti-colonial resistance to be expressed in a variety of forms, in which the biographical dimension of the narrators is to be taken into consideration. This interweaving of life stories has the objective of highlighting interactions between people, and the reality of exchanges (rather than the classic ethnographic identification of cultural specificities). As such, accounts of anti-colonial resistance come in a variety of narrative forms. They may take the form of an enigma, a rumour, or a legend even perhaps, one that is not always corroborated by facts such as they are understood by the scientific community. This article proposes a narrative approach to the topic of restitution, of restoring to Africa goods that were looted during colonisation. In this case, the objects in question are human remains. Thumbs to be precise, the severed thumbs of Konkomba archers (Togo/Ghana) allegedly amputated by militias, first German and then French, during the anti-colonial revolts of 1884 and 1934. Accounts of such torture continue to be passed down to this very day, yet they are rejected as ›legends‹ by historians who can find no trace of them in the colonial archives. Should such accounts thus be denigrated?

Seeking to examine the ramifications of such accounts as well as following up a childhood memory (I had myself heard this account in 1976), I revisited Konkomba territory in 2006, then again in April, and finally July of 2018. Though I did, I believe, find evidence tending to confirm the reality of this practice, my research – which is still ongoing – revealed certain surprising and disconcerting ways of retelling colonization. In this paper I argue that the debate on the restitution of looted objects cannot take place without taking into account the symbolic trauma engendered by colonization. Restitution, then, ceases to be simply a problem of museum conservation. As this specific story from Togo, which is part of my own biography, shows, the restitution debate is situated in a narrative knot which is currently precisely in the process of being unravelled. Can or

ZfK – Zeitschrift für Kulturwissenschaften 2|2021
urn:nbn:de:hbz:6:3-zfk-2021-41962

should the museum be the place where these stories are transmitted? If so, what status should be given to these accounts and how should they be transmitted?

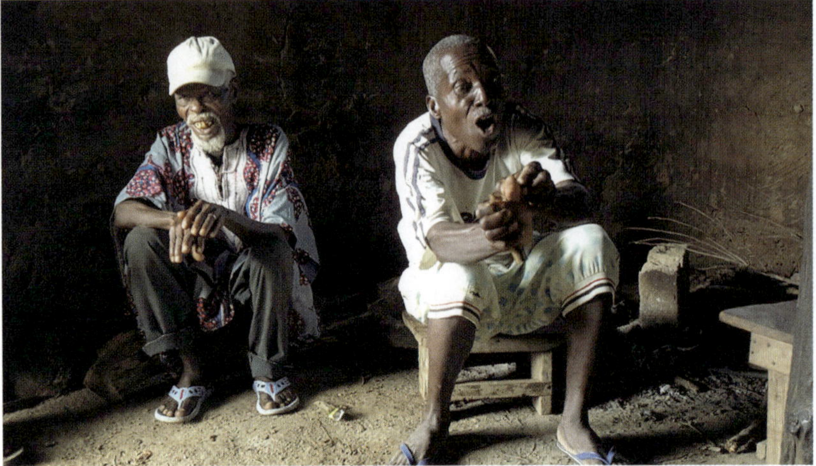

Fig. 1: A Bapuré elder showing how and why Konkomba archers' thumbs were amputated by German militias in the colonial period. Photo: Bernard Müller, May 2018.

The Anecdote

In Ghana and Togo, the image of Konkomba archers' amputated thumbs, severed by militias during the colonial conquest, is still raw in popular memory. The practice was first attributed to the Germans, and thereafter the French, though there is currently no formal, or rather scientific, evidence to support these claims. These accounts have spread well beyond the Konkomba region, yet there is no corroboration to be found in the military archives. The Konkomba are an unassuming people, and though they are certainly combative, they are modest peasants. Still, their stories are taken for mere fantasy. And yet the persistent transmission of this account poses certain questions. What if this was not just about verifying the oral sources (Gayibor 2011b) that allow us to understand the colonial phenomenon and its contemporary implications on a less factual but more symbolic level? To this end, we should have to relieve ourselves of the weight of the written tradition and, as in theatre, explore fiction in order to find the truth. We do so in the hope that such a step might finally reveal to us the ways in which history transforms the men who transform history, and the stories that constitute it.

But let us first ask how it is that this story has reached you, the reader of this text (taking an interest in the interstices of biographies and oral transmission).

The »Barrière de Pluie«: From One Memory to Another

It so happens that I was confronted with this story in 1976 when I was ten years old. We were living with my parents at the time, not far from Lomé, the coastal capital of Togo. We would occasionally visit friends living further inland, availing of the opportunity to discover the country. The road network was almost non-existent back then. Apart from a central axis that was more or less asphalted, the roads were rapidly deteriorating into mere tracks, more frequented by bicycles or warthogs than cars. We knew we were in the heart of Konkomba country, in the Dankpen, but no one remembers the name of the village where we stopped. Accompanied by a certain Kpakpatrou, a colleague of my father's, we arrived in a village that had been indicated to us as Konkomba country, and proceeded to introduce ourselves to the elder of the locality, as was customary. As my mother recalled:

> »the Germans brought Togo under their control around 1885 in a belated effort to find territories to ›protect‹. But they did not go unresisted, certainly not by the Konkomba. So sure were the latter of their invincibility while battling on their own territory that they came rushing into battle, claiming many of the aggressors' lives. Ultimately, however, they were mowed down by European weaponry. Victorious but embittered, the Germans enacted a cruel revenge on every young man deemed capable of taking arms. They severed the thumbs of their right hands, making it impossible for them to hold a bow. The man we went to greet with Kpakpatrou was very old, dressed as an authentic Konkomba should be, that is, in a simple animal skin. He had personally survived those sinister times and Kpakpatrou discreetly drew our attention to the missing thumb of the revered old man's right hand« (Denise Müller, interview on 25.04.2018).

In 2006, 30 years later, I revisited the Dankpen. It was one leg of a trip with the Togolese writer Kangni Alem, as part of preparations for an exhibition on colonial memory (the ›Broken Memory‹ project). We had decided to travel the old colonial route traced by the Germans up from the Atlantic Ocean. A light account of this journey was first published in 2009 (Alem 2009), earlier developed in a more detailed version in a blog (Alem 2006). I returned once again in July 2018.

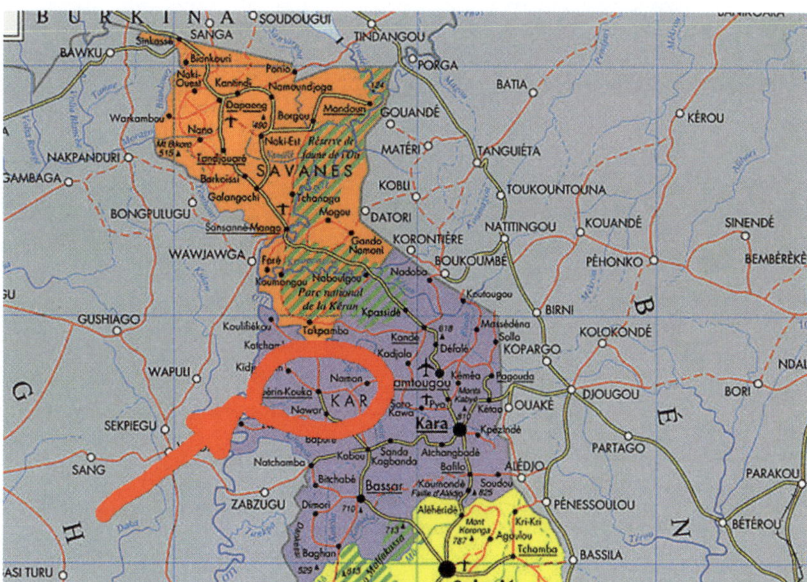

Fig. 2: Konkomba. Map: Bernard Müller, 2021.

Bernard Müller

Dankpen Rebellious

»The entire Konkomba army is coming for me. I cannot possibly escape.«
Dr. Gruner, cited by Peter Sebald[1]

It is quite possible that this elderly man, who, it seemed to me in 1976, was no longer of any age, knew how to use a bow in 1896 when the German Valentin von Massow invaded his country. In the entirety of the German colony of Togoland at that time (which currently straddles present-day Togo and Ghana), it was in the Dankpen region that the greatest resistance to conquest took place, such as to inflict heavy losses on the invader. On 14 May 1895, a German troop stationed at Katchamba, and led by the German von Carnap-Quernheimb, was violently attacked by Konkomba warriors armed with poisoned arrows. But we should leave this turbulent military chronicle aside for a moment to consider the events of 1896, the extreme violence of which has left its mark on the popular memory of the region's present inhabitants. Even the children here can trace the sequence of events, can point out where it happened, not, albeit, without indulging their imagination by adding a little twist of their own. At the end of November 1896, the expedition left Kete-Kratschi and headed toward Yendi. It consisted of four German officers or *chargés de mission*, 91 soldiers, 46 ammunition carriers and 231 simple porters. Massow and Heitmann directed military operations, while Dr. Gruner was in charge of the general, and political, coordination of the expedition as well as the signing of treaties. A fourth German, Lieutenant Gaston Thierry, would later join from Sansané-Mango.

Hans Gruner (1865–1943) is a key figure in the internal conquest of Togoland. Arriving in 1892, he was head of the ›colonial station‹ of Misahöhe for more than twenty years. Proudly bearing the title of *Doctor of Philosophy*, he was appointed head of the German expedition to the Togoland hinterland (›Togo-Hinterland-Expedition‹) from 1894 to 1895, and thus became the initiator of most of the treaties signed with rulers in the country's interior. These, in turn, would give rise to the negotiations for the territorial formation of the German Togo. Despite his doctorate in philosophy, he published surprisingly little about Togo, where he lived almost uninterruptedly from 1892 to 1914. He would never publish his travel journals in his own lifetime, indeed, it was not until 1997 that these were edited under the title *Vormarsch zum Niger: Die Memoiren des Leiters der Togo-Hinterland-Expedition 1894/1895*. The memoirs provide detailed documentation of the methods and means used by the Germans in the conquest of the Togo hinterland from 1894 to 1895. There is no mention of amputating thumbs.

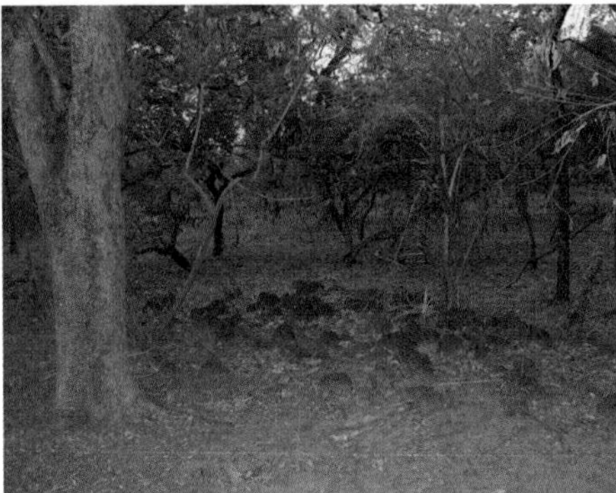

Fig. 3: Iboudjo Cemetery, Dankpen (the site was presented to me as the final resting place of Konkomba archers killed in combat with the German militia). Photo: Bernard Müller, 2006.

1 Original quote: »Das gesamte Konkombaheer will mich hier angreifen. Ich kann nicht fliehen.« (Sebald 1988: 192, then note 109 on page 706 (ZStA = Zentrales Staatsarchiv der DDR, Potsdam, Nr. 4392, Bl. 90). Translation by Bernard Müller.

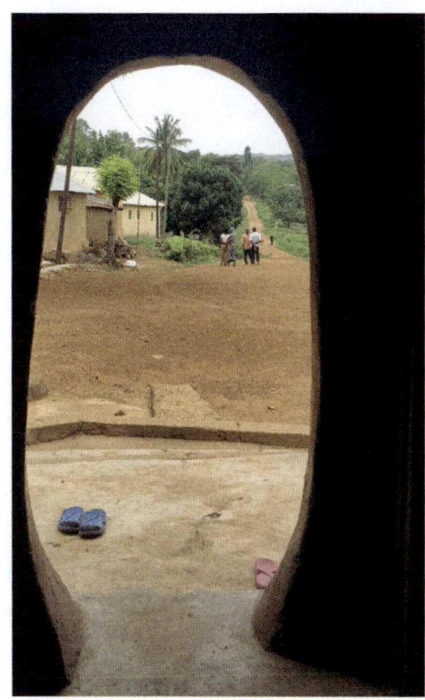

Fig. 4: Room with a view, Bapuré. Photo: Bernard Müller, 2006.

While returning from the famous battle of Adibo on 4 December 1896, which precipitated the fall of the Dagomba kingdom and, on the following day, the capture of the capital Yendi (present-day Ghana), German troops found themselves surrounded by an army of 7.000 Dagomba and Konkomba archers on »roughly 7 December 1896« (Gbandi 2009: 19). Despite their technological superiority, the conquerors suffered heavy losses. Rebel positions, in turn, were subjected to hails of machine gun fire and it is here that the thumbs of the young Konkomba would have been cut off to prevent them from firing their bows. It was this the thumb that would serve as support when firing an arrow, such as had set the Konkomba apart for their »determination and valour« (Cornevin 1962). There were heavy losses on both sides and Sergeant Heitmann, who was wounded on the battlefield, died of a poisoned arrow a few days later, on 28. December 1896, as did five other militiamen.[2]

The troupe accompanying the expedition consisted of ›police‹ that were stationed at Lomé. It was led by German officers (such as the ill-fated Heitmann) while its executors, policemen, civil servants and auxiliaries were all recruited elsewhere in Africa as local populations refused to enlist in the repression of their own. Following these battles, the Germans launched several campaigns following the simple principle of complete devastation, with a view to definitively imposing themselves. Writing in December 1897 after a fresh incursion into Konkomba country had put a temporary end to the revolts, von Massow stated: »basically, I reduced 40 to 50 villages to ashes, destroyed as many farms as possible, scattered nearly 300 head of cattle and 100 to 200 sheep…« (Von Massow/ Sebald 2014). In the context of such extreme violence, amputating thumbs is unlikely to have been mentioned at all, as it would have seemed derisory compared to the other exactions, more brutal and deadly as they were.

From von Massow to Massu

A few decades later, the French sent in Lieutenant Massu in the rather unreasonable hope of putting an end to the chronic refusal of the Konkomba to submit to administrative rationalism. He would remain from April 1935 to July 1936. According to the historian Nicoué Gayibor, Massu »took the opportunity to strengthen the power of the canton chiefs, which was frequently contested, and to remind people of their duty to render taxes, it was to be the cause of significant unrest« (Gayibor 2011a: 508). He confiscated and burned

2 »Mitteilung« from the German archives DKB 1895: Sergeant, Police master, born 01.03.1869 in Rüete, district of Hamm, »auf einer Expedition mit Eingeborenen gefallen« on the 28.12.1896 (294; 1897, 166), cited in Sebald 1988 : xxx.

nearly 300.000 arrows and arrow tips, as well as other war accessories (knives, finger tabs). The *strophantus*,[3] which were used to poison the arrows, were systematically destroyed. A renowned public figure in France, Jacques Massu was a general officer in the military. A *Compagnon de la Libération* and former commander-in-chief of the French forces in Germany, he had distinguished himself in the Leclerc column in particular, as well as in the 2nd Armoured Division during the Second World War. He was the subject of some controversy for his roles in colonial conflicts in Indochina and, in particular, in Algeria, given his open acknowledgement of the use of torture during his time there. Concretely, he was accused by Algerian FLN veterans of having endorsed and even participated in acts of torture during the war in Algeria. Freshly graduated from the Saint-Cyr military academy in 1930, he first cut his teeth as a second lieutenant in the colonial infantry during this operation of pacification, as well as other missions in Morocco and Chad. Though he would later go on to confirm the thrust of prior statements concerning his military activities in his book *La Vraie Bataille d'Alger* (*The True Battle of Algiers*), he at no point claimed to have participated in the amputation of Konkomba thumbs. Perhaps the manuscript of *The Real Konkomba Battle* will one day be found and published. To share one further anecdote, Massu returned to Konkomba country in 1979 and was »received with great pomp and circumstance [...] The Konkomba offered him, not without humour, a magnificent empty quiver (without arrows!)« (Gayibor et al. 1997: 22).

Irrespective of the particulars of each soldier's brutality, the presence of the two men has gone down in local history as exceptionally violent. Yet the similarity in their names provided the Konkomba with a chance to articulate the archetype of European military behaviour during the conquest: they are referred to as »masy« (phonetic transcription), meaning, simply, European soldiers. Whether this occurred in 1896 or 1936 makes little difference, given that the logic is the same. With thumb or without, on this point the Konkomba analysis is entirely correct. Of course, there's something shocking about this crude chronological rendition, but what offends an historian may well fascinate the anthropologist, because, for the latter, an anecdote does not have to be true to be relevant.

From the Archive to the Ethnographic Object

To value the narrative drifts of oral history in no way implies an invalidation of the historian's method. Instead, it invites us to read between the lines. The same is true for ethnographic collections; since the publication of Sarr and Savoy's report in November 2018 – *Restoring African Heritage: Towards a New Relational Ethics*[4] – the historical conditions under which they were acquired is once again on the agenda. Thus, if we were to rely solely on the written evidence provided by museum inventory sheets, the real conditions of their acquisition would escape us. This was the case with the flute allegedly ›bought‹ by Gaston Thierry during an ongoing conflict.

3 The highly toxic seeds of *strophanthus gratus* were once commonly used in the preparation of poison for arrows: they were ground with the sticky juice of the plant and the tips were dipped in this mixture.

4 Presented by Bénédicte Savoy and Felwine Sarr to the President of the Republic, Emmanuel Macron, on 23 November 2018.

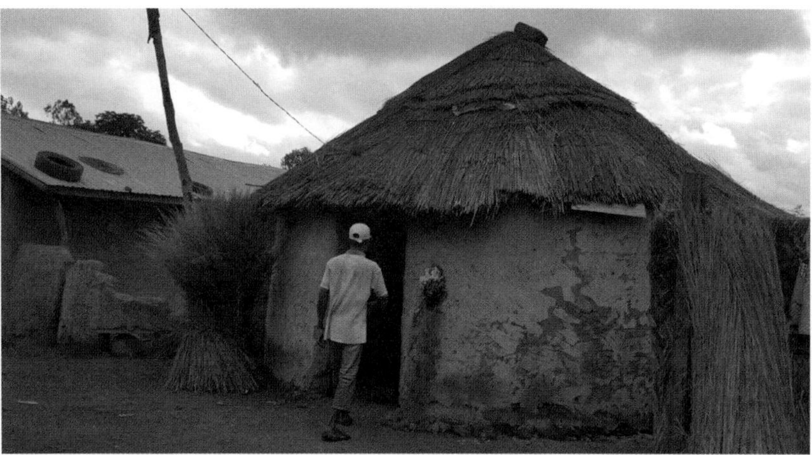

Fig. 5: Entering the family house, Bapuré. Photo: Bernard Müller, November 2018.

In the ethnographic collections in Saxony, Germany (Staatliche Ethnographische Sammlungen Sachsen im Verbund der Staatlichen Kunstsammlungen Dresden), one object in particular caught our attention: a signal whistle (»Signalpfeife«, inventory number MAF 1268). Insignificant though this may at first appear, it actually facilitated the Konkomba in challenging German soldiers, as is attested in the archives (Klose 1906). Known to hunters, it functions by way of coded sounds indicating directions. The whistle was supposedly ›purchased‹ – there are grounds to doubt this – and integrated into the collection in 1900. Seemingly banal, it most likely provided Konkomba warriors with a means of taking their enemy by surprise given that the sound, which is similar to that of a particular bird, was unknown to the Germans. This function, militaristic so to speak, explains why it was seized by agents of Lieutenant Gaston Thierry when he came to the rescue of Gruner's so-called scientific expedition.

Indeed, though no human remains resembling the Konkomba thumb phalanx can be found, German and French ethnographic collections are not lacking in Konkomba bows and arrows, nor are they short on flutes. The case of the severed thumb may not be a classic example of an object looted during the colonial era, but it nevertheless allows us to put our finger on an essential dimension of this debate, namely the aura of an absent object and the sheer quantity of strategies mobilized for its reinvention, even if it is thereby transformed. Objects live their own lives in a certain way, and the issue of the severed thumb testifies in this sense to the sheer volume of objects looted during the colonial era. Such objects are now housed in ethnographic museums in Europe and beyond. Such objects, like ghosts, can seem all the more present, paradoxically enough, by virtue of their absence. In any case, these objects become the accessory of an account for which their non-existence is the very condition of its possibility.

With German military archives supplying no documents to prove this practice, there are some who have concluded that this story was the result of an overactive imagination, that of a peasant and illiterate population, which has always been insubordinate and whose accounts ought not be taken literally. Without wishing to excessively probe that which is essentially an enigma, it remains the case that in Ghana, on the English-speaking side of Konkomba country, this matter is taken quite seriously. This is attested by the claim that

> »old Konkomba men could show the severed thumbs of their right hand, a fool-proof method [sic!] to restrict their armed resistance as they could no longer use bow and arrow […] The left toe of the Kokomba was usually severed, for the Germans believed that they used the left toe on the ground to gather momentum while the right arm released the dangerous arrow from the bow that caused havoc« (Maasole 2006: 185, cited after Kachim 2013: 168).

As far as Togolese historians go, they are content to claim that »there is, effectively, an erroneous legend circulating in schools and according to which Lieutenant Massu […] ordered that Konkomba warriors' thumbs be severed, so as to put a definitive end to the Konkomba revolts. This is not at all the case«. At most, they may also concede that it is not impossible that this »legend of the ›severed thumbs‹ […] was born of its quasi-homonym, 36 years earlier« (Gayibor 2011b).

A Touch of Theatre at the European Cemetery of Sokodé

On our journey to trace German colonisation in Togo in 2006, we left Konkomba country and arrived 100 km and two hours later in Sokodé, capital of the plateau region. Kangni Alem writes in his diary that

> »the welcome at the hostel was simple and the grilled chicken excellent. A man approached us while we were nibbling our skewers and sipping our beers. Friendly and talkative, he soon came to understand the purpose of our stay in Sokodé – the search for traces of the German conquest of Togo – and offered to be our guide for the next day. Or at least, he acted as though he had understood, he swore he would take us to Mango (another town altogether), to show us the cliff from which, he explained, sorcerers and other great criminals of the community were thrown into the void in ancient times. I asked him if it was true that there was a place in Sokodé where one could see chains sealed in the cement of the tombs… ›yes, yes‹ he said, brimming with excitement ›tomorrow I'll show you the prisoners buried with their chains‹. I was positively hopping with excitement: was the story true? Who were the men buried in this cemetery? What had they done? Our friend was hesitant to recall. In a very elegant gesture, he had the honesty not to speak any further, and we decided to meet the next day« (Alem 2006).

It was there in Kotokoli country, far from the Konkomba, that our investigation was to take on another dimension. It was an opening, one which – as we had set out on this parallel road, almost abandoned by the living but host to more ghosts than we could possibly have imagined – had not been foretold.

As we entered the cemetery, we saw a young man perched on the fence with whom we spoke, explaining the reasons for our visit. A whole group of youngsters in khaki school uniforms soon joined, followed by other onlookers. There then followed, in the middle of the cemetery, an erratic discussion as to how the colonial past ought to be discussed today, and the nature of its impact on the current state of Togo and the world. The ideas flowed freely; colonial violence was broached with a mix of condemnation and the regret of still living under a dictatorship that basically operates under the same principles, the same apparatus. »The only thing that's changed is the administrator's skin colour«, one secondary school student said.

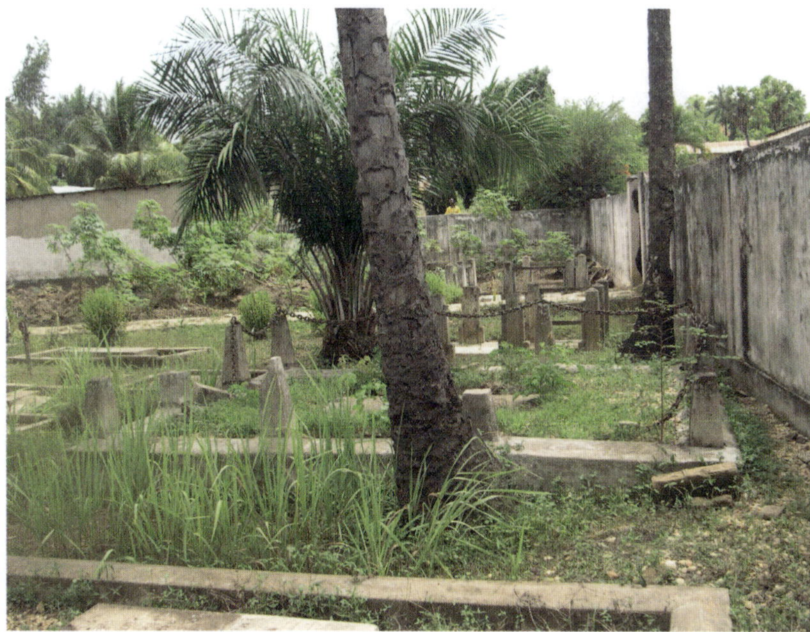

Fig. 6: The broken chains of the European cemetery of Sokodé, capital of the province of Centre and the prefecture of Tchaoudjo. Photo: Bernard Müller, May 2006.

An impromptu school class occurred and just as we were about to visit the graves, one of the schoolchildren remembered that he had an old magazine with an article on the cemetery. Convinced that the text contained information that would aid the discussion, he went to look for it. He returned with issue 99, dated May 1985, of the now defunct *Togo Dialogue* magazine, in which the French sociologist Jean-Claude Barbier had written an interesting article entitled »A cemetery amongst the green«.

Over the course of the discussion, a surprising turn of events occurred, whereby the children of yesterday's victims sat at the bedside of their persecutors' remains. As Kangni Alem recalls:

> »Bernard took out his camera to film Mr Dehée's grave. I asked one of the youngsters if, by any chance, he knew why there were chains around the central monument. Without hesitation, he answered that the white man buried in the tomb was a prisoner, so the chains were put there to distinguish him from the others. A splendid explanation, but the other school kids were not convinced. Another student corrected him: no, the man in the grave was a prisoner, true, but he hadn't served all his years in prison, so they put his soul in chains so that he could finish his sentence in the afterlife. Naively, I replied: ›his crime must have been horrible for them to punish him like this, even in death.‹ When did he die? How many years did he have left to serve? How can he now be unchained, beyond death? Is there a ritual for doing so?« (Alem 2006)

Against all expectations, the youngsters seemed to be interested in the fate of those Europeans, some of whom were not much older than they were. They wondered what sense of respect Europeans could have for their dead, given that, according to the rumours in the neighbourhood, the children's graves were never visited by their parents. The rituals required were never performed, leaving the souls of these ›whites‹ in a perpetual state of wandering, the effects of which could prove dangerous for everyone. There was no doubt in the mind of the young audience that if the ceremonies had been carried out, the chains would have been broken and the souls of the prisoners thus freed. In chorus, they wondered: »don't the families over there in Europe know about this? Aren't they suffering the consequences of this abandonment?«

Beware of Anecdotes...

The poet-philosopher Emil Cioran once stated: »doctrines vanish, anecdotes remain« (Cioran 1997). We are thereby reminded that the very stories that circumvent the facts are often those that come closest to them. In praising the anecdote (ἀνέκδοτα; ›unpublished/unprecedented fact‹), it is not that I wish to pontificate on the virtues of the rumour, nor do I wish to problematize the very objectivity that I share with historians as an anthropologist. Rather, it is a question of demonstrating that these narrative convolutions, which account for facts that evade our evidence-based system, provide us with a truth nonetheless. The anecdote refers to a detail, to a secondary aspect that is not stated in the main account, and which is also ›unpublished/unprecedented‹ in this sense. Paradoxically, it allows us to articulate its core components, at times to expose its most genuine of components. The imaginary at work in this narrative energy reacts to the aphasia generated by colonial epistemic conditions, the extensions of which are still with us today. The very transmission of the present narrative attests to this. It is very much this present form of a certain past with which we are now faced, and it is also undoubtedly to this very same end that it is transmitted to us in this particular manner. It is in keeping with Achille Mbembe when he states that »Europe has taken something from us that it will never be able to give back« (Mbembe 2018). Nevertheless, the void thus created cannot so much be compensated with financial compensation as with

> »a symbolic re-establishment through a demand for truth. Compensation here consists in offering to repair the relation. The restitution of objects (having become the nodes of a relation), also implies a fair and just historiographic work and a new relational ethics; by operating a symbolic redistribution repairing the ties and renewing them around reinvented relational modalities that are qualitatively improved« (Sarr/Savoy 2018: 40–41).

The current debate on the restitution of goods looted during colonisation appears to be just the tip of the iceberg, there is an ocean of stories hidden beneath. In so far as it highlights epistemic violence, this contribution also seeks to highlight the symbolic dimension of the restitution of goods looted during colonisation, the stakes of which go well beyond the simple movement of objects from one place to another. It seeks to call attention to other forms of knowledge production, highlighting the diversity of explorations of the world »with, against and beyond the heritage of Western epistemologies« (Mignolo 2000: 9). These regimes of truths (Foucault 2001) do not preclude one another, they are intertwined. They »archipelagise« one another (Glissant 1997) by crystallising various traditions of thought, aesthetic modes or heuristic regimes that refer to social and historical contingencies, and which we would do well to consider in their narrative creativity and their propensity for the anecdote.

What becomes of the memories that evaporate? How are they sublimated? The colonial enterprise continues to be steeped in ambiguity. This, and whatever meaning it is we should give to it today, are illustrated all too well in the Dankpe, through the enigma of the thumb and all the vagaries that surround it. To this extent, the Konkomba are asking themselves pertinent questions, through which colonial history is reflected as an enigma, to be seen more or less everywhere. It is met with a mixture of condemnation and intrigue for all the change that it has caused in the world, and of which we would do well today to take stock; for we are asking ourselves the same questions.

Conclusion: a Point of Honour?

The case of the severed thumbs – an atypical example of colonial plunder though it may be – tables one essential dimension of this debate on which we can now definitely lay a finger. Specifically, that of the aura of absent objects and the sheer quantity of strategies by way of which they are reinvented, though this may mean their transformation.

Akin to what in neurology is known as pseudohallucination or phantom pain the severed thumbs continue to feel. It is a finger that touches us. The reactions provoked by its mere evocation go to show, in their own way, that it moves still, detached though it is from its previous body. Objects live their own lives one might say, and it is in this sense that the case of the severed thumb testifies to the existence of the many objects looted during the colonial period, sitting now in so many ethnographic museums in European and beyond.

It seems, in certain cases, that these objects continue to act. Like so many ghosts, their presence is all the greater – paradoxically – now that they are absent. At any rate, they become the accessories of a narrative for which their non-existence is the condition of possibility.

The touch of theatre at the Sokodé cemetery shows us a way forward: colonial history can only be overcome if it is done through a collective work involving both the victims and the colonisers of yesterday, through an exchange of ghosts, a barter of traces, a bazaar of stories… As people reinvest in colonial history ever anew, they articulate events into accounts that decompose with each passing day, without ever really disintegrating. They will always know, albeit confusedly, that colonization was decisive in the history of their family and their community, in the history of humanity. What status should be given to these narrative drifts? What status should be given to this oral history? By making a fool of academics, museum professionals or restitution specialists and all those who

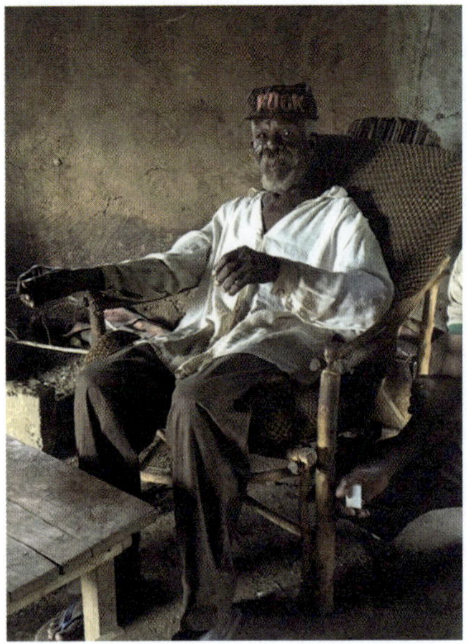

Fig. 7: An old Konkomba. Photo: Bernard Müller, May 2018.

today refuse to give credit to the story of amputated thumbs, the people who today perpetuate this narrative, like this old man with a cap with the astonishing graffiti…

How can these accounts be heard? And, if it should turn out that ethnographic museums, the main holders of colonial collections, could indeed become appropriate sounding board – what kind of structural reforms would have to be undertaken, what operations of decentralisation and decolonization would have to be carried out so that this institution, born of colonization, could become a theatre for a dynamic recomposition of the imaginary, rather than a cabinet of ethnography gone rotten?

Translation from French by Michael Dorrity.

Literature

Alem, Kangni (2006): *Carnet de route* ›Togoland‹*: un cimetière à Sokodé (Inch'Alem, le blog de Kangni Alem,* http://kangnialem.togocultures.com/carnet-de-routetogoland-un-cimetiere-a-sokode/ (25.03.2021).

Alem, Kangni (2009): *Dans les Mêlées – Les Arènes Physiques et Littéraires*, Yaoundé: Editions Ifrikiya-Collections Interlignes.

Borges, Jorge Luis (1970): *Le Rapport de Brodie*, Paris: Gallimard.

Cioran, Emil (1997): *Cahiers 1957–1972*, Paris: Gallimard.

Cornevin, Robert (1962): *Les Bassari du Nord Togo*, Paris: Berger-Levrault.

Foucault, Michel (2001): *Dits et* Écrits II, 1976–1988, Paris: Gallimard.

Gayibor, Théodore Nicoué (2011a): *Histoire des Togolais: Des Origines aux Années 1960. Le Refus de la Colonisation, Volume 4*, Paris: Karthala.

Gayibor, Théodore Nicoué (2011b): *Sources Orales et Histoire Africaine. Approches Méthodologiques, en Collaboration avec Moustapha Gomgnimbou et Komla Etou*, Paris: L'Harmattan.

Gayibor, Théodore Nicoué (Ed.) et al. (1997): *Le Togo sous Domination Coloniale* (1884–*1960)*, Lomé: Presses de l'Université du Bénin.

Gbandi, Adouna (2009): *Description Phonologique et Grammaticale du Konkomba, Langue Gur (voltaïque) du Togo et du Ghana – Parler de Nawareé*, Université Rennes 2, Université de Lomé, https://tel.archives-ouvertes.fr/tel-00416375 (14.04.2021).

Glissant, Édouard (1997): *Traiteé du Tout-Monde*, Paris: Gallimard.

Kachim, Joseph Udimal (2013): »African Resistance to Colonial Conquest: The Case of Konkomba Resistance to German Occupation of Northern Togoland, 1896–1901«. In: *Asian Journal of Humanities and Social Studies*, 1:3, 62–72.

Klose, Heinrich (1906): »Musik, Tanz und Spiele in Togo«. In: *Globus, Illustrierte Zeitschrift für Länder- und Völkerkunde* 89:5, 69–75.

Maasole, Cliff (2006): *The Konkomba and their Neighbours*, Accra: Ghana Universities Press.

Massow, Valentin von/Sebald, Peter (ed.) (2014): *Die Eroberung von Nordtogo 1896–1899*, Bremen: Edition Falkenberg.

Mbembe, Achille (2018): »La Vérité est que l'Europe Nous a Pris des Choses Qu'elle ne Pourra Jamais Restituer«. In: *Le Monde*, 01.12.2018, https://www.lemonde.fr/afrique/article/2018/12/01/achille-mbembe-la-verite-est-que-l-europe-nous-a-pris-des-choses-qu-elle-ne-pourra-jamais-restituer_5391216_3212.html (14.04.2021).

Mignolo, Walter (2000): *Local Histories/Global Designs. Coloniality, Subaltern Knowledges and Boarder Thinking*, Princeton: Princeton University Press.

Sarr, Felwine/Savoy, Bénédicte (2018): »The Restitution of African Cultural Heritage. Toward a New Relational Ethics«, http://restitutionreport2018.com/sarr_savoy_en.pdf (14.04.2021).

Sebald, Peter (1988): *Togo 1884–1914. Eine Geschichte der deutschen »Musterkolonie« auf der Grundlage amtlicher Quellen*, Berlin: Akademie-Verlag.

Table of figures

The Museum of Black Civilisations, between History and Utopia

Sabrina Moura

Introduction

The idealisation of the Musée des Civilisations Noires (Museum of Black Civilizations, MCN) is attributed to Senegalese activist Lamine Senghor (1889–1927). It was in 1926, with the creation of the Comité de Défense de la Race Nègre (CDRN)[1] that the pan-African luminary firstly mentioned a museum for the preservation of African dignity and heritage. Forty years later, after the successful completion of First World Festival of Negro Arts (1966), president Léopold Sédar Senghor revisited this idea. The museum, designed to be »the most important cultural centre of its kind in West Africa« (Senghor *apud* Camara 2014: 40), was to be built on the Atlantic coast of Dakar, integrating a vast cultural complex accompanied by an arts and crafts village, a conference room, and a national library, among others. Then named Musée d'art négro-africain, the venue was to house pieces safeguarded by the Institut Fondamental d'Afrique Noire (IFAN), along with new ones to be acquired by the Senegalese state. Its galleries were to be guided by thematic and chronological itineraries, from prehistory to the present, and its mission was to challenge that of European museums built on the colonial experience (Camara 2014: 40).

Despite Senghor's efforts, the museum would not come to fruition during his mandate (1960–1980), nor those of his immediate successors. Indeed, the Musée des civilisations noires, as it is now, is a result of more than four decades of negotiations that would come to a conclusion in 2015, due to the funds leveraged by Chinese soft-power strategies in West Africa.[2] »The development of the museum is part and parcel of an intellectual and cultural history of modernity«, claims Senegalese curator and scholar Malick Ndiaye (2019). »Reinterpreting that history in light of the profound changes it has entailed is therefore a challenge to the whole museological system« (Ndiaye 2019).

1 »The first black popular movement that brought together hundreds of members in France through the ports and major cities of the Hexagone« (Murphy 2015: 55, emphasis in the original).

2 For a deeper analysis on Chinese foreign policies in Senegal see Gehrold/Tietze 2011.

urn:nbn:de:hbz:6:3-zfk-2021-41972

In this article, I examine the *Musée des Civilisations Noires* throughout three moments of its existence. Firstly, as an aspiration; secondly, as a project in the making; thirdly, as a fact. In the first section, I confront the expectations behind the project of the museum by positioning the institution in a broader geopolitical and historical context. This extends from the 1970s Mexican project of a cultural park, to the so-called »Seven Wonders of Dakar«, advanced during Abdoulaye Wade's mandate (2000–2012). Following this contextualization, I demonstrate how the museum's current public form grapples with ancient and current dilemmas on African art history and museology, with an emphasis on the »restitution debate« of 2018, initiated by Bénédicte Savoy and Felwine Sarr. Finally, I delve into the highlights of the museum's parcours and curatorial narratives in order to demonstrate how the MCN seeks to foster a vision of pan-Africanism that positions Dakar and *négritude* as the organizing tropes of Black history, assuming a central role among Africans and the diaspora.

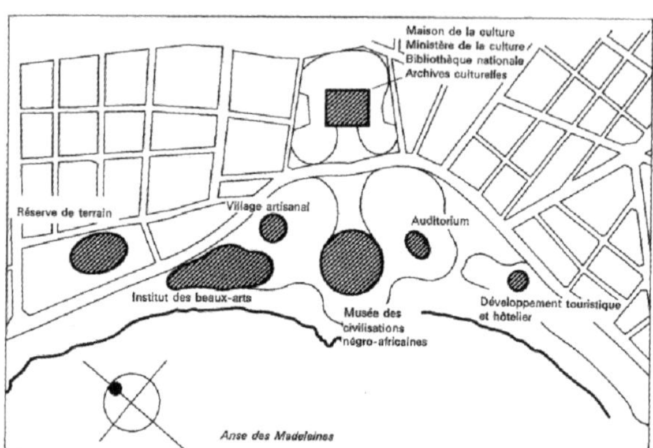

Fig. 1: Musée des Civilisations Négro-Africaines in relation to the Dakar Ensemble Culturel (Lehmbruck/Rautenstrauch 1974: 155).

Museum Politics, Past and Present

The history of the museum's building starts in 1972, soon after UNESCO assumed the project's sponsorship. It was then entrusted to the same architect who had signed the National Museum of Anthropology in Mexico City, Pedro Ramírez Vázquez (1919–2013).[3] Senegalese curator and museologist Ery Camara was one of the key witnesses of such developments, as he closely followed the conception of the MCN from the beginning. At the age of 22, he was still finishing university in Dakar, when he was invited by the government of Senegal to study cultural heritage in Mexico City. It was intended that he joined the museum's staff in the future. »My arrival in Mexico, in 1975, was prompted by the project of the Museum of Black Civilizations«, explains Camara (2014: 41). Throughout his training in Latin America, Ery Camara established a close relationship with Pedro Ramirez Vasquez.

The construction of the building did not see light under Senghor's mandate, and was consigned to his predecessors. However, during Abdou Diouf's term in office (1981–2000) the project was undermined by the implementation of structural adjustment plans (SAPs). Many records related to the original project were lost; »the collections were left vulnerable

3 Assisted by Jorge Campuzano and Thierry Melot, and having the Swiss ethnographer Jean Gabus as its scientific advisor.

in these uncertain conditions and many pieces were lost due to deterioration and theft« protests Camara (2014: 41). In 2003, with the arrival of Abdoulaye Wade to the presidency, the idea of the museum was re-established. Wade then contacted Ery Camara in order to resume the Mexican project for the museum, an invitation that the Senegalese curator promptly accepted. With still no feedback from Wade in 2010, Ery Camara travelled to Dakar to attend the second edition of the World Festival of Negro Arts. He came across a publication that featured the Museum of Black Civilizations as a creation of Senegalese architect Pierre Goudiaby Atepa: »an adaptation, or rather a plagiarism, of the original project« he stated (2014: 43). Camara then decided to bring public attention to the subject. As a result of this imbroglio, the Senegalese state put Ramirez Vasquez's project to the side, and the MCN was then entrusted to the Beijing Institute of Architectural Design (BIAD).

Camara's account[4] was published in the Mexican magazine *Gaceta de Museos* (2014), four years before the opening of the MCN, and is remarkable for a number of reasons. Firstly, because it revisits floor plans, mock-ups and principles that guided the initial project for the museum. Secondly, because it points to fundamental aspects of post-war cultural relations between West Africa and Latin America, still little explored by academic literature. Finally, because it complexifies the well-polished narratives of cultural and artistic institutions nurtured by strong political positions, such as that of the MCN. As we shall see, the latter is absent from many of the public debates celebrating the birth of this important African museum.

As in the 1970s, the idea of a cultural park guided the ensemble of facilities retaken during Abdoulaye Wade's mandate. Broadcasted on national television, the new constructions were dubbed the Seven Wonders of Dakar. In addition to the MCN, the project featured a new national theatre (opened in 2011), a national library, the national archives, a museum of contemporary art, the school of fine arts, the school of architecture, a music palace and the legendary statue entitled Monument de la Renaissance Africaine (Monument of African Renaissance).[5] »They are wonders in the sense that through their

4 In the 10th issue of the magazine *Something We Africans Got* (2019), Ery Camara elaborates on a second account which he names »the other story of the MCN«. Here, he overtly testifies to the contradictions between its curatorial project and political character. He states that he was initially part of the museum's scientific committee, being invited to participate in the International Planning Conference of the Museum of Black Civilizations (*Conférence Internationale de Préfiguration du Musée des Civilisations Noires*), held in July 2016 in Dakar. »I had the opportunity in my communication to recall the original history of the project and its initiator. My intervention was in the direction of a deep reflection on the museum, its identity, its discourse, its program, as well as its anchoring within the territory. But I quickly understood that the main actors of the project were not in this perspective but rather in the urgency of responding to a well-established political agenda« says Camara (2019).

5 Since its conception, the monument signed by Pierre Goudiaby Atepa – the same architect who had been accused of plagiarizing Ramirez Vasquez's project, and who was now being charged by Senegalese artist Ousmane Sow – was shrouded in a series of controversies. From its production costs, which ran in the millions, to its being commissioned to a North Korean art production studio, to the representation of a ›normative‹ vision of the African family. »May the symbol that [this monument] embodies and the message it conveys inspire, throughout the centuries, the peoples of Africa and the Diaspora, in our common search for a better destiny in a fraternal humanity« stated Wade (2010) in his inaugural speech.

architecture and their meaning, they transmit messages through time to future generations« said Wade (*apud* Drame 2011).

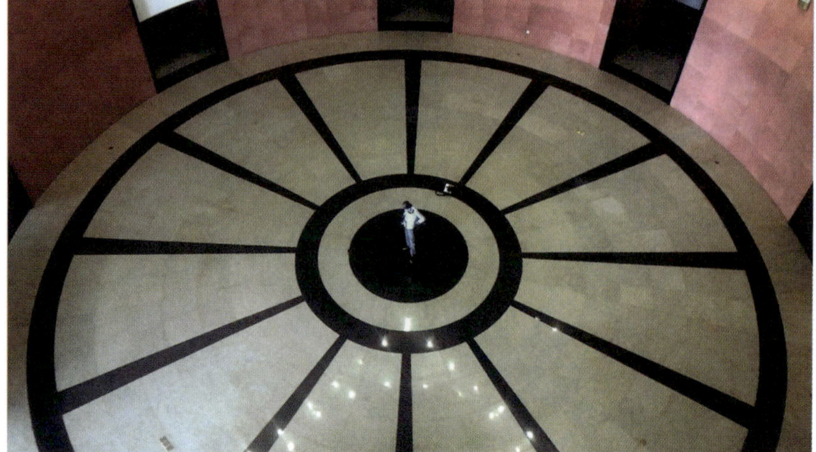

Fig. 2: Atrium of the Musée des Civilisations Noires (Dakar) three months before its opening (September 2018). Photo: Sabrina Moura.

Art Histories, Empty Rooms

I had the opportunity to first visit the Musée des Civilisations Noires a few months before its public opening[6] (September 2018), while its galleries were still uninhabited. On that occasion, I was in Dakar working on my PhD dissertation, which focused on the notion of diaspora at the Dakar Biennial[7]. I was attending the third edition of the Condition Report symposium series – Art History in Africa – convened by curators Ugochukwu-Smooth Nzewi and Koyo Kouoh, in partnership with the independent art space Raw Material Company. The gathering sought to foment a discussion of subjects, perspectives, and methods emerging from an art history written on, and from within, the African continent.

»The history of African art« declared Kouoh (oral communication, 2018) in her opening speech, »continues to be dominated by Western academics who set the tone for the subject. Their frames of reference, posed as universal, play on the interpretation of African art, social conditions, and cultural milieus. Besides, the audience for this kind of production is usually not in Africa«.

The call »to reconfigure the parameters and potential of art history in Africa«,[8] as posed by the symposium, is not a novelty in African art theory and curatorship, being part of recurring impasses in the field since the second half of the last century. Indeed, it unpacks a series of paradoxes that encompass the Western origins of art history as a discipline, and are inscribed in the very concept of Africa, and its forms of writing. »We cannot think of an African-based art history from a dichotomous point of view, which isolates Africa from the rest of the world« stated Salah Hassan (oral communication,

6 The museum was opened to the public in December 2018.

7 Sabrina Moura. *De volta para onde nunca estive: pensar a diáspora africana a partir da Bienal de Dacar (1992–2012), PhD Dissertation*, Universidade Estadual de Campinas (Unicamp), Brazil, 2020.

8 See http://www.rawmaterialcompany.org/_2237?lang=en; date of pageview 23rd March 2022.

2018) in his keynote speech for this symposium. In quoting historian Robin Kelley (2000), Hassan asserted that Africa and its diaspora were produced in contact with the West, in the same way that they have altered the artistic expressions of Western culture.

As these lively discussions unfolded throughout the meeting, speakers and members of the audience were having parallel conversations about what would be displayed in the vast empty galleries of the museum programmed to open in only a few months. At the end of the second day, a long-awaited conversation between Malick Ndiaye, Curator of the Musée Théodore Monod, and the MCN's general director Hamady Bocoum introduced some aspects of the museum's history and mission, without clearly defining the scope of its collections. Essentially, the debate concentrated more on the concept than the practicality of the museum.

»Why is this project coming back today, when it has been neglected for all these decades?« Ndiaye asked Bocoum (2018). After briefly drawing on some guidelines that framed its institutional and scientific project,[9] Bocoum positioned the MCN as an experiment for the utopian reinvention of the African museum. He argued that its contemporary relevance relates both to the new place of Africa in global cultural geopolitics – which translates into an African-based museum that refuses to uphold a subaltern position regarding its Western counterparts –, and the epistemological reassessments of art history, ethnography and social sciences recently seen in the humanities.

> »We have often been seen as subalterns, as a resonance chamber [...]. I think that what can make the interest of this museum today is to see things differently. [That means] that it is very, very likely that if this museum had been built about thirty years ago, it would have been an ethnographic one. When we look at the trajectory of ethnographic thought – the study of the other – and ethnographic museums, [they] are copies of World Expositions that were presented to us a bit like saddle beasts, the other thing is that no one goes to ethnographic museums in Africa because precisely these museums are the reflection of a subaltern Africa.« (Bocoum, oral communication, 2018)

Just as Senghor had done in the past, Bocoum introduced the 15 thousand square metre museum as one of a kind. It was intended as a museum that would undergo constant change, with no permanent exhibitions or fixed narratives; it should find a balance between social interaction and artistic fruition in its circular Casamance-inspired architectural style; it should not fall prey to the traps of ethnography and othering; nor be exclusively dedicated to black people, but instead acknowledge the contributions of black civilizations to the »universal heritage of humankind«; it should honour the legacy of the First World Festival of Negro Arts... The list is long, and the stakes are high.

Once the debate had come to a close, the attendees and speakers went with Bocoum on a guided tour through the vacant galleries of the museum. However, instead of unravelling the museum's mystery, that is, how those massive exhibition spaces would be inhabited in such a short time, the visit seemed only to aggravate the air of doubt that had filled the rooms.

9 These guidelines were drafted during the International Planning Conference of the Museum of Black Civilizations (Conférence Internationale de Préfiguration du Musée des Civilisations Noires), held at the King Fahd Palace in Dakar, between July 28–31, 2016.

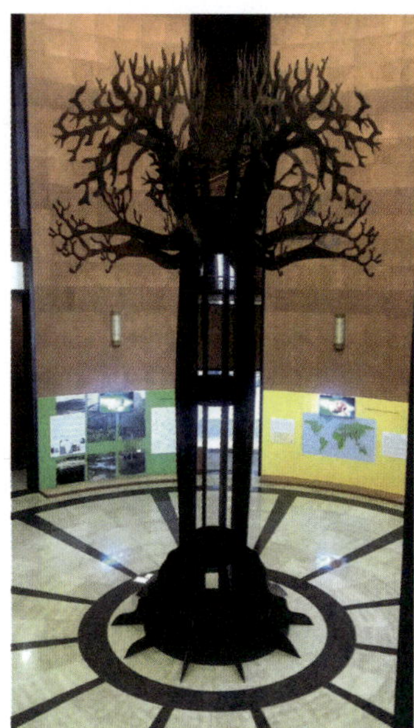

Fig. 3: Baobab, Édouard Duval-Carrié Atrium of the Musée des civilisations noires (Dakar 2019). Photo: Sabrina Moura.

During the Q&A session, one of the most poignant questions was posed by a young Senegalese art teacher in the audience. »What place will be given to contemporary African production, labelled as crafts (*artisanat*), in these new African museums? How will these institutions read, deal with, and preserve such practices?« she asked. Simply put, these questions summarize a number of issues regarding African museology and art history addressed by the symposium. On the one hand, they encompass an art perspective that challenges the logic of value attribution based on the primitivist (and formalist) legacy. On the other, they problematize the very concept of art that guides the foundational narratives behind this long-awaited museum.

With the MCN's opening,[10] in December 2018, I came across the following headline in a local Brazilian newspaper: »The Senegalese Museum that wants to ›decolonize‹ African culture« (*Nexo Jornal*, December 8, 2018). The French *Le Monde* (December 5, 2018) stated: »the opening of the institution defeats the argument of the lack of adequate infrastructure in Africa, often opposed to requests for the restitution of works of art«. Like much of the international press, the inauguration of the MCN gave way to a series of celebrations, which indiscriminately mingled the political interests behind its execution and the high expectations around it. Before embarking on further considerations, however, I should note that the sceptical tone of the following lines in no way seeks to invalidate the significance of the MCN in the African and international museum landscape. Rather, it refers to the imperative of drawing a critical analysis of the self-laudatory discourses that underpin not only state-led institutions of this kind, but also Western anxieties regarding its own role in changing the course of African cultural structures in the current context of the debate on restitution.

In the introduction of his keynote speech for the colloquium Museotopia. Réflexions on the avenir des musées en Afrique (Museotopia. Reflections on the future of museums in Africa), June, 2019, the Senegalese philosopher Souleymane Bachir Diagne stated »today, the question of the return of objects to the continent where they were born [Africa] questions the very meaning of such return, as well as the need to re-imagine the museum that would host them, in Africa and around the world«. Guided by the engaging word play that gave rise to the name to the meeting, organized by Bénédicte Savoy and Felwine Sarr at the Collège de France (Paris), Diagne and his colleagues sought to reassess museological narratives, collections and structures, forecasting the future of these institutions. Such an exercise of critical imagination led to a radical interrogation of the relevance and the nature of museums in the 21st century. As one of the speakers, French anthropologist Philippe Descola (2019), would elaborate in one of the colloquium sessions: »What should museums be actually made of? And how should they be named?«.

10 The museum was inaugurated by president Macky Sall, in power since 2012.

Diagne's initial take sheds light on his perspective on the translocation of African PPobjects to European museums. As he put it, these objects migrated from their »homeland« to Europe where they changed their status, from curiosities to ethnographic samples, and later from scientific to aesthetic pieces, widely intersecting with the visual grammar of modern Western figuration.

»A word about the radical rupture that most often would have been the forced migration to the museums of the colonial scientific expeditions, the ethnographic museums and, finally, the museums of the primitive arts. However, this is only a mutation whose possibility was indeed carried by the work in its infinite plasticity. These transplanted objects did not become mute in spite of this. Their mutant quality was expressed in the language of the ›negro revolution‹. Who will say that it was a misappropriation, that these works were made to speak against the intention that gave birth to them? The term primitivism renders them inert by making them the creation of Europeans who, weary of ›their ancient world‹, sought out a primitive that was in part their own invention. No, these objects acted as mutants and found their own way into a modernity they helped to create« (Diagne 2020: 109–110).[11]

It is not surprising that, in light of these considerations, the recently-inaugurated Musée des Civilizations Noires epitomized Diagne's idea of a »mutant museum«, making it the highlight of the Museotopia (2019) conference.

With a view to explaining the importance I attribute to this excerpt of Diagne's speech, let us turn, for a moment, to the report on restitution prepared by Felwine Sarr and Bénédicte Savoy in 2018, at the request of French President Emmanuel Macron. As art historian Zoë Strother (2019) reminds us, one of its most-cited passages, within the public debate, refers to the observation that »almost all the material heritage of the African countries to the south of the Sahara is *preserved outside the African continent*« (Sarr/Savoy 2018: 3, emphasis added).[12]

The perspective of art and heritage sustained by the report, and the restitution debates *vis à vis* the MCN curatorial scope, must be subject to scrutiny. Especially when the theories underpinning recent revisions to art history point to a redefinition of its objects and subjects. In fact, Strother (2019) was one of the voices questioning the notion of »art« that permeates some of Sarr and Savoy's arguments. For this, she took as an example her own research with the masked performances among the Eastern Pende. Described by the author as a complex chain of actions that encompass the memorization of music and proverbs, the learning of dance techniques, as well as the mastery of ritualistic protocols, the value of these practices is not restricted to the materiality of the artefact. By focusing on the object, only the masks used in these performances are considered to be art. »Such

11 This reflection was first presented in a conference at the Collège de France organized by Bénédicte Savoy on June 11, 2019 and later reproduced in a written essay published in the journal *Esprit* (2020).

12 According to Strother (2019): »The authors of a recent report on restitution prepared for Macron attribute this statistic to Alain Godonou, who estimated in 2007 that the ›inventories‹ of individual African museums ›hardly ever exceeded 3,000 cultural heritage objects‹.«

a selective view of what constitutes cultural heritage continues the colonialist paradigm that African cultural achievement should be defined by European criteria« Strother claims (2019: 5).

Malick Ndiaye, in turn, acknowledges that the gestures of restitution »must be considered in both political and scientific terms« (Ndiaye 2019), and highlights the necessity to challenge the paradigm of the ›work of art‹ when addressing this agenda. »This tendency distorts the terms of the debate, insofar as it leads certain actors rejecting this legacy for the simple reason that it is a product of the history of Western taste, and therefore, should no longer be considered a proper African heritage.« (Ndiaye 2019: 5)

As previously mentioned, this debate was cleverly enunciated by the arts professor who was part of the audience of the 2018 Condition Report symposium, and is by no means a novel contention. In the 1990s, authors and curators like James Clifford (1988), Susan Vogel (1989), Christopher Steiner (1994) and Alfred Gell (1996) – supported by the contributions of contemporary art, performative and conceptual practices – already discussed the paradoxes related to the ties between art and artefact, art and matter, art and figuration. Their analyses gave rise to a series of experiments on the ways of exposing ethnographic pieces and the primitivist wave among European modernists, demonstrating that a non-object-based view of art offers important clues to fostering the establishment of collections in new African museums.

A Walk through the Museum Galleries

In March 2019, I was back in Dakar and keen on revisiting the MCN, now open to the public. My initial take was to follow the museum's suggested path in order to underscore the narratives advanced by its scientific committee. According to the viewing sequence, the museum sections establish a *parcours* that begins at the centre of a circular-shaped atrium, occupied by a 12-metre-high bronze baobab, commissioned to Haitian artist Édourad Duval; allegedly, the only permanent piece on view (Bocoum 2018). Around the metal tree, the multiple galleries encompass a range of displays, from the so-called ›tribal arts‹, through the echoes of Abrahamic religions in Senegal, to contemporary arts.

The imposing bronze tree and its surrounding rooms emphasise the idea of Africa as the heart and the cradle of humanity, and marks the beginning of the visitation route. Here, a reconstituted version of the Toumaï skull is displayed along with explanatory panels on the continent's contributions to architecture, agriculture, mathematics, and other sciences. This narrative inscribes Africa in a worldly perspective and in the *longue durée*, and was exhaustively discussed by a number of stakeholders in 2016 during the International Planning Conference of the Museum of Black Civilizations (Conférence Internationale de Préfiguration du Musée des Civilisations Noires). In attendance was historian and dean of the Cheikh Anta Diop University (Dakar) Ibrahima Thioub (2016: 13), who affirmed that »[…] humankind owes an immeasurable debt to Africa.« Indeed, the MCN opening galleries are a powerful statement in light of the continent's position in the history of modernity, the transatlantic slave trade, and neoliberal capitalism. What follows, however, is a missed opportunity to confront this positioning with Souleymane B. Diagne's (2019; 2020) idea of a mutant museum.

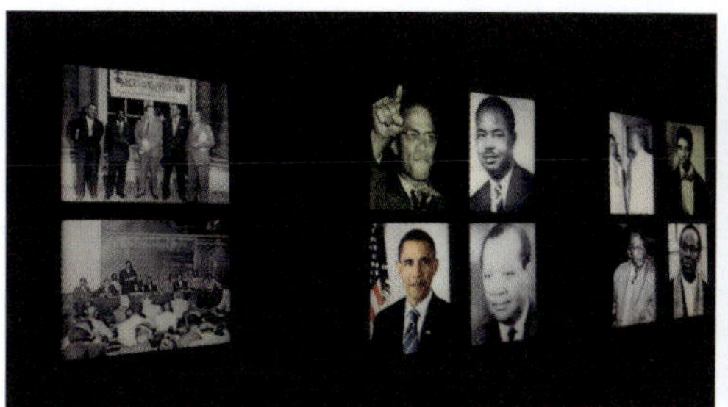

Fig. 4: Les Lignes de Continuité and Femmes Noires et la Production des Savoirs Installation shots, Musée des civilisations noires (Dakar 2019). Photos: Sabrina Moura.

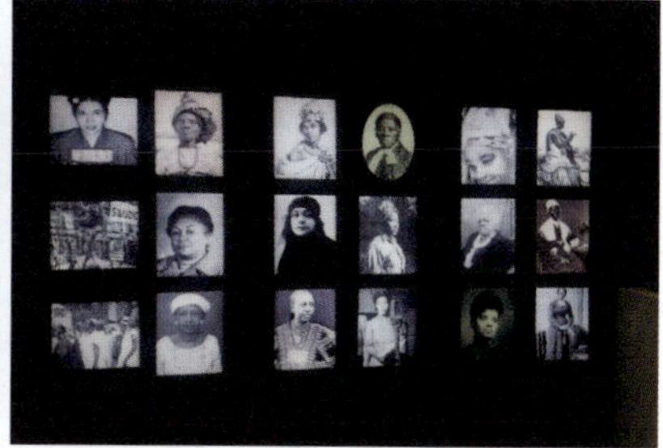

Fig. 5: Les Lignes de Continuité and Femmes Noires et la Production des Savoirs Installation shots, Musée des civilisations noires (Dakar 2019). Photos: Sabrina Moura.

Pursuing the *parcours* of the lower left-side galleries, a section entitled Civilisations Africaines (African Civilisations) features a series of masks, statues, tunics, and other objects, presented as a sign of »African ancestry and authority«.[13] While lacking contextualisation, this gallery proceeds without further addressing the pieces' meanings (be they copies or originals) within the museum, or their role in Western and African art historiography. As the visitor continues to walk along the ground floor, a set of illuminated portraits emerges against a dark background. Titled Les Lignes de Continuité (The Lines of Continuity), it shows a number of black leaders, from Kwame Nkrumah to Barack Obama, and Frederick Douglass to Nelson Mandela. On the first floor, a similar display is dedicated to women: Femmes Noires et la Production des Savoirs (Black Women and the Production of Knowledge). Among the series of portraits, a photograph of American activist Rosa Parks (1913–2005)[14] stands out. The representation of Parks and the great figures of pan-Africanism in the installation, included in the *parcours* of the MCN, immediately led me to associate it with one of the works exhibited in the seventh edition of the Dakar Biennial (2006), where the Senegalese artist Ndary Lo (1961–2017) chose to celebrate »the refusal of Rosa Parks«.

Speaking in a radio interview in 2013, the artist explained that his interest in Rosa Parks began in 2005, right after her death: »I felt very moved by that lady. I started by making a portrait of hers, then a second, then a third… and, suddenly, I thought, I'll make portraits of all the Rosa Parks of the world.« His words show that for many Africans based on the continent, the experiences of racial segregation linked to the black population outside Africa are an important subject of solidarity and political mobilization, just as for the diaspora. In the name of these connections, Lo included in his installation, in addition to Parks, a selection of portraits of other Black personalities, born in and outside Africa. Among them were Mandela, Angela Davis, Léopold Sédar Senghor, Bob Marley and even Okwui Enwezor (Andriamirado 2009, n.p.). »This work is entitled *The Refusal of Rosa*

13 Citation retrieved from the explanatory panels in the galleries of African Civilisations' section (2019).

14 Known as a forerunner of civil rights movements in the United States, Parks refused, at the age of 42, to stand up from the bus seat on which she was sitting after being approached by James Blake (1912–2002), the white man driving the vehicle.

Parks, but I could have called it a ›*pantheon*‹. When I visited the Pantheon [in France], I reacted like a Black man, coming from Africa, and I said, we also need our Pantheon« claimed the artist (Lo *apud* France Cultures 2013). Be it a coincidence or not, MCN's portrait galleries seemed to emulate Lo's Black Pantheon.

In a third visit to the museum, still in 2019, I decided to take a guided tour with one of its mediators. The young guide was proud to present the city's colossal museum to a foreigner visitor, and knew the curatorial *parti-pris* of each gallery extremely well. One of his favourites was, in fact, the illuminated portrait section, where we stood for almost half an hour discussing the current echoes of each figure.

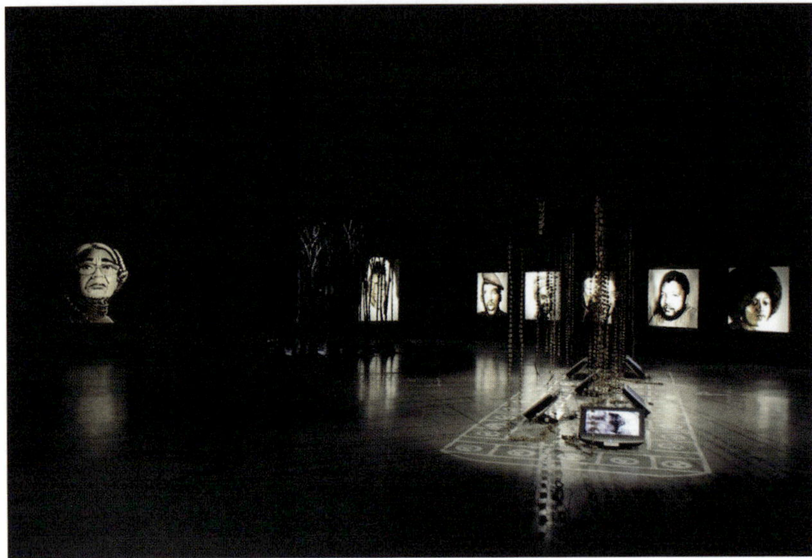

Fig. 6: The Refusal of Rosa Parks (2009), Ndary Lo, Fondation Blachère, Paris. Work recreated from the artist's installation at the Dakar Biennial in 2006. Photo: Laure Tarot.

Nonetheless, it is at MCN's second-floor galleries that the museum actually honours its promise to be »one of its kind«. The first of these galleries, in a sequential order, is dedicated to the »African appropriations of Abrahamic religions« and is especially noteworthy as it offers elements representing a key dimension of Senegalese daily life. It includes reliquaries, Ayahs and portraits of spiritual leaders, such as Sufi saint Amadou Bamba or marabout Serigne Babacar Sy. Here, »Islam is Sufi – it is the Islam of sects and brotherhoods, presenting itself as a non-conformist, mystical tendency. [...] It is a patient search for the union of the soul with God« states one of the exhibition panels. As one leaves this gallery, a corridor immerses the visitor in a video installation of moving waves in a deep blue sea. The principle, my guide explained, was to recall the Middle Passage and the forced African dispersions. On the occasion of my visit, at the other end of this passage, a temporary exhibition on Cuban contemporary art featured works by Marta María Pérez Bravo, Roberto Chile, Leandro Soto, and other artists, reinforcing the idea of reaching out to the Transatlantic diaspora. Following this sequence, the exhibition Maintenant l'Afrique presented the award-winning works of the Dakar biennial (Dak'art), including pieces by Fodé Carama, Soly Cossé, Dory Lo, Abdoulayé Konate. This was a veritable feast for those seeking a fine selection of African contemporary art hosted by an African institution.

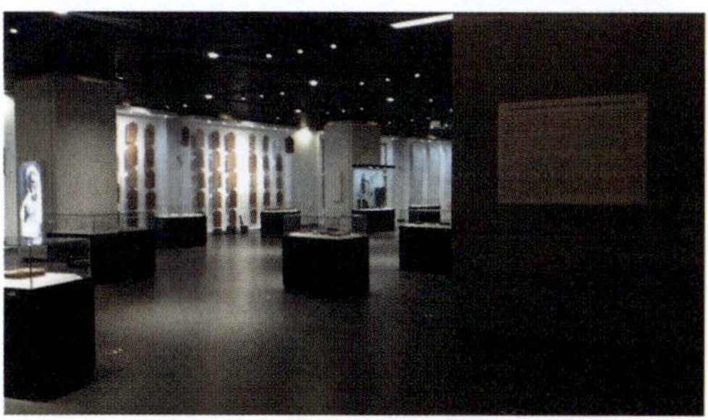

Fig. 7: Les appropriations africaines des religions abrahamiques, installation shot, Musée des civilisations noires (Dakar 2019). Photos: Sabrina Moura.

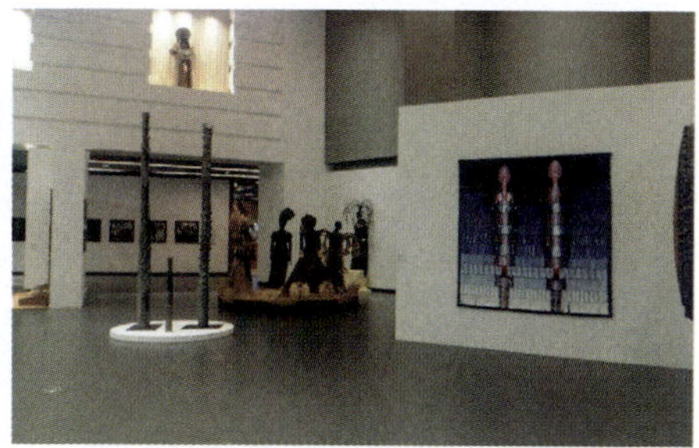

Fig. 8: Maintenant l'Afrique Installation shot, Musée des civilisations noires (Dakar 2019). Photos: Sabrina Moura.

Final Considerations

This time, I left the museum convinced that the MCN should not be read solely by *what it contains*, but also by *what it claims* to represent in the landscapes of the continent and the diaspora. As Senegalese historian Iba Der Thiam (*apud* Bocoum & Ndiaye 2016: 21) stated, »the Museum of Black Civilizations must be […] a museum that reconstructs man (from Abel to Obama) and allows him to look into the future«.

Five years past the museum's first public announcement, a report on Senegalese cultural policies, by diplomat and journalist Mamadou M'Bengue (1973), described it as an ambitious long-term project aligned with the nation's future:

> »Senegal is, of course, continuing to look ahead, since its cultural action concerns both the present and the future: as far as the present is concerned, it takes the form of constantly readjusting and developing the existing cultural structures, including training machinery and the necessary facilities for implementing the cultural policy drawn up by the government; for the future, it involves drawing up and carrying out cultural development projects forming an integral part of the national four-year plans and the long-term overall plans for economic development, which extend over a period of several decades.« (M'Bengue 1973: 64)

One should also note that the *look toward the future* is a key principle for the different expressions of Black emancipation, such as the African Renaissance. This conceptual and historical framework guided the gestation of Abdoulaye Wade's »wonders« and included the Musée des Civilisations Noires, and its surrounding cultural park. The notion emerges between the end of the 19th and early 20th centuries amidst a circle of black intellectuals in the diaspora. Its early uses refer to the speech *The African Regeneration*, given by South African lawyer and politician Pixley ka Isaka Seme at Columbia University in 1905. »The giant is awakening!« proclaimed Seme. Later, in 1956, in the speech *L'esprit de la civilisation ou les lois de la culture négro-africaine*, presented at the Paris congress of black artists and writers, Sédar Senghor announced the African cultural »Renaissance« by overcoming the physical and symbolic losses caused by the Atlantic slave trade (Senghor 1956: 51).

Part and parcel of these debates, the contemporary version of the Museum of Black Civilizations recalls the glory of those intellectuals who rethought the meanings of Africa in history. As with the pan-African mobilizations in the past century, what is at stake with the MCN is an idea and a sense of Africa, its place in history and its position in the current global order.

I cannot end this analysis, however, without evoking the questions and positionings enunciated in the initial sections of this article. While the decolonization agenda or the recent restitution claims point to necessary debates related to the foundation of the MCN, the task of collecting should also be placed under the spotlight. Why has the MCN not been engaged in the establishment of its own collection? Which contemporary cultural expressions have not yet been validated by its gallery walls? How could they challenge an approach to art, which is focused on objects? And why are they not seen in this museum? If the MCN is to fully explore its institutional ambitions, it must put an emphasis on consistent curatorial research leading to long-term collection practices and new display strategies. All together, these initiatives can build a foundation from which the MCN can be positioned as a groundbreaking museum in the global landscape, as its precursors once dreamed.

This article has undergone a double-blind peer-review.
All the translations in this article were made by the author.

Literature

Andriamirado, Virginie (2009): »Le refus de Rosa Parks«, http://www.ndary-lo.com/textes/rosa-parks/ (25.03.2021).

Bocoum, Hamady (2018): »Le Musée des Civilisations Noires: une vision d'avenir«. In: *Présence Africaine* 197: 1, 183–194. https://doi.org/10.3917/presa.197.0183.

Bocoum, Hamady/Ndiaye, El Hadji Malick (2016): »Rapport de la Conférence de préfiguration du musée des Civilisations Noires«, https://mcn.sn/wp-content/uploads/2020/12/RAPPORT-CIP-1.pdf (30.03.2021).

Bocoum, Hamady/Ndiaye, El Hadji Malick (2018): »Le Musée des Civilisations Noires et l'histoire de l'art«, *Condition Report 3: Symposium on Art History in Africa, Dakar*, 20.-22.09.2018, https://www.mixcloud.com/RawMaterialCompany/session-55-musée-des-civilisations-noires-and-art-history/ (25.03.2021).

Camara, Ery (2014): »Museo de las Civilizaciones Negras de Dakar: el proyecto de un lugar de memoria«. In: *Gaceta de Museos* 57, 38–43.

https://www.revistas.inah.gob.mx/index.php/gacetamuseos/article/view/546.

Camara, Ery/Sy, Fatima Bintou Rassoul (2019): »Ery Camara et l'autre histoire du Musée des Civilisations Noires«, Interview, December 2019. In: *Something we Africans got*: 10, https://avril27.com/art-community/ery-camara-et-lautre-histoire-du-musee-des-civilisations-noires-interview-f-b-rassoul-sy/ (26.03.2021).

Clifford, James (1988) : *The Predicament of Culture: Twentieth-Century Ethnography, Literature, and Art*, Cambridge, MA/London : Harvard University Press.

Descola, Philippe (2019): »Table ronde«, *Museotopia. Réflexions sur l'avenir des musées en Afrique, Collège de France*, https://www.college-de-france.fr/site/en-benedicte-savoy/symposium-2019-06-11-10h30.htm (25.03.2021).

Diagne, Souleymane Bachir (2019): »Musée des mutants (Keynote)«, Museotopia. Réflexions sur l'avenir des musées en Afrique, Collège de France, https://www.college-de-france.fr/site/en-benedicte-savoy/symposium-2019-06-11-10h30.htm (25.03.2021).

Diagne, Souleymane Bachir (2020): »Musée des mutants«. In: *Esprit* 7, 103–111. https://doi.org/10.3917/espri.2007.0103.

Drame, Oumou Sidya (2011): »Projet architectural des sept merveilles de Dakar: Me Wade présente la maquette«, *Xibar.net - L'oeil critique du Sénégal*, https://www.xibar.net/PROJET-ARCHITECTURAL-DES-SEPT-MERVEILLES-DE-DAKAR-Me-Wade-presente-la-maquette_a32281.html (25.03.2021).

Gell, Alfred (1986): »Newcomers to the world of goods.« In: *The Social Life of Things. Commodities in Cultural Perspective*, ed. by Arjun Appadurai/Cambridge/London: Cambridge University Press, 110–138.

Gehrold, Stefan/Tietze, Lena (2011) : »Far From Altruistic – China's Presence in Senegal.« International Reports, November 13, 2011. https://www.kas.de/en/web/auslandsinformationen/artikel/detail/-/content/kein-altruismus-die-chinesische-praesenz-im-senegal.

Hassan, Salah (2018): »In and Out of Africa: African Art History as a Paradox!«, *Condition Report 3: Symposium on Art History in Africa, Dakar*, 20.–22.09.2018, https://www.mixcloud.com/RawMaterialCompany/in-and-out-of-africa-african-art-history-as-a-paradox-keynote-by-salah-hassan/ (25.03.2021).

Invité Culture (2013): »Ndary Lo, artiste sculpteur sénégalais«. In: *Radio France Inter*, 03.10.2013, https://www.rfi.fr/fr/emission/20131003-ndary-lo-artiste-sculpteur-senegalais (25.03.2021).

Kelley, Robin D. G. (2000): »How the West Was One: On the Uses and Limitations of Diaspora«. In: *The Black Scholar* 30: 3–4, 31–35. https://doi.org/10.1080/00064246.2000.11431106.

Kouoh, Koyo (2018): »Opening speech«, *Condition Report 3: Symposium on Art History in Africa, Dakar*, 20.–22.09.2018.

Le Monde (2018): »Le Sénégal inaugure un Musée des civilisations noires à Dakar«, 05.12.20218, https://www.lemonde.fr/afrique/article/2018/12/05/le-senegal-inaugure-un-musee-des-civilisations-noires-a-dakar_5392879_3212.html (25.03.2021).

Le Monde (2018): »Le Sénégal souhaite la restitution de ›toutes‹ ses œuvres d'art« 28.11.2018, https://www.lemonde.fr/afrique/article/2018/11/28/le-senegal-souhaite-la-restitution-de-toutes-ses-uvres-d-art_5389814_3212.html (25.03.2021).

M'Bengue, Mamadou Seyni (1973): *Cultural policy in Senegal*, UNESCO.

Murphy, David (2015): »Tirailleur, facteur, anticolonialiste: la courte vie militante de Lamine Senghor (1924–1927)«. In: *Cahiers d'histoire*. Revue d'histoire critique 126, 55–72. https://doi.org/10.4000/chrhc.4122.

Ndiaye, El Hadji Malick (2019): »Musée, colonisation, et restitution«. In: *African Arts*, 52:3, 1-6. https://doi.org/10.1162/afar_a_00473.

Ramirez Vazquez , Pedro/Campuzano, Jorge/Melot, Thierry/Gabus, Jean (1974): »Musée des Civilisations Négro-Africaines« In: *Musée et Architecture*, UNESCO, 155.

Rocha, Camilo (2018): »O museu do Senegal que quer ›descolonizar‹ a cultura africana«. In: *Nexo Jornal*, 08.12.2018, https://www.nexojornal.com.br/expresso/2018/12/08/O-museu-do-Senegal-que-quer-%E2%80%98descolonizar%E2%80%99-a-cultura-africana (25.03.2021).

Sarr, Felwine (2016): »Rapport général de la Conférence internationale de Préfiguration du Musée des Civilisations noires.« In: *Rapport de la Conférence de Préfiguration du Musée des Civilisations noires*, ed. by Hamady Bocoum/Ndiaye, El Hadji Malick, Dakar, 28.–31.07.2016, https://mcn.sn/wp-content/uploads/2020/12/RAPPORT-CIP-1.pdf (30.03.2021), 105–113.

Sarr, Felwine/Savoy, Bénédicte (2018): *Rapport sur la restitution du patrimoine culturel africain. Vers une nouvelle éthique relationnelle*. France, Ministère de la Culture, http://restitutionreport2018.com/ (25.03.2021).

Sarr, Felwine/Savoy, Bénédicte (2019): »*Opening remarks*«, Museotopia. Réflexions sur l'avenir des musées en Afrique, Collège de France, 11.06.2019, https://www.college-de-france.fr/site/en-benedicte-savoy/symposium-2019-06-11-10h30.htm (25.03.2021).

Senghor, Léopold Sédar (1956). »L'esprit De La Civilisation Ou Les Lois De La Culture Négro-africaine.« Présence Africaine, Nouvelle Série, no. 8/10 (1956): 51–65.

Simbao, Ruth/Kouoh, Koyo/Nzewi, Ugochukwu-Smooth/Sousa, Suzana/Koide, Emi (2019): »Condition Report 3: Art History in Africa: Debating Localization, Legitimization and New Solidarities«. In: *African Arts*, 52: 2, 10–17. https://doi.org/10.1162/afar_a_00456.

Steiner, Christopher (1994): *African Art in Transit*. Cambridge: Cambridge University Press.

Strother, Zoë S. (2019): »Eurocentrism still sets the terms of restitution of African art«. In: *The Art Newspaper* 308, 5.

Thioub, Ibrahima (2016): »Discours du Professeur Ibrahima Thioub, Recteur de l'université Cheikh Anta Diop de Dakar.« In: *Rapport de la Conférence de Préfiguration du Musée des Civilisations noires*, ed. by Hamady Bocoum/Ndiaye, El Hadji Malick, Dakar, 28.–31.07.2016, https://mcn.sn/wp-content/uploads/2020/12/RAPPORT-CIP-1.pdf (30.03.2021), 11–17.

Vogel, Susan (Ed.) (1989): *Art, artifact: african art in anthropology collections* (second Edition), Munich, New York, Prestel.

Wade, Abdoulaye (2010): »Inauguration à Dakar du monument de la ›Renaissance africaine‹«, 04.04.2010, https://www.youtube.com/watch?v=rbLXplepoxw (25.03.2021).

Table of figures

The Post/Colonial Museum: Rethinking the Past, Collecting the Present

A conversation with Dr. Silvie Memel-Kassi, former Director of the Musée des Civilisations, Abidjan, and currently Directrice Générale de la Culture de Côte d'Ivoire, Nanette J. Snoep, Rautenstrauch-Joest Museum, Cologne and Martin Zillinger

Nanette J. Snoep (N.J.S.) & Martin Zillinger (M.Z.): In your work you've always stressed that the museum is a space of memory for communities and individuals alike. Museum objects are meaningful objects, they affect, as you once put it, the soul of the community and relate to questions of identity. Perhaps we should start our conversation by thinking about the mnemonic function of the museum.

Silvie Memel-Kassi (S.M.K.): The museum is indeed a place of memory. I think it is quite clear, considering the definition given to us by the International Council of Museums (ICOM). The museum is this truly permanent institution, a non-profit institution, in the service of society and open to the public. It acquires, preserves, studies, displays and transmits material and immaterial world heritage to provide for study, education and delectation.

Beyond this definition, we must also understand that the museum is the site par excellence where one goes to discover and learn about history, traditions, civilization, and the ways of life of peoples in their evolution. The Musée des Civilisations, which I direct, is an ethnographic and archaeological as much as an iconographic museum. It contains 15,000 pieces, from every region of Côte d'Ivoire. They form a testimony to the four cultural areas of the country and deal precisely with the material and immaterial culture of Côte d'Ivoire. The history of the peoples that preceded us is gathered together under one roof.

It is important to see how the people that come to the museum can not only discover themselves as specific and distinct entities, enriched at the sight of their diversity, they can also find inspiration for themselves as artists in the creation of traditional artwork. The museum is at once a catalyst both for creative potential and for a change in mentality for groups that are unaccustomed to visiting this space. Running an institution that has suffered violence and numerous crises over the last 20 years, we are quite aware of

urn:nbn:de:hbz:6:3-zfk-2021-41985

the magnitude of our project. This is why the permanent exhibition that we have at the moment was devised to engage with the topics of pride, symbolism and identity. Pride, because the different traditional, artistic creations exhibited essentially constitute the pride of the people of Côte d'Ivoire. Symbolism, because the artefacts – given their intrinsic value on an historical, archaeological and anthropological level – are themselves symbols. They symbolise the cultural foundations of Côte d'Ivoire. Identity, for its part, speaks to the identity of Côte d'Ivoire.

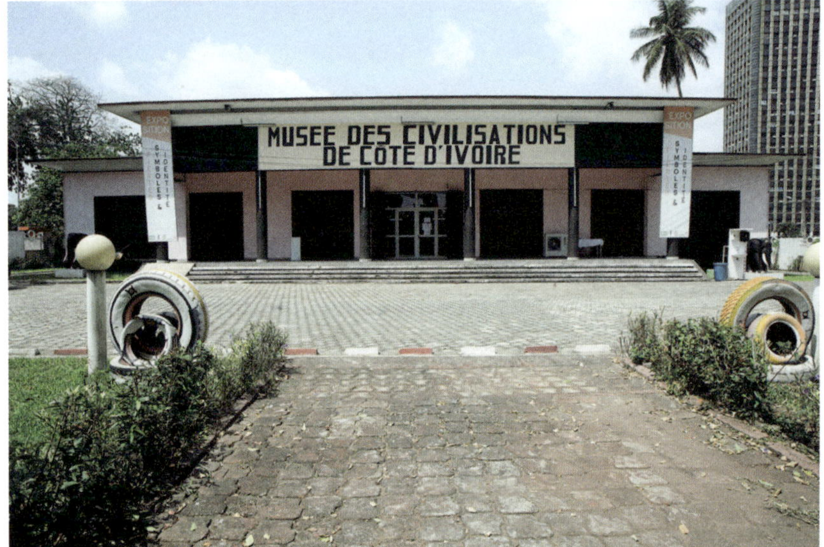

Fig. 1: Main Entrance of the Exhibition Hall. 2021. Photo: Museum of Civilizations, Abidjan.

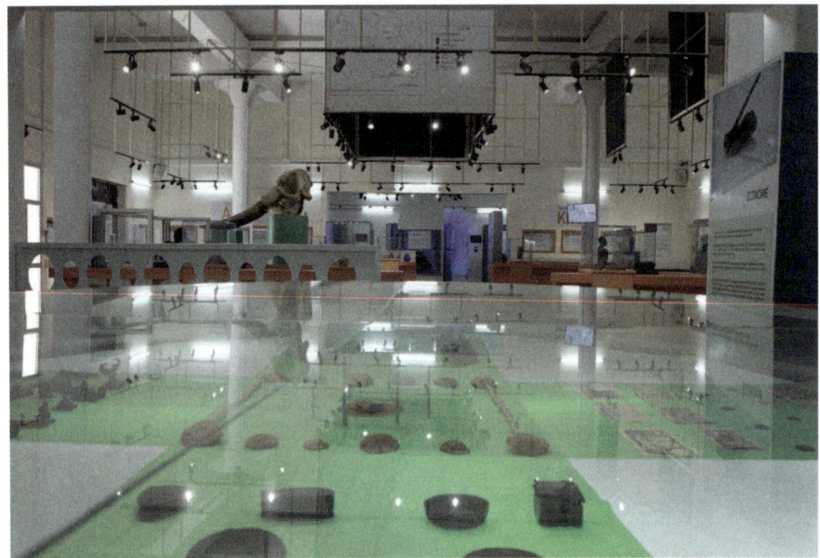

Fig. 2: Objects in Showcases, Permanent Exhibition. 2021. Photo: Museum of Civilizations, Abidjan.

We put this exhibition together in collaboration with all of the actors concerned and with the universities in Côte d'Ivoire. We included anthropological, technical and archaeological expertise in the making of the exhibition, in order to create a space in which people realise that their way of life depends on the choices that they make. For that reason, we also decided to include the Ivorian constitution in the exhibition. As you know, constitutions are a controversial subject in Africa. We displayed the text of the 2016 constitution so that Ivorians can genuinely understand its essence and its importance, but also to have the museum play a stabilising role in Ivorian society. We also wanted to put an emphasis on royality in Côte d'Ivoire in this exhibit, that is to say, on traditional political management in our communities. For that reason, I would say yes, we do discover our identity in all of these material and immaterial expressions.

N.J.S & M.Z.: Perhaps it is fair to say then, that the museum is not only a space of memory, of archiving and memorizing a past, but a mnemonic space, which lends itself both to remembering a past and to remind us of our positionality in the present. It seems that the importance of Macron's speech in Ouagadougou speaks to the importance of the past as well as the powerful discourse in postcolonial societies that demands a re-definition of the present.

S.M.K: The museum has often been a theatre of anti-humanist acts, when we consider the theft and pillage involved. As far as President Macron's speech goes, we could call it an historical speech because the issue of returning objects is of central importance for former colonies. The speech at the University of Ouagadougou was grounds for general euphoria; it was a central concern for African people. Everybody was waiting for that moment, which is why – once the euphoria had passed – African states started organising themselves. They did so individually and collectively, that is, at both national and regional levels, with the Economic Community of West African States (ECOWAS), which is composed of 15 member states, including Ivory Coast. First, there was a summit in December 2018 attended by certain members of governments and the heads of state who had decided to speak together with one sole voice and to combine forces against the complexity of the issue of restitution. This was followed in July 2019 by a meeting in Cotonou, Benin, organised by the ECOWAS Commission, which brought together the ECOWAS Ministers of Culture, who reflected on a plan for the return of cultural goods. The meeting resulted in the elaboration of two tools. Firstly, a regional cultural policy, i.e. a sort of white paper in which major axes regarding the return of objects – as the points on which all member states should speak as one – were defined. Secondly, the 2020–2022 action plan. The action plan is a kind of road map that was given to each country so that, on both a local and national level, concrete action could be taken with a view to preparing for the return of cultural goods.

Any conversation about Côte d'Ivoire should clearly state that the issue of restitution neither emerged nor took shape with President Macron's speech. The issue of return has always preoccupied African states. As early as 1987, Amadou-Mahtar M'Bow provoked public outcry when he spoke of African states' need to recover symbolic objects being kept in the West. The same issue was addressed in correspondence between Ivorian president Félix Houphouët-Boigny and his Senegalese counterpart Président Senghor in 1977. Indeed, the despoliation of cultural goods is an ethical and moral issue because people have the right to enjoy their heritage as they see fit. For me, restitution is, as such, a work of justice and humanity. We need our objects because of the purpose they served and which is crucial for the balance and stability of our societies.

N.J.S. & M.Z.: You are the director of a museum which was founded by French colonial officers. The collection was part of the colonial project to administer Côte d'Ivoire, similar to other places on the continent perhaps, whether it was German, English or French policies that framed the endeavour of collecting, documenting and classifying humans, artefacts and objects of nature. But despite the rhetoric of salvaging culture for educational purposes and for the people of Côte d'Ivoire, thousands of objects were brought to France during and after colonial rule. How does this problematic and violent history impact your work in the museum?

S.M.K.: To give you a concrete example, there is a sacred drum belonging to the Ebrié community, that is to say, to the people in the department of Abidjan, which is the economic capital of Côte d'Ivoire, where we currently find ourselves. The sacred drum is considered a cultural asset by the Ebrié. The talking drum was stolen by the colonist in 1920 while he was looking for workers to build the railway lines in the colony. What happened is that every time the white man came to the area, it seemed no one could be found, it was deserted; because of the drum. The instrument was used as a means to communicate, to sound the alarm that the colonist was about to arrive. It wasn't until some time later he realised that this drum, measuring three and a half meters in length, was the informer. So it was that the drum was torn from the community in 1920. Some years later, in 1930, it was found in the collections of the Musée de l'Homme. Today, it's part of the collections of the Musée du Quai Branly.

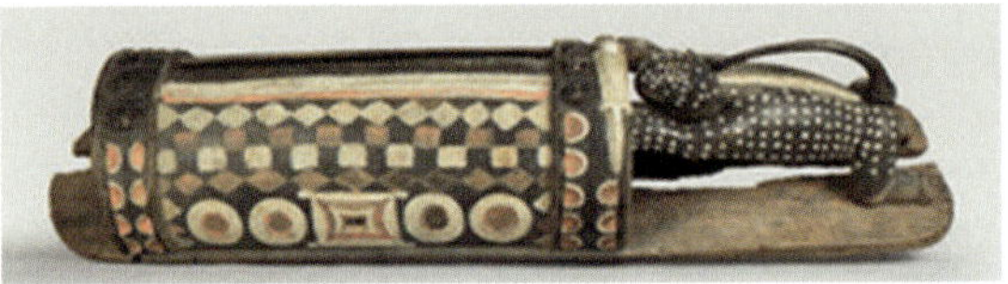

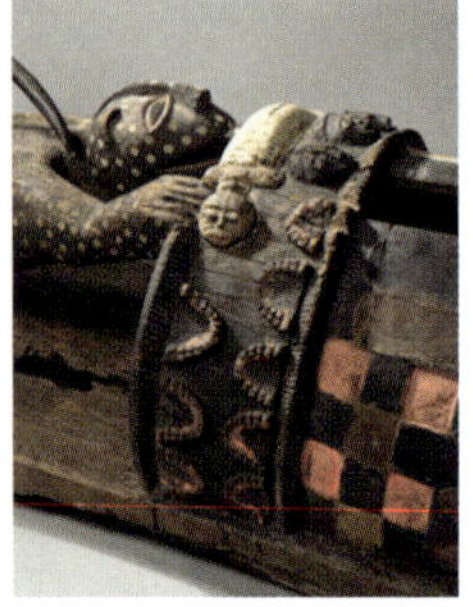

Fig. 3: Djidji Ayôkwè Ébrié Drum in the possession of the Musée du Quai Branly. 2021. Photo: Musée du Quai Branly, Paris.

Fig. 4: Djidji Ayôkwè Ébrié Drum in the possession of the Musée du Quai Branly, Detail. 2021. Photo: Musée du Quai Branly, Paris.

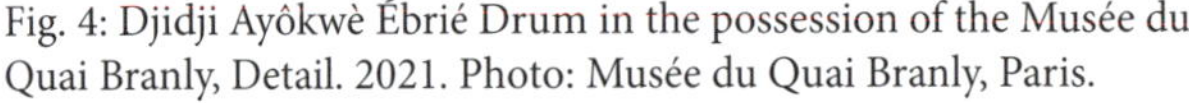

Museum management was exclusively carried out by European conservators during the colonial period and even during the first years of African independence. The men were adept at creating networks through which the museum collections from colonised countries would flow. In that business of dispossession, it is not difficult to remember the quite significant role played by French ethnologist, and former director (1947–1978) of the Abidjan Museum, Bohumil Holas who helped transfer collections from the Musée National d'Abidjan (which was the former name of the Musée des Civilisations de Côte d'Ivoire). During one of our visits to the Musée du Quai Branly in June 2007, we were shocked to see an impressive donation of a thousand objects from Côte d'Ivoire to France, for which Holas was responsible.

N.J.S. & M.Z.: What do you think restitution would look like?

S.M.K.: The restitution of cultural goods is a complex issue. What form of advocacy should be used? What strategy should be put in place in terms of an official demand for the reinforcement of the legal framework? What approach should be adopted to successfully meet the challenge of restitution? Up until a few months ago, one could speak of two blocks in Africa regarding this question. There was a block in favour of immediate and unconditional restitution and another advocating a consensual approach based on diplomacy. Today the states at the heart of the ECOWAS have come to understand that the process adopted by the French government, where each country's request is examined case by case, could well take some time, hence the need to consider a strategy through which member states do not emerge as losers. I agree with Bénédicte Savoy's emphasis on the need for cooperation between all parties involved in the process of restitution. This is not an issue for state agencies alone. In point of fact, restitution demands cooperation between experts and others, such as conservators at museums, people working on heritage, academics, legal experts, representatives of traditional communities, artists, and so on. The other main difficulty is undoubtedly that of the precise number of cultural goods currently stored overseas, which is difficult to ascertain given that African museums did not keep inventories of their collections during colonial times. This, in turn, has grounded the need for bilateral or multilateral cooperation to encourage the creation of formal chains of exchange.

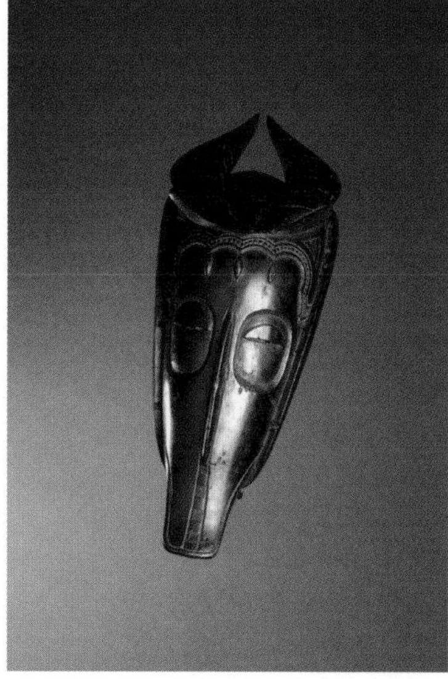

Fig. 5: Masque Zamblé (Gouro). No. Inv. 50.2.918. 2021. Photo: Museum of Civilizations, Abidjan.

For our part, we enjoy positive relations with the Musée du Quai Branly whom we know well and with whom we have shared experience. We should not forget, however, that it is thanks to the tremendous work of Bénédicte Savoy and Felwine Sarr that we are aware of the 3,951 pieces from Côte d'Ivoire at the Musée du Quai Branly.

N.J.S. & M.Z.: How do you evaluate these objects, how do you classify what it is that you want to recuperate?

S.M.K.: President Macron was right to suggest that we first give priority to symbolic objects. These are landmark objects that have gone with worlds, that have gone with wisdom, that have gone with lives, and so you understand that having gone, these objects have created a void in their communities of origin, in their original setting, and this has structurally disrupted the life of these communities. Take the Krou Wê people as an example. Unlike other peoples of Côte d'Ivoire – such as the Akan, Gour, or Mande, who organise around court cultures and the institution of the king at its centre – the Krou Wê have no central power. Authority in the village is linked to the mask, which is handed down from father to son. In times of crises, it is the mask that intervenes to regulate the life of the community, it therefore functions as a guardian, a protective mask. Hence, to the extent that these objects have been removed, you understand that the power of the customary chiefs and the overall established order has also taken a blow. The mask was feared because it had power, when the mask appeared, everyone was reminded of the need for coherence, to re-adjust. If there was a wrongdoer who didn't respect the established rules, the mask had the power to send a disease, even death. As long as the mask was there, order was respected, and once it was removed there was an imbalance. So if we talk about choosing objects for restitution, we need to talk about these landmark objects, these symbolic objects. Also, for the Musée des Civilisations, there is concern around the fact that we do not currently represent all the cultures of Côte d'Ivoire. We call it the Musée des Civilisations and yet there are entire regions that remain unrepresented in the museum's collections. It should be clear – precisely because the Musée des Civilisations is a vestige of the colonial administration – that the regions, which came into contact with colonial administrators early on, are precisely those whose cultural goods were taken. Our main concern is for the lagoon regions and the south of Côte d'Ivoire, which do not have enough traditional objects in the national collections. In my opinion, works from these regions ought to reappear.

N.J.S. & M.Z.: Thank you Silvie! Let us please talk about the wonderful project that you have put in place called *La Collection fantôme*. What is a *Collection fantôme*? And how do you make it tangible through an exhibition?

S.M.K.: La Collection fantôme, that was our way of reacting to the looting of the Musée des Civilisations. The creation of this multifaceted cultural project allowed us to de-dramatise the acts of violence committed against the country's national collections. *La Collection fantôme* is, as such, a collection of artistic responses to the issues raised by the phenomenon of illegal trafficking of cultural goods, of which the Musée des Civilisations was a victim in 2010. *La Collection fantôme,* and the manifesto accompanying it, aim not only to address and prepare mentalities as regards the return of original goods that had been kept overseas, it also seeks to establish an impulse among the communities for the preservation of cultural goods. French and Ivorian schools alike have seen the implications of the pedagogical content. So what really happened?

Our museum is located besides the Ministry of Defence and was hit by a shell that shook all of the buildings. We only just had the time to close the doors and run. 121 pieces were stolen, including the gold collection of the first president Félix Houphouët Boigny. The gold of the Akan people is sacred. It also a precious good for distinguishing certain individuals (generally royal families) and corresponds to social, political and economic power. Hence, when the looting occurred, it was really quite disastrous. With the disappearance of the objects, a part of the culture was erased. We spoke a lot about the subject in the media. Unfortunately, the investigation hasn't gone anywhere.

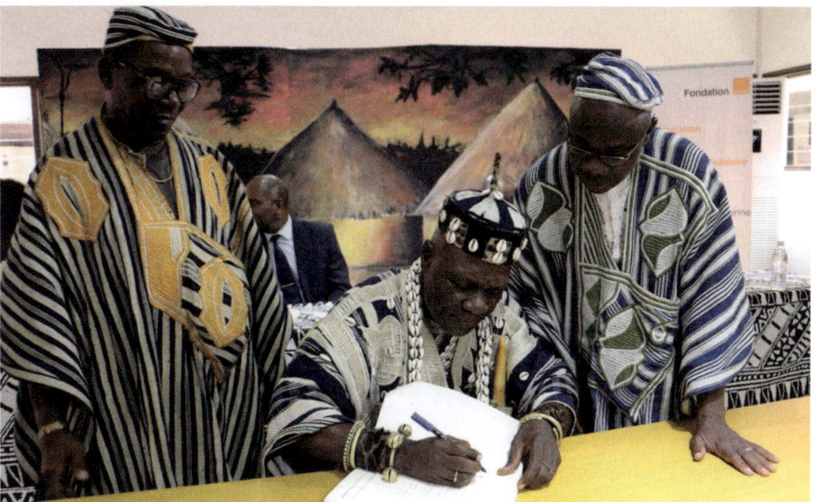

Fig. 6: Signing of the manifesto *La Collection fantôme* by His Majesty Toubo Taho Maurice, Supreme Chief of the Wê, surrounded by his notables. 2018. Photo: Museum of Civilizations, Abidjan.

La Collection fantôme, or the collection of disappeared objects, is both a cry from the heart and a lament, because neither the country nor the communities that produced the objects will be able to forget. This project exists to remind us that the objects will always remain in memory, even if they have disappeared. It's like losing a limb. Even if you amputate an arm, you can still feel its absence when you move the remaining one. We thought that the best place for this project to germinate was in schools. This would give it an educational and pedagogical dimension. We turned our attention to schools so that the children of tomorrow could grow up with a museal awareness, defending their culture. In Africa, you often have the impression that no one is interested when you talk about culture. For my part, I am convinced that this is largely the result of the fate inflicted on Africa since the disastrous geographical division imposed on the African continent at the Berlin Conference.

It is for this very reason that we need to raise our voices as much as possible, so that not one single person in Côte d'Ivoire can avoid hearing about the *Collection fantôme*. The project has brought together representatives of the cultural world, local partners, Interpol's National Central Bureau, the UNESCO bureau in Abidjan, the Ivorian National UNESCO Commission, prefects, mayors, police, customs, regional directors of culture and customary authorities, in short, all those concerned with the issue of heritage preservation or the security of museum collections.

For the next step in seeking to fight illegal trafficking, it was important to make the campaign international. On Kader Attia's invitation, we went to *la Colonie* in Paris, with the *fantôme* collection under one arm. Kader Attia later joined us in Abidjan, as well as the French artist Sébastien Rémy, who was in residence at the museum for two months to work on the *Collection fantôme*. All within the framework of this project, there were exchanges with the Ivory Art Centre, which led to a partnership with the Bingerville School of Applied Arts and the Art Department of the Félix Houphouët-Boigny University.

The theme of the work for the Paris group was *Ceux qui nous regardent* (those who watch us). It was about inverting the colonial gaze. Know that Africa is watching you! Let's just talk about your so-called universal museums that are filled with our cultural goods. The question on the African's lips is this one: These collections, – preserved in public collections in the West – for whom are they important? For the countries of origin or for those who took them? The campaign for Côte d'Ivoire is *Non à la culture du vide* because the mobility of cultural goods on the continent is our responsibility too.

We hope that in time these efforts will culminate in a major exhibition on the Collection fantôme. When the project was launched in 2017 in Abidjan, we dressed mannequins in white cloth with holes in the eyes to look like ghosts. We set up empty showcases and convinced visual artists to provide contemporary creations, while other artists recited poetry. We would love to work with musicians for this project too. We need to get people to come together so that the issues of return and the preservation of heritage are shared by everyone, and so that looting and trafficking can no longer occur as they do today.

N.J.S. & M.Z.: In Germany, the institution of the anthropological museum, with its enormous collections, has come under siege. As we know, only a fraction of the collections are ever exhibited, not to speak of the research. More and more people talk about de-collecting, opening up the archives, releasing objects from the depots. The repatriation of objects is only one element in your reflections on linking the Museum of Civilisations, comprehensively, with the different communities. You also mentioned issues of representation, which are important for how you manage the collections and exhibitions in the context of Côte d'Ivoire. Does the question of collections also extend to the present, is there a collection of the present – or, in short, what might a postcolonial collection look like?

S.M.K.: It's an important issue. How do we create a post-colonial collection now that we're the ones running things, rather than those Western anthropologists from the pre-independence period? Well, when I arrived at the museum, I had my own idea of museum management I have to say, and it's not necessarily one shared by other Africans. Once I'd made my way to the top of the museum in 2006, I realised that an awful lot was missing. The state budget for the museum, which is a public museum, was really quite insufficient for its status. What's more, there was no protocol for the acquisition of objects. Apart from

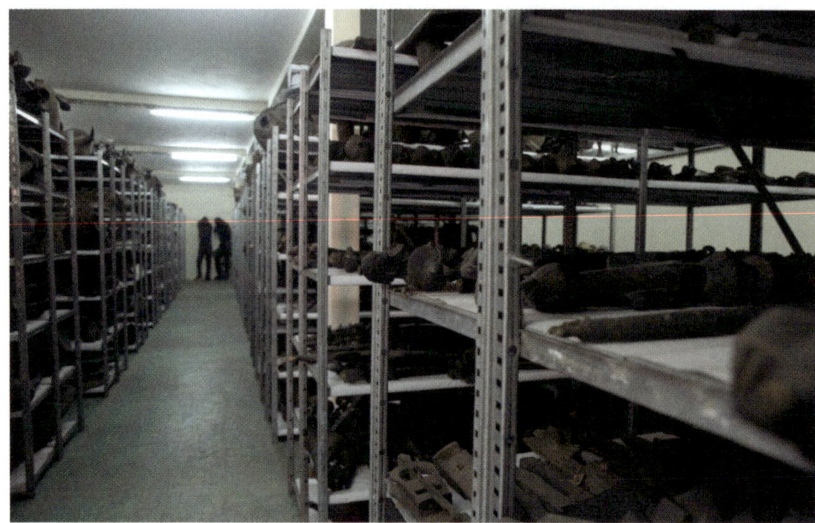

Fig. 7: View into the Depot. 2021. Photo: Museum of Civilizations, Abidjan.

that, it was clear to see in the inventory that certain regions were nowhere to be seen in the museum's collection. We decided to identify those regions and start classifying their cultural and artistic wealth. We turned to academic researchers and started working a lot with archaeology and history departments in the universities here. We drew up a list of objects that ought to be integrated into the museum.

How was the collection carried out? When we identify a region, we send a letter to the customary administrative authorities and do what's called a pre-collection, a pre-project, we go out and meet with the community we're interested in. You know, of course, that speaking with a community means speaking with the chief, with the nobility. You cannot simply go see some individual or other and say: »this is what I'm interested in«. Well, we typically go there and meet with the relevant authorities and explain the situation to them. We talk to them about the merit of the project, that the museum is this place where they and their children will be able to come and see the objects that are in the museum. We emphasis the risk of losing these objects, due to illegal trafficking or corruption, if the objects remain there with them. The fact is that wherever people are poor in Africa, there's an elevated risk of illegal trafficking.

Let me tell you about something that happened to me not so long ago and that is significant in this respect. In 2015, we received a visit from Mr Kouamé who came from the Toumodi region in the centre of the Côte d'Ivoire. He came to tell us about two men who'd come to his village during the night. They had arrived at two in the morning, went straight to the oldest man in the village and said: »We want you to give us the sacred mask that is in your house«. This sacred mask emerges every seven years for atonement ceremonies or whenever the eldest person in the villages passes away. When the old man refused, they took out their phones to talk to someone who knew the house and who told them the location of the sacred mask, which was kept in a suitcase under the bed. Once they'd committed their crime, they left. To this day, the mask has never been found. For us, it was a clear sign that we cannot work alone. We must work collectively if we're to curb the scourge of theft.

As such, working with communities means alerting them to the risks of losing their objects, letting them know they do have a choice. The objects we offer to safeguard are authentic objects, if it's a mask, it must be a mask that has actually danced. But we certainly don't ask for the central mask, we don't say »give us the mask that is the subject of all the libations, all the incantations«. Instead, we suggest another that goes along with it. To be sure that one has also its importance and may be crucial for the community. But the practice of simply demanding the most valued object was at the centre of museum work in colonial times, and continued well after the colonial period.

In terms of the history of the museum, I can remember the institution that houses the Musée des Civilisations being a festival hall originally. During the World War, the governor at the time made the space available to Ivorian artisans so they would come and display the best samples of their artistic works. After the war, the disused festival hall was turned into a museum and those best samples were kept there, as well as authentic objects collected in the communities. We explain all this to the communities who then generally respond: »We understand, yes, we've taken careful note, and it's our wish that the names of our communities be perpetuated through our cultural goods, for posterity«.

I think it's important that we don't impose our will, and we let the communities decide for themselves. Generally speaking, this policy works exceptionally well, given that after some time and reflection, the communities themselves give you the best of their artistic works. They'll tell you, for example, that such and such an object is very important because it belonged to the greatest of the warrior chiefs or to the founder of the community. After that, once weve agreed on which works are to be taken, we go on to the next phase. We go back out with the technical team, equipped with all the necessary equipment and in certain cases with payment for the purchases.

This cooperation in collecting is equally important as an epistemic practice, so to speak. Certain ancient works in Western collections contain erroneous information. The fact is that in certain traditional societies during colonisation, the white man was considered a stranger. He did not have access to accurate information. They would respond to his questions with fake answers that would have the whole community giggling as soon as he'd turned his back. It's clear to see from the names that were given to certain villages or towns of African peoples. Essentially, when a stranger comes, we don't give him all the information, we just tell him what he wants to hear. I realised that while I was visiting two great museums in ›the West‹. A significant part of the information displayed on the labels or in the explanations was inaccurate.

That is also why we prefer the communities to tell us »here, we want you to take this«. Often it is also the first generation objects that they give us. They tell us »no, there is no problem, we will take this, take the major object, if you have it, we can rest assured«. And the advantage of this kind of collaboration is that these communities are involved in everything we do here at the museum. When we have openings or other kinds of activities we involve the customary authorities. They also frequently come to our houses. Descendants of the communities come to see the objects from their homes that are stored in our collections. For what may be called ›scientific documentation‹ we work together with history departments and archaeology departments, which send us their doctoral students, for example, who help us in doing the documentation work.

N.J.S. & M.Z.: Do you see this as a new form of cooperation with the communities in the country? It seems to be redefining the task or the mission of the museum, don't you think? It is about building a museum that is there for the communities.

S.M.K: Well yes, but there is still a long way to go. Material and financial resources are really crucial here. You may have the most wonderful ideas, but if you can't get them off the ground there's no use at all.

When I arrived at the museum, I wanted to think the museum differently. For me, the ideal museum would be one in which communities recognise themselves. It thus needs to differ very much from the classical museum in its colonialist conception, which we've gotten used to in Africa. Museums were institutions for receiving elitist populations, spaces dedicated to whites only. Excuse me when I say white, in Africa we understand very well that, traditionally, these spaces are dedicated to Westerners only. When I arrived in 2006, I drew up entrance statistics to see how many people attended the museum.

The statistics showed that it was mostly Westerners, followed by Africans, and then the local public – and to me, that was not normal. The museum is established, first and foremost, for the people to whom it belongs. For me, running a museum without the local public is a failure, so what should be done? We've always been told that in Africa, Africans do not visit their museums, perhaps because Africans have not yet thought of a purely African museum. For me, an African museum should be one which people are proud to visit. The ideal museum is the museum that responds to the daily concerns of the communities, of the audiences that surround it, this is a museum in which the objects speak directly to those who visit. Wherever the objects are silent and there is no communication, however, I'd call that plain failure. Whatever it may be elsewhere, in the context of Côte d'Ivoire, the populations must recognize themselves in this museum. As such, the museum must be inclusive, even if it looks outward, it should be inclusive above all else. That's very important for me. But to achieve this, it's really a question of political, financial and cultural support.

N.J.S & M.Z.: This is an important issue for all museums. How were you able to build this kind of support?

S.M.K: Thanks to a concept that we created, and baptised *LA NOUVELLE VISION*, our activities have benefited from diverse support. It was a policy that took every aspect of the development of the museum into account. I think that the development of fundraising, as well as the placements that occurred at museums in the United States, were also decisive. It was in the U.S. where we learned how to put together funding projects. The last thing to mention is the Tapa Foundation, an NGO we created at the suggestion of some American friends in 2002. And they were right: in Africa, private donors don't give much money to state institutions, they prefer to fund NGOs. I created the foundation to gather funds for African museums, and the Musée des Civilisations in particular. Companies would normally close their doors to me because I direct a national museum, but the same companies are quite accepting when I come in my capacity as president of the Tapa Foundation. We are thus funded from both the public and private sector. In terms of strategies, we began by choosing a museum ambassador who worked in an international financial institution. It was thanks to him that the museum was first renovated. We took over the lighting of the permanent collection in 2006 and went on to set up the permanent exhibition *Identité et brassage des cultures*. The ambassador put his address book at our disposal.

We looked for other partners, got the media involved, and drew up a partnership with the national press, so that every three months we were on the 8 o'clock news. Plus, all the museum's activities were publicised, which meant that everybody started hearing about it. There was equally an historic partnership (which is still ongoing) with a mobile phone company (Fondation Orange Côte d'Ivoire). Either annually or every two years, according to the programme, the foundation we created to support museums gets funding from our partners at Orange. We were thus able to furnish every museum in Côte d'Ivoire with IT and technical equipment (dehumidifiers or thermo-hydrographs). The Tapa foundation also works with several embassies including those of France and the United States, who funded the digitization process. At an international level, the NGO has enjoyed, and continues to enjoy, the financial support of organisations that work on cultural heritage.

We launched the project *La visite des élèves premiers de classe* to reach a wider audience. With the support of local partners who provided transport, every primary school class in Abidjan came and visited the museum. I see the children that came as their parents' ambassadors to the museum. They thus managed to have their parents come as well. There have been other projects such as the *Le musée vient à vous* which saw the museum head out to meet the public, to organise exhibitions outside the museum walls, in schools and in other public spaces. It is quite encouraging that there are schools from the country's interior that come to visit the museum now. We've gone from 8,000 admissions in 2006 to over 50,000 today in the main hall, and on the museum site itself over 120,000 visitors before COVID-19. The museum also receives more than 200 students of diverse nationalities on placement each year. Today, we receive requests for the museum space to be used for weddings and other social events. So, you see, the museum is becoming indispensable in the lives of groups and companies. In my opinion, this is what a museum should be ideally; a museum that is nourished and enriched by diverse contributions.

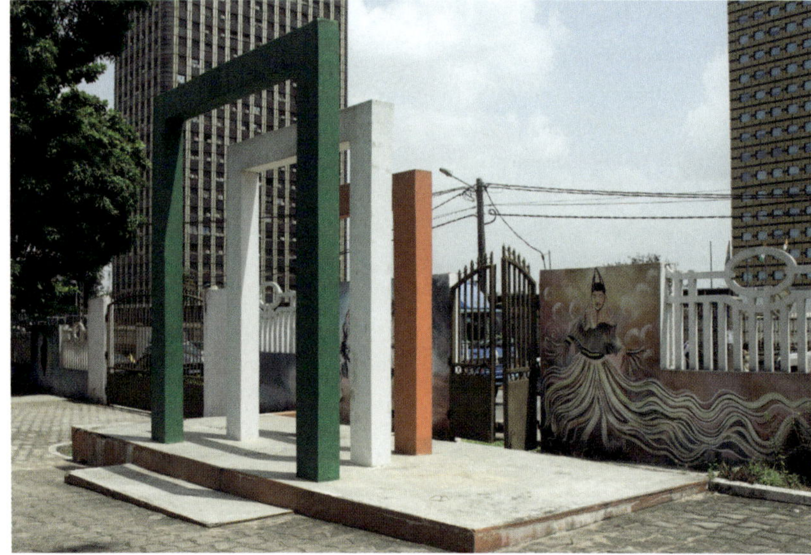

Fig. 8: Pedestrian Entrance to the Museum of Civilizations. 2021. Photo: Museum of Civilizations, Abidjan.

One last point on collaboration: we collaborate with the musée du Quai Branly at the moment, but I dream of opening our museum up to others as well. In the 38th UNESCO Recommendation concerning the Protection and Promotion of Museums and Collections, as well as their diversity and their role in society, provisions are made for cultural bridges and mutual assistance between museums in depository countries and those in countries of origin. As far as I'm concerned, objects that were deported no longer belong exclusively to one country. Today, those objects have double nationality, whether we like or not, and we should endeavour to establish collaboration. Museums in Africa are very young and we should co-operate to make them grow. After all, the objects we have, the collections we manage, the works we have, they're all part of world heritage. If we want to pass on the history of the world tomorrow, and have better balance for the well-being of all our populations, we have an obligation to work hand in hand.

The conversation took place on February 19, 2021. After the transcript of this exchange was revised by the interlocutors, the subsequent translation into English underwent a thorough copy-editing. We thank Michael Dorrity for the latter, and Manon Raynaud for her meticulous transcription of the conversation.

Table of figures

Fig. 1: Main Entrance of the Exhibition Hall. 2021. Photo: Museum of Civilizations, Abidjan.

Fig. 2: Objects in Showcases, Permanent Exhibition. 2021. Photo: Museum of Civilizations, Abidjan.

Fig. 3: Djidji Ayôkwè Ébrié Drum in the possession of the Musée du Quai Branly. 2021. Photo: Musée du Quai Branly, Paris.

Fig. 4: Djidji Ayôkwè Ébrié Drum in the possession of the Musée du Quai Branly, Detail. 2021. Photo: Musée du Quai Branly, Paris.

Fig. 5: Masque Zamblé (Gouro). Inv.Nr. 50.2.918. 2021. Photo: Museum of Civilizations, Abidjan.

Fig. 6: Signing of the manifesto *La collection fantôme* by His Majesty Toubo Taho Maurice, Supreme Chief of the Wê, surrounded by his notables. 2018. Photo: Museum of Civilizations, Abidjan.

Fig. 7: View into the Depot. 2021. Photo: Museum of Civilizations, Abidjan.

Fig. 8: Pedestrian Entrance to the Museum of Civilizations. 2021. Photo: Museum of Civilizations, Abidjan.

Beyond the Museum: The Bandjoun Station

An Interview with Barthélémy Toguo, conducted by Anna Brus and Bernard Müller

This conversation focuses on the local activities and community work of the visual arts centre and museum of contemporary art Bandjoun Station in the West-Cameroon highlands. The project that is run by the Cameroonian artist Barthélémy Toguo goes far beyond the model of most Western museums, combining culture and agriculture, dinner gatherings, festivities, music, and education for children with contemporary art. Its residency programme brings global artists as well as technicians, physicians, economists, agriculturalists, and a variety of other experts into conversation with the local community. Toguo reports on the benefits of this mutual exchange, but also on the initial struggles to install an ›art space‹ in a region where, for many people, art is part of a sacred practic.

Addressing the prospect of the restitution of African art, Toguo makes it clear that this decision should be made along with the artists' ancestors and the local population, and he offers Bandjoun Station as a place where such debates can take place.

Anna Brus (A.B.): Since 2007, when Bandjoun Station was opened in a rural area near to the city Bafoussam, in the West Region of Cameroon, it has become a centre for visionary, community-oriented museum practice. How does your approach differ from the standard Museum? What does the work you are doing there look like?

Barthélémy Toguo (B.T.): Yes, it's a very different approach from Europe because we have the name of a museum, which is certainly a Western name, but how it functions, its approach or practice, is not the same as in the West. Very early on, we associated an agricultural project with our museum project. The museum has its own plantation. It produces food for the public because we understood that to put on art events in Bandjoun, it would be necessary to build up cohesion. Food and festivities are at the centre of our preoccupations, for giving something to the people, so that they eat and embrace the culture that we offer. Therefore, we had to acquire land, and on this land we planted banana trees, maize, manioc, coffee. Imagine the Tate Modern having a potato plantation in London! During the harvests, we distribute to our community what we have cultivated,

ZfK – Zeitschrift für Kulturwissenschaften 2|2021
urn:nbn:de:hbz:6:3-zfk-2021-41999

to the population of Bandjoun, and we associate cultural projects with this result, for example music festivals like the Goldstar Festival. The Goldstar Festival was created for young rappers and young slammers to come inside the museum, to eat, to party, and to discover what we do. So, you can see that our museum becomes a multiplicity of things that we embrace simultaneously and has a different approach from the West. That's how we were able to get the population to take hold of our project, because if we had come just with contemporary art, it would have been very difficult. Not only is contemporary art difficult to understand, just like it is for most Westerners, but we also didn't want to copy a Western museum model. Rather, we moved it around; we wanted to take a more abundant, more expanded approach to embrace the population and to bring them back to our cultural project as well. That's how we operate.

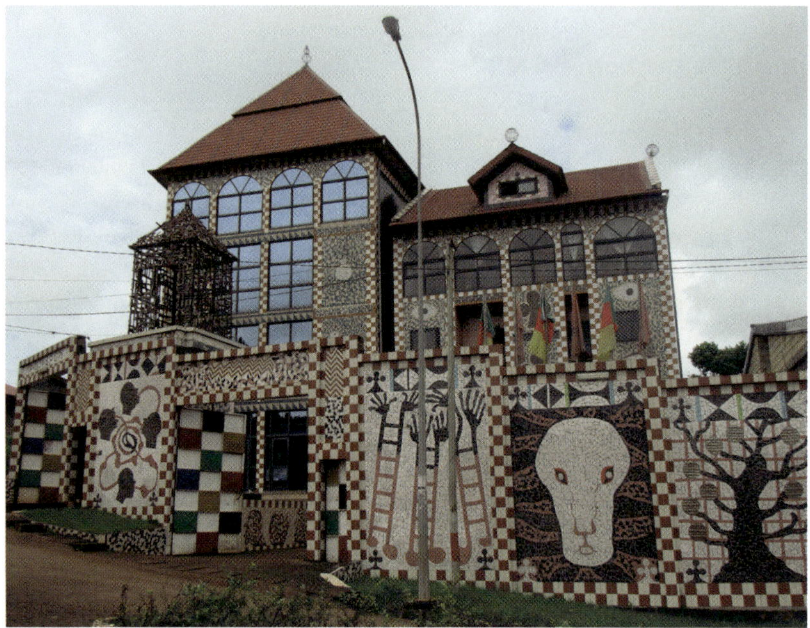

Fig. 1: Bandjoun Station, front side with wall paintings. Copyright: Barthélémy Toguo.

Bernard Müller (B.M.): What happens when someone comes to the residencies? Are there programmed meetings for when an artist comes?

B.T.: When an artist first arrives in Bandjoun, we first set up meetings in the high schools and we organize a presentation of his or her work at Bandjoun Station. We keep it down to earth; we go to the neighbourhoods to tell the head of the blocks that we have an artist who has arrived and that they should come and listen to what he is going to say because he will also come to them. So, there is this communication work that we do before, so that when he arrives he can go to the public, go to the local leaders, to the villages, and meet the people; and he involves them in his project. Above all, the idea is that each time an artist arrives in Bandjoun Station, he or she must have a project in which he or she will involve the local community. There was a photographer who arrived and he wanted to do a work with the women who break the stone in the Bandjoun quarry. He first went to church on Sunday to introduce himself and, on Monday, he went to the quarry to meet these women, the stone-breakers, and chatted with them for weeks, built a trusting relationship before making portraits. So, he doesn't come with a camera and the very next day start shooting the photos. To go straight to the people and take photos is seen very badly there.

So the work of communication is, first, we approach, advance, and trigger in the neighbourhoods, in the churches, and also in meetings. We are in an environment where the Bamiléké are the ethnic group and they really like to hold meetings and *tontines*,[1] and so we try to go to these meetings, these *tontines*, as well as additional time meetings that still exist there, to announce that an artist is coming.

A.B.: The Bandjoun Station website stresses that the place not only fosters artistic exchange but also theoretical and practical exchange on environmental and social issues…

B.T.: Yes, Bandjoun Station is a multi-sided and diverse place. It is not only for the field of art, it's for the field of agriculture, health, and professional training, too. When someone useful, someone with a special skill, arrives in Bandjoun, we look for the sector where we will bring this person. It may be in the field of agriculture, in the field of automobile mechanics, in carpentry, or in the health field. In this case, we bring him to the Bandjoun hospital, if they are an ophthalmologist or a dentist, we present him to the head of the department of medicine or to a doctor. This is a little bit how we work promoting exchanges and ideas in the region. We receive all the competences coming from abroad, from Germany, France, Denmark, and we place these people in fields in a useful way, so that they will train the people everywhere in Bandjoun. We put the residents at the service of the people, of the community.

A.B.: What is the relation between your museum and other cultural institutions like the Musée de la Civilisation in Dschang, and the little palace museums nearby? Is there any kind of exchange and collaboration going on?

B.T.: We meet regularly with Sylvain Djache, who founded the Musée de la Civilisation in Dschang, with Mr. Nchare, who manages the Musée du Palais de Foumban, or with Albertin Koupgang, who manages the Museum of the Bandjoun chiefdom, in order to exchange ideas. We have a project with Sylvain Djache from the National Museum in Yaounde to receive an exhibition that they organized. We also have an agreement with the University of Dschang and organize workshops and symposiums with international professionals and with the Fine Arts Institute of Foumban. We have only been in existence for seven years. We are at our beginnings, but we have very good relations with the

1 In a *tontine* several people join together and pay a regular contribution; the sum is collected in turn by one of the partners. The members of such an association, which can vary from ten to one hundred, determine the amount of regular contributions and the frequency of the meetings. The *tontine* allows each member to easily make use of a large sum of money, which he or she can use as they see fit: launch a business, pay for a hospitalization, organize a wedding, or make an important purchase.

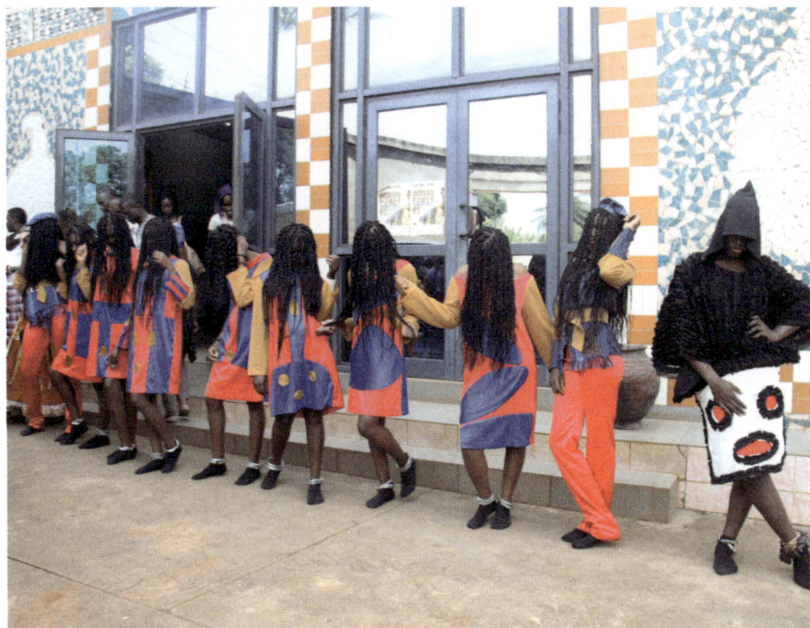

Fig. 2: Fashion show and performance by the stylist Yvy Gisleine Mbianda. Copyright: Barthélémy Toguo.

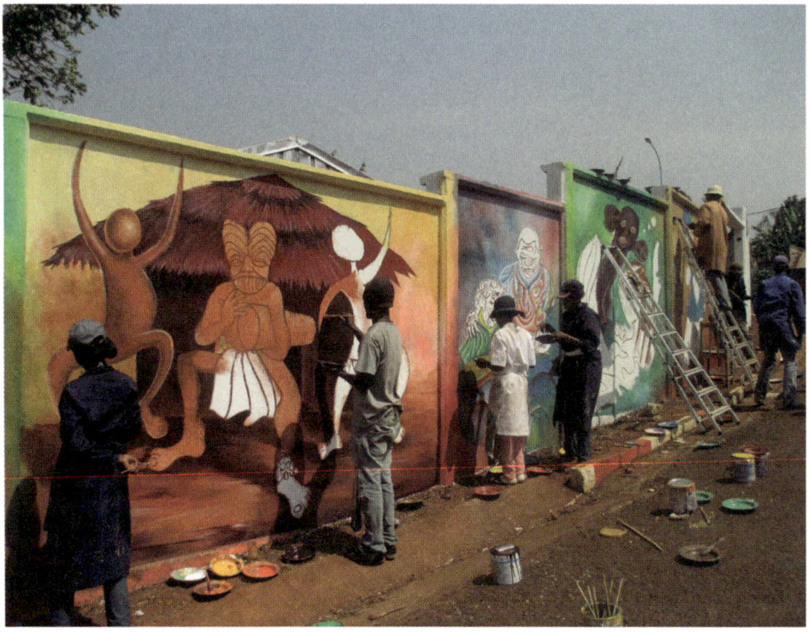

Fig. 3: Drawing workshop with the students of the Institute of Fine Arts of Foumban and the professors Pascal Kenfack and Olivier Tima. Copyright: Barthélémy Toguo.

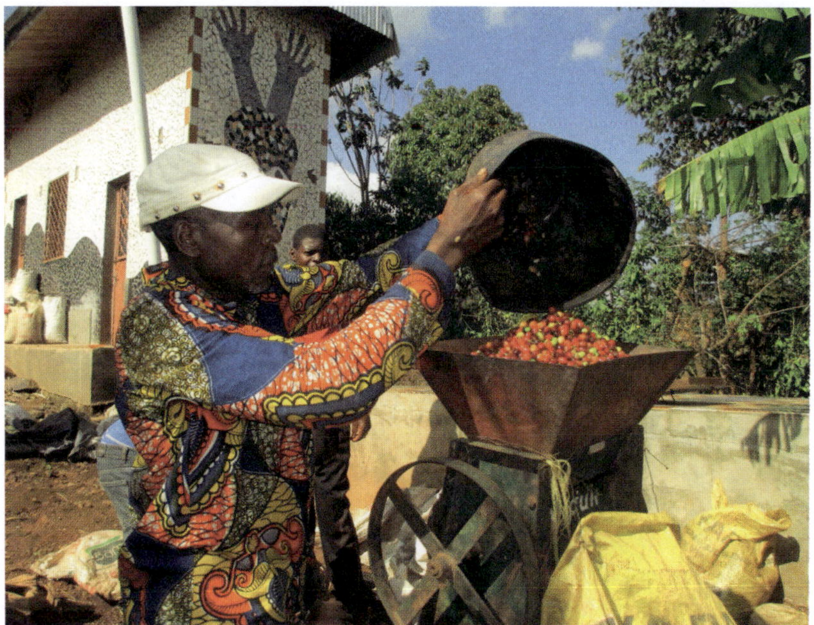

Fig. 4: Talla Zaché, planter in Bandjoun. Copyright: Barthélémy Toguo.

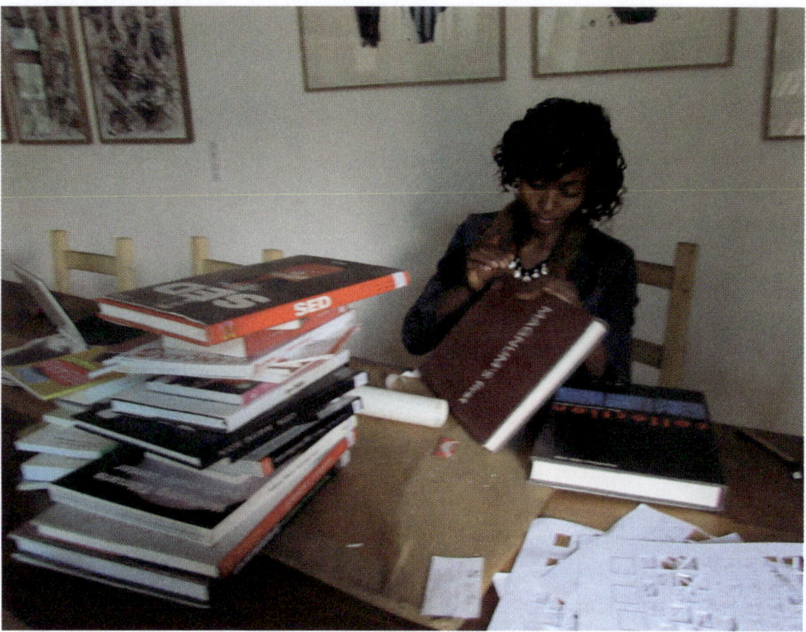

Fig. 5: Floriane Kuitche in the library. Copyright: Barthélémy Toguo.

Museums of Foumban, Dschang, and the Royal Museum of Bandjoun. We don't have a project on our hands that we could set up, but we are open with these places because we collaborate well.

B.M.: In a 2014 magazine article, you talked about the school project, creating a school of visual art, but at the time it was suspended. Is something taking shape? Is it this concept of a school or is it rather, as you just said, something that you practice in a periodic way with each person who comes, each contributor? Or is there an idea of creating a space for teaching visual art?
B.T.: For the moment, we operate in a more informal way and we do training. We also exist as a school, but periodically, not with a new school year and each year training for a diploma. We have just invited a Danish curator, a Senegalese, an Ivorian theorist, and teachers from art schools in France. We brought them to Bandjoun a year ago to organize a training course for managers of cultural institutions. We invited managers of heritage museums in West Cameroon because there are about 120 traditional chiefdoms that exist in the West Cameroon region and these chiefdoms have small museums with trained guides working in them. They were invited to a training course in Bandjoun Station for a fortnight, together with Jacob Fabricius, from the Aarhus Museum in Denmark, and Hafida Jemni di Folco, from Ivory Coast, who runs a curatorial study program in Paris, and Laure Malécot, who is an artist and journalist in Paris and Dakar. So there is a school, but it is periodic, it is at a certain point in time. When we find a small budget, we organize a training course in a specific field. It can be in the medical field, in the economic, or in the cultural or agricultural field.

A.B.: What were the main problems you encountered beginning with the involvement and activation of the community? How did you pave the way in the very beginning for the acceptance and welcoming of your practice?

B.T.: In the beginning, there were some misunderstandings. The walls of the Bandjoun Station were covered with mosaics designed from my graphic universe. The imagery can frighten people because they think it's magic. Art is magic. An artist who creates, who draws, who invents something new, for many, it is magic. People in the area thought, at the beginning, that it was a house where occult practices were taking place. So, we have this local problem, which is very important, that people flee from cultural spaces because they think there are occult practices behind it. It is necessary to explain to people what a museum is, and the ideas from my graphic universe, which is all around Bandjoun Station, can be misleading.

When we started our work, we cooperated with a Christian school and the priest that teaches there liked the project and he brought the children to Bandjoun Station. When the children came home in the evening, they told their parents what they saw, where they were taken. The families were very upset and went to church in the evening to interrogate the priest, threatened him, and asked him why he had brought their children to this place of magic, this sect. We understood that there was an educational problem that we had to meet with the parents first. Members of the Catholic Church came back to the school to have a meeting with the parents to tell them that it is important for the children to discover the culture in the museum. It was really the regional Catholic Church that came to calm the situation down!

What we learned from that is that we must be able to create a conversation to reach out to parents, to even go to churches and local meetings, to go to canteens, to neighbourhoods to talk about what we do. We have to establish communication work that must be done at the grassroots level. So, we have this problem with the public on a daily basis; we are in a rural area, too, and it is not easy for people to understand these things. We understood that we had to associate – as I said at the beginning – agriculture, restaurants, food, and music with embracing contemporary art.

A.B.: Your online collection database shows that you not only have a collection of contemporary art but also a collection of classical African art, figures and masks from Cameroon, the Congo region, Nigeria, etc. I was wondering where these objects came from, where you collected them, in Europe or on the Continent? Regarding what you just said, do these objects contribute to making people think that it's a place of magic? Doesn't the presence of this type of object contribute to – as you were saying earlier – the association of Bandjoun Station with occult activities, with a sect that would come and take traditional objects?

B.T.: The classical objects come from the exchange I have had with African collectors – from Bafoussam, Foumban, Yaoundé, or Douala. The contemporary art in Bandjoun Station also comes from exchanges that I made with contemporary artists during their lifetime, or from their galleries or collectors, as well. That's how we built up our two collections, which are a mix of classical and contemporary art.

This idea that Bandjoun Station is an occult place is also connected to an installation I created in 2010, when we had just started our cultural work. I had been living in Bandjoun since 2000. When I arrived, we didn't see too many coffins and, in 2002 and 2004, little by little, I saw shops opening where coffins were being made. In 2005 the area where I bought planks was transformed into coffin shops and, in 2010, a whole street, a whole district, the Bafoussam district, became the industrial coffin factory. I told myself as an artist that there is a problem in Africa. Why are people dying? Why are all these things made, these coffins that I see everywhere in the street, on motorbikes, on people's heads! I arrived in 2000 and I didn't see this atmosphere! By 2010 it was becoming incredible! I said, it's not normal, there's a problem. I was also doing a tour in Benin, Senegal, and Kinshasa, so I need to work with that. So I decided to have a carpenter in Bafoussam make 54 coffins that would speak about what Africa is going through at the moment, this visual hecatomb. And so, the carpenter made 54 coffins for me, and they had to be moved from Bafoussam to Bandjoun Station for storage. For a whole day I transported coffins with my car and everybody in Bafoussam, which is the third largest city in Cameroon, saw how the gentleman who lives in Europe, who is building the museum, is moving coffins. It frightened everyone that I could build this house to put coffins in. That's what created the atmosphere of fear. This marked Bandjoun Station. The installation called

Time was shown at the Biennale in Lyon, so the coffins were transported from Bandjoun to Lyon, but not everybody saw the coffins coming out of Bandjoun, the same people who saw them returning were not there. So until today, there are some who think that inside Bandjoun Station, there are coffins. This is the problem we had.

But it's true; the fact that we have classical art can frighten people. Classical art in Africa is also considered sacred because it's part of the culture and we have used it for sacred ceremonies as well. When you see someone who has it, you're going to say: »This is someone who believes in sacred worship practices, in magic«, and that can be taken badly. But I think the basic problem is literacy, from the start. We are among a somewhat illiterate people and the problem of education is very important. In Africa, education must be accelerated, we must call for the education of people, culture, school, and dialogue as well.

To get back to the story of the unsettled parents, when the school children came to visit the museum, we had put a bucket of water at the entrance with gel where the children had to wash their hands first, so as not to dirty the museum. They washed their hands, wiped them with towels and went inside. Inside they were given a presentation of vases made by the women potters in the town of Foumban. Twenty kilometres from the town of Foumban, there is a quarry where the bricks for the construction of the Royal Palace were made. That's how I was able to acquire about twenty gigantic vases. The children were fascinated by their grandeur and when they came home, they told their parents that they washed their hands at the entrance and that they discovered the vases, and there was this misunderstanding that the parents thought they had washed their hands in the vases or in gourds. In Africa, washing hands in a gourd is a sacred act because we put the skulls of our ancestors and grandparents in the gourd to be buried in the family home. So, the parents thought that the owner of Bandjoun Station used magic to take the knowledge, the brains, of their children and that it was the priest who brought them to me so that I could take their knowledge. So you see, there is a problem of education in the region that needs to be solved, through conversations, through meetings.

B.M.: It's interesting how it's said, how it's formulated. This symbolism, this fear of being robbed, of having a spiritual part of oneself taken away. Sometimes it's healthy to be wary, but why be wary of yourself and not of certain sects. Did you grow up in Bandjoun?

B.T.: I grew up in Yaounde, but my family is from Bandjoun and I came back to settle where my family comes from.

B.M.: Do you remember having lived through experiences like the ones you tell us about as a child? Being taken to places where there were strange objects and then you were told it was a museum?

B.T.: In the region of Mbalmayo where I was born, there is not the cultural strength and continuity that the Bamilékés have. Among the Fangs, among the Ewondo, the traditional chieftaincies have mostly disappeared. I was born over there, I came back to Bandjoun at the age of 25 or 30, just because my parents live there. Unfortunately, during my youth in Mbalmayo, there was no museum and there was no culture to be found anywhere like in the West of Cameroon, where until today there are still chieftaincies which are respected. This is something else! The West region of Cameroon is culture! Since they are in the inland they were less affected by colonisation. Those inhabitants who are on the coast, on the sea like the Douala have been very much affected by the West, which asked them to destroy their cultural practices. The Bamiléké on the mountains in the interior of Cameroon are more remote and have been able to preserve their traditions and culture. Among them, seeing something cultural in the home, sculptures or drawings, you say: »Here is someone with a strong mind, a strong spirit and a belief system«. But, of course, sometimes this is scary, you're a little bit suspicious of someone who draws because he's a scholar, he has strong spiritual knowledge and you might be afraid of the artist, even spiritually.

B.M.: Precisely in relation to the impact of colonialism, how does the debate on decolonisation, decoloniality, this awareness that there is this symbolic and physical violence from colonialism, how does this debate take place in Bandjoun? Does it translate into a desire for the return of certain objects? Concerning the royal paraphernalia of Njoya, for example, I think that people know that these objects are in Europe. Is there something being said – not only in intellectual circles – about a desire for the return of colonial objects? In fact, I have two questions, for one, is the debate on colonialism, that is everywhere today, happening in small towns like Bandjoun? And, secondly, what about the restitution debate?

B.T.: People talk less about it and those who are informed about it think that when these objects are returned, they shouldn't be put in a museum, as they were in the West. They think they should be redistributed to the cultures from which they came, so that they can continue their daily work, the usual work they used to do. So if an object arrived and it was an object from Batcham or Bangangté or Foumban, which was used for a ceremony, it would have to go back to that culture and continue to serve. It should not return to a closed, glassed-in space, such as a museum, because from the outset it was not intended for museums. Such an object was intended for ceremonies, for practices, for acknowledgements by a chief who wanted to appreciate the arrival of his host, offer him a stool and ask him to sit. So put the stool back there, in the chiefdom. That's what they think, they don't think about returning these objects to museums, they want them to be able to return to their usual functions in society.

A.B.: Could you imagine Bandjoun Station as being an intermediate place for the return of certain objects coming from Europe? Would it be a place that enables thinking about restitution as an evolving process that helps to identify spaces of return – as spaces that are created by the people who are going to receive the objects?

B.T.: A place for debate and exchange, of course!

B.M.: And for the physical transition of the objects? That is to say that at some point the objects would pass through there, surrounded by debate and discussion?

B.T.: Yes, of course. That's our role, that's the function we want to occupy, we want to exercise, to be a place of passage. It would really be ideal, not to welcome the pieces and lock them up in Bandjoun Station, but to have a dialogue on which approach to follow, because it is necessary to prepare well and build up procedures, to understand the steps that the work will follow. We are a cultural space and we want to exercise this with the museum curators, to create a link between the museum and the community, between the museum and the inhabitants. We really need to weave this, this rapprochement between these two worlds.

B.M.: This is very interesting. One could imagine a kind of forum to which one could bring from the region about ten objects, objects that are potentially returnable. At this forum the discussion takes place with local chiefs, with the guides you were talking about, the potters, and all the people concerned, and at the end of this discussion one would come to a conclusion of what to do.

B.T.: We could not only invite representatives of the places where some of the works come from, we would certainly also invite the chiefs, the inhabitants of the towns and villages that surround Bandjoun Station. Everybody invited would think about how to develop a project of return and imagine together with the curators from abroad how the works can be restored. The chiefs, too, will tell us how they are going to welcome the work in their community, because the idea is not only to give without knowing what they are going to do with it, but to invite new imagining about what they are going to do with it, how they are going to receive it, where they are going to put it. Bandjoun Station is in the field; we know who are the people to invite for a conference.

That's an essential and current project that we must set up, we must talk about it. It's current, it's our moment, our period, and we need projects in this field!

We are grateful to Manon Reynaud for the transcription of the conversation. Translation from the French: Anna Brus, copy-editing: Michael Dorrity.

Table of figures

Fig. 1: Bandjoun Station, front side with wall paintings. Copyright: Barthélémy Toguo.

Fig. 2: Fashion show and performance by the stylist Yvy Gisleine Mbianda. Copyright: Barthélémy Toguo.

Fig. 3: Drawing workshop with the students of the Institute of Fine Arts of Foumban and the professors Pascal Kenfack and Olivier Tima. Copyright: Barthélémy Toguo.

Fig. 4: Talla Zaché, planter in Bandjoun. Copyright: Barthélémy Toguo.

Fig. 5: Floriane Kuitche in the library. Copyright: Barthélémy Toguo.

Trafficking Vague Cosmological Boundaries: Towards Knowing Experiential Relationality in Museum Epistemics

Helen Verran

This article seeks inspiration in engaging with African art works displayed amongst sculptures and paintings from European pasts in Berlin's Bode Museum 2017–2019. Concepts at play in designing that exhibition, deriving from both history and philosophy of art and anthropology, expressed a modern spacetime cosmology. As is the modern way, it focussed on what it took to be various cultural and social qualities of the art works assumed to be objects, ›real lumps of matter set in spacetime‹ – universal common sense. I offer a reading of the exhibition that arose in knowing otherwise than in this modern common-sense way. Reading the displays as enacting a multiversal relationality, I aim to inspire museum curators to develop an alternative epistemic demeanour as they face challenges of decolonising. I propose this will involve curatorial analyses and interpretations that begin in incommensuration, and work through knowing experiential relationality.

Opened in 1904, Berlin's Bode Museum keeps largely to its original design. Apart from the temporary exhibitions display space in its basement, the building houses a series of period rooms with the decor of each designed to show artworks from Europe's classical, byzantine, gothic, renaissance, and baroque periods, each in the unique context of its emergence as named art form. The concept of this museum, originally called the Kaiser-Friedrich-Museum, was developed by Wilhelm von Bode (1845–1929) who is recognised as carrying on the work of previous imperial European museums, for example »the papally sponsored Museo Pio-Clementina and [particularly the work] of Vivant-Denon, the Director of Napoleon's imperial museum« (Eisler 1996: 23).

Taking up the position of director of royal museums in Berlin in 1883, the display techniques Bode pioneered have been systematically developed for over a century now (Backer 1996). The collection of the Bode Museum is renowned. Neil MacGregor, former director of the British Museum, has celebrated the sculpture collection of the Bode Museum as offering »the most comprehensive display of European sculpture anywhere« (MacGregor 2006), adding that through the sculptures a visitor to the Bode Museum can witness Europe's history – aesthetic and religious, intellectual and political. The displays in the Bode exhibit the multiplicity of what historian of European art, Henri Focillon, has termed »the life of forms« in the histories of European cosmologies (Focillon 1992).

urn:nbn:de:hbz:6:3-zfk-2021-42006

The African art with which art works inhabiting some of the Bode's rooms sang in glorious concert between October 2017 and November 2019, had been brought in from another, and much larger collection of items owned by a different branch of Berlin's powerful Staatliche Museen zu Berlin, the Ethnologisches Museum, which temporarily had no access to display space. It seems that the brief ›louding‹ of African voices that the Bode exhibition afforded, had mundane institutional origins and motivations. Notwithstanding, in this essay I recognise the exhibition as a unique and significant happening in museum history.

Such a concert of art works as that which could be experienced in a few rooms of the Bode Museum across 2018 and 2019 is a unique opportunity. Of course, it is a very different affair than the concert that happened for a few months in 1884–1885 in a building that was situated just a twenty-minute walk from the Bode Museum. That unique ›happening‹ planned

> »the European partition and conquest of Africa [...] perhaps the greatest historical movement of modern times [...] [a] phenomenon, usually associated with the rise of a ›new imperialism‹, [which] was given concrete expression [...] when the Concert of Europe assembled at Berlin, the capital of the newly-formed nation-state of Germany« (Uzoigwe 1984: 9).

I use the occasion of the so-called *Beyond Compare. Art from Africa in the Bode-Museum*[1] exhibition to attend to a much needed, and long overdue, redesign of museum epistemics. What happened when displays in galleries designed for, and dedicated to European art were interrupted by introducing African art objects? One might attend to this question in many registers and genres of judgement and critique. Here I ask the question in the light shed by the idea that museums, like all modern institutions, collectively enact themselves in expressing a modern spacetime cosmology,

> »the official physical cosmology of modernity [...] culturally marginalised at the heart of the social system by the contrary pressure exerted [...] by a progressive sensibility that sought certainty in cosmological closure. Cosmological openness was redacted [in modern institutionalisation] « (Abramson/Holbraad 2014: 11).

In the past decade or so philosophers, practitioners of science studies, social theorists, and anthropologists have been gradually ›outing‹ this formerly sealed off modern spacetime cosmology, its formerly solid socio-cultural framings are beginning to dissolve. With Karen Barad's skilful bringing of physics' relational metaphysics to the fore (Barad 2007), and the emergence of the new materialisms, a move is underway to devise and tell stories of new modern relational cosmologies. The problem of course is that on the ground – in the complicated workings of modern institutions, places like, say schools in Nigeria, or museums in Europe – it always takes more than having a new story; developing new on-the-ground epistemic practices and methods takes work. Many years ago, I found myself

1 Despite the title the epistemic design of the exhibition was comparative through and through.

struggling with the issue of the pervasive modern spacetime cosmology in Nigerian classrooms, although at first, I could not name my struggle in that way. My book *Science and an African Logic* tells how I came to ›see‹ and ›see through‹ the translating figure of matter set in spacetime, in conceiving numbers as uniquely different conceptual expressions of disparate cosmologies (Verran 2001: 150). Different epistemic demeanours than modern epistemics are possible, and they involve conceiving of our concepts differently and recognising how we might use concepts in negotiating vague and flimsy boundaries of cosmologies (Verran 2018: 112).

In contemporary institutions the unmarked and sealed off modern cosmology at the core of institutional functioning, is mobilised by what we might name a ›modern epistemics package‹ which gives particular answers to epistemic questions: axiological issues, ›Why is our knowledge valuable?‹; and teleological, ›What are the purposes of our knowledge making and doing?‹, for example. It involves the doing of particularly configured knowns, by particularly configured knowers, who collectively make and do modern knowledge, in answering to taken for granted ontological and epistemological standards. In operationalising museums' missions as dealers both in ›the cultural heritage of world civilisation‹ with its undergirding universalism, and in ›the national patrimony‹ with its enabling relativism this, by now past its use-by date ›modern epistemic package‹, has proved its worth for museums in the colonial and postcolonial eras.

In developing an epistemics that has utility in the period of decolonising that has now hit museums like a tidal wave (Maples 2020), here I elaborate the claim that museums must undertake substantial epistemic renovation. In this makeover, different sorts of answers will need to be found in negotiation with ›others‹. Of course, this will require some tricky work in recognising who or what ›the others‹ are, and how they might be negotiated with. In particular, I argue that, ontologically speaking, the entities museums know through and with, need to be explicitly recognised and attended to. Ontologically, the entities museums need now are *not* objects that have the property of being universal in expressing a state of cosmological universalism in their being, as is necessitated by claims of world civilizational heritage. Nor, alternatively, are objects with the property of being culturally relative in expressing a state of a different, hermetically sealed cosmological specificity, or historical uniqueness, as required by arguments of national patrimony, suitable for museum operations nowadays. Rather, museums need to devise ways and means of ›happening‹ knowns as expressions of relationality in embedding a multiversal relationism in their being (Verran in preparation). Such an epistemics would befit museums as liminal multiversal institutions in beginning to live up to their task of negotiating boundaries of cosmologies in doing a canny cosmopolitics, opening up possibilities for inventing new worlds.

Unvergleichlich. Kunst aus Afrika im Bode-Museum/ Beyond Compare. Art from Africa in the Bode-Museum

Bode Museum displays have expressed a contradictory approach towards cosmologies from its inception. Inheriting the imperial mantle, the universalistic side of the modern constitution has been the natural domain of its operations since the beginning. Indeed, in

1995, while celebrating the 150-year anniversary of Bode's birth, such ambitions, along with an unwillingness to take on a relativist epistemic ethos more suited to a postcolonial world were made obvious. »The cosmic goals [of the institution for which] only an ensemble of universally accepted ›master- pieces‹ from all over the [...] world was uniquely adequate, [were] the ambitions of Bode's employer« (Eisler 1996: 32), the implication being, that such cosmic goals were still valid in 1990s. This institutional ethos in its period displays proposes its art objects as expressions of the many diverse cosmologies that historically have animated the past polities of Europe. Yet, these cosmologies can only ever be mere steps on the way to a triumphant European modernity, with its powerful but backroom, instrumentalist spacetime cosmology, which the Bode Museum as a whole represents.

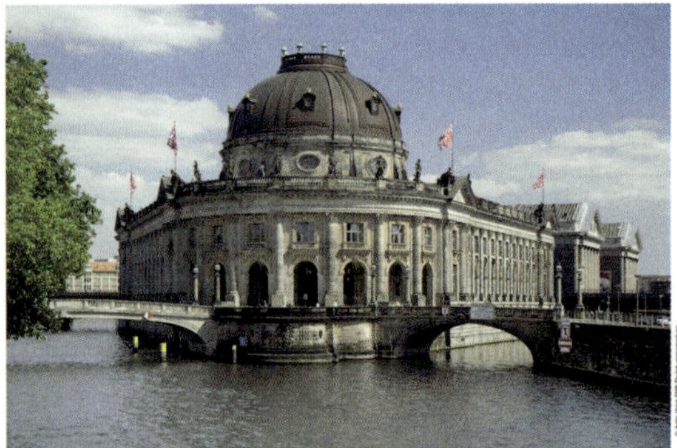

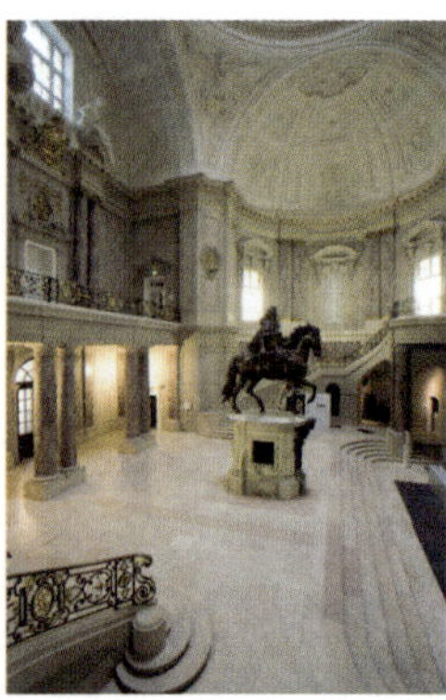

Fig. 1 and 2: The Bode Museum enacts modernity's cosmic goals. Staatliche Museen zu Berlin–Preußischer Kulturbesitz. Skulpturensammlung und Museum für Byzantinische Kunst. Photo: Antje Voigt, Berlin.

Across the two years of the *Beyond Compare* exhibition, the very first display case that most visitors to the museum would come across, located in the Museum's Grand Basilica entrance hall, explicitly performed the museum and its modern ethos. Two bronze/brass figures sat side-by-side in a single display case: »Putto with a Tambourine«, by fifteenth-century Italian artist Donatello, sat beside »Statue of the Goddess Irhevbu or Princess Edeleyo«, made in the Kingdom of Benin sometime in the seventeenth or eighteenth century. In this display, visitors were instructed through engagement in an institutionally reflexive exercise.

The explanation provided for this display contrasted the institutional accessionings of the objects by two separate museum collections, evidenced in the African art object carrying its accession number and other markings on its shoulder and back, in a spidery white-ink tattoo. At the beginning of the twentieth century one object was categorized as art object, the other as ethnographic object. The explanatory text accompanying the display uses the juxtaposition to comparatively describe how each item was treated by the institution of the state museum: the one as art, and the other as cultural artifact exemplifying ›otherness‹, infused with the ›less-than-ness‹ implicit in European imperialism and colonizing – as ethnographic object.

Despite being delighted by the juxtaposition of these objects I had three critical reactions to this display. First with this exhibition threshold display, the museum as modern

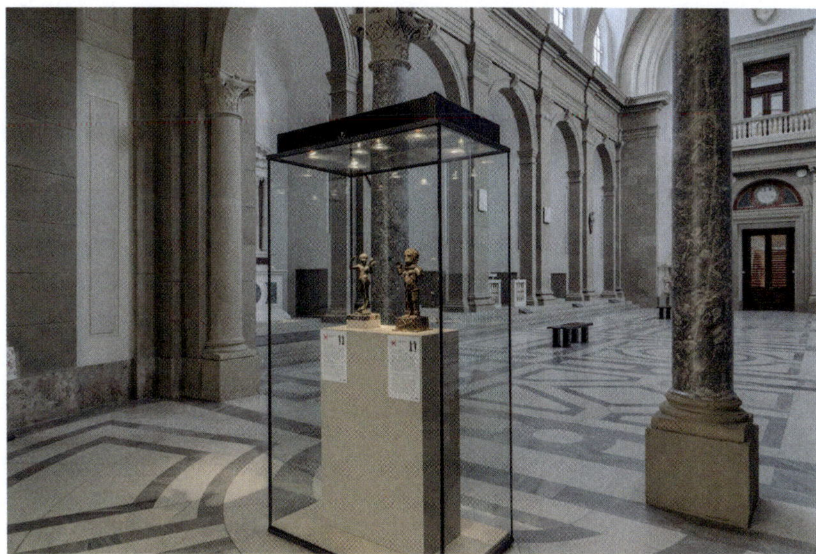

Fig. 3: *Putto with a Tambourine*, by fifteenth-century Italian artist Donatello, sits beside *Statue of the Goddess Irhevbu or Princess Edeleyo*, made in the Kingdom of Benin sometime in the seventeenth or eighteenth century. Staatliche Museen zu Berlin–Preußischer Kulturbesitz. Skulpturensammlung und Museum für Byzantinische Kunst. Photo: Wolfgang Gülcker, Berlin.

institution proposed itself the main focus of the exhibition; second, it is yet another rehearsal of the old modern science progress story: we used to think we knew the truth, but then the true truth emerged, and we realized we were mistaken back then; and third the display papers over the assumption that both objects remain the cultural property of the German State, despite implicit recognition of the dubious morality of the exchanges that enabled passage of the Benin goddess/princess from Benin City to Berlin. I come back to this display – the art objects deserve better than this.

In the substantive elements of the exhibition, the curators of *Beyond Compare, Jonathan Fine and Paola Ivanov* developed two different display frameworks (cf. Chapuis/Fine/Ivanov 2017) mobilising what in the modern cosmology are proposed as universal cultural categories, arising in what modern analytic philosophy names as »universal canons of thought and action« (Wiredu 1996: 1). The museum's special exhibitions gallery on the ground floor assembled a large number of both African and European sculptures, dating from the sixteenth to the twentieth century, in rather a small space. The accompanying interpretive material listed and explained the groupings: »The Others«, »Aesthetics«, »Gender – or the multiplicity of the person«, »Protection and Guidance«, »Performance«, and »Taking Leave«. In this way they elaborated a conceptual framing which connected. These conceptual categories then became the means to compare and contrast. This is a top-down application of categories assumed as universal. The second element of the exhibition consisted of twenty-two displays scattered in sixteen separate galleries across the first and second floors of the building. Here the terms of comparison were said to arise from universal properties embedded in works themselves. Some pairs were compared and contrasted on aesthetic criteria, others on social grounds. Here the universal categories work, so to say, bottom-up.

In this essay I read against the grain of the of curators' intentions. While they take an empirical approach in a deliberative attending to the artworks as objects that might be indexed, I experience the artworks in alternative mode. Mobilizing the typology of experiential possibilities developed by American philosopher C. S. Peirce, I take the artworks as expressions of iconicity. To experience the iconic, one must develop capacities to experience prior to conceptualising, learning to trust ontic experience of experience (Christie/Verran 2013: 304). In proposing this approach, I do not seek to replace, but to expand the epistemic repertoire of curators.

In beginning I acknowledge the brilliant artfulness of Bode's display techniques as in large part affording my (mis)reading. In recognising their artful display techniques, I discern that the curators seem to know more than they know they know. In suggesting that museum curators need to renovate museums' epistemic practices I am proposing that curators learn to make explicit in epistemic talk, what it is they already seem to know about the lives and ways of forms in art objects. In the past I have made explicit some different ways and means in working with numbers; museum curators can make explicit different ways and means of working epistemically with museum objects.

Later in this essay, I offer an ethnographic narrative of experiencing the exhibition within an explicitly translating cosmology that expresses a multiversal relationality (Verran 2018). This reading does not pretend to review the exhibition, the voice here is not that of the ›every-visitor‹; on the contrary. Taking multiversality seriously, the reading enacts the claim that ours is, and always has been a world of many worlds. In both subsuming it and revealing it as just one possibility, in this framing the modern epistemics mobilising universals enacted in expressing modern spacetime cosmology, through which the exhibit has been deliberatively designed, is parochialized. Rather than the usual approach of adopting a demeanour of epistemic good will afforded by unremarked epistemic bad faith, the multiversal relationality mobilised in narrating my experience of the exhibition, amounts to an expression of epistemic good faith enabled by initially and explicitly indulging a transient, knowing epistemic bad will (Blaser/de la Cadena 2018: 11; Verran 2018: 113). Featuring explicit and minimalist metaphysical commitments, this translating cosmology is nothing more and nothing less.

Bringing to the fore art works' existential relationality refuses to begin in a postulated conceptualised sameness. Ontic distinction is acknowledged as framing experience, while recognising possibilities for experience of partial and oscillating connection. Epistemics expressing this posited general multiversal relationality, involves relations enacted knowingly outside of/without universalism and relativism which are epistemics packages precipitated within the modern spacetime cosmology (Verran 2001: 32). Recognising that there are many ways to experience any exhibition, and that eisegesis is both legitimate, and an expression of profound respect both for the art works displayed and the art of the display work, in my idiosyncratic reading of the effects of the constellation of artworks assembled in several rooms of the Bode Museum given over to the *Beyond Compare* exhibition, I offer an auto-ethnographic narrative; a story of experiencing which I propose as ethnographic data. The experiencing has been purposefully contrived as experiencing outside a modern spacetime cosmology which ontologically prescribes particular forms for knower, known and knowledge (Verran 2001: 34). Instead, it is experiential knowing contrived within a cosmology of multiversal relationality.

I made four visits to the exhibition across a year, each visit taking up the better part of a day. Downloading the exhibition app, I devised a means to attend to the items, and experience the displays in ways that, while cognizant of the curator's categories, simultaneously actively sought to evade them. In this way I contrived to develop a sort of multiversal double vision (Verran 2021a). Such contriving is always particular to a situation, and when it comes to application of this experiential methodology, the beauty of museum exhibition spaces is that replications are possible. The story of epistemically experiencing the exhibition, which I present here, can be understood as making particular passage out of apory (aporia) felt as infernal chaotic confusion that only deepened across the year of my visits. I tell my story here insisting that such a contriving of one's own experience of a museum exhibition, is analogue to museum staff setting about explicitly designing ›visitor experience‹. Mobilising a modern spacetime cosmology they contrived comparison between the objects understood as modern objects, lumps of matter with particular attributes and 'qualities, I choose to know otherwise (Verran 2014).

Beginning in Knowing Experiential Aporetics

Institutionally it is difficult to insist that epistemics begins in recognizing difference because it amounts to insisting on beginning in a ›not knowing‹, in the experience of apory. Experientially apory is singular, particular and situated; one always begins off balance, on the back foot.

To experience apory is to recognise that passage, going on, is blocked; we are epistemically disconcerted, suffering negative affect when it comes to epistemics. Knowing experiential aporetics is the name I have coined for the first step towards the knowing otherwise of multiversal relationality. The *aporía* of the Meno in Plato's Socratic dialogue is an epistemic emptiness; at that moment, a knower knows nothing, does not know what to think or say or do next; a paralysis, numbness results. There is no path in sight. But, a different kind of aporia, or apory to simplify the English term, is to recognise that one has lost one's way, and is confused; there are too many paths from which to choose. Different still is apory experienced when one cannot see a path, but acknowledge that others do. Of course, there is also apory in which the path is apparent, but most knowers are not willing to follow it, perhaps because the destination is unknown, perhaps because it is known and unpleasant. Any or all these experiential apories might come into play in knowing experiential aporetics.

The first step in knowing otherwise than through the epistemics package of the modern spacetime cosmology, and in beginning to enact a multiversal relationality, is becoming comfortable with epistemic apory, learning to relax and not panic. In chapter one of *Science and an African Logic*, I tell of such panic, and how narrating the experience of epistemic disconcertment turned out to be a form of therapy (Verran 2001: 23). I contrived this shift in ›doing difference‹ in social sciences many years ago now, and since then I have been developing my skills in this regard, a knowing experiential aporetics lies at the core of a multiversally competent epistemics. This story of participants struggling to do difference together and experiencing apory in the field might help here, in that it offers some terms needed to develop a path together and to muddle a way out of apory (Verran 2008).

The arcane concept of the ontic, what ontology studies, is part and parcel of knowingly working with experiential apory. But note ontic here is quite other than the concept as used by other philosophers. The ontic of multiversal relationality is certainly not the ontic of phenomenologists with their commitments to the universalism of a modern cosmology. One way to introduce the ontic of multiversal relationality is to connect it with the puzzling comments Wittgenstein made about knowing-doing in his very last writings.

> »[…] I meet with someone whom I have not seen for years; I see him clearly but fail to know him. Suddenly I know him, I see the old face in the altered one […] Is this a special sort of seeing? Is it a case of both seeing and thinking? Or an amalgam of the two, as I should like to say? The question is: *why* does one want to say this?« (Wittgenstein 1958 IIxi: 197e).

My answer to Wittgenstein here would be this. »I say this because this ›thinking-seeing‹, or ›knowing-looking‹ points to the actuality of an experiential ontic relationality: I know I know the face before I conceptualise the manifestation as the face of my friend«. Here Wittgenstein is presenting us with a case of a conceptual ontic knowing (Verran 2021b).

In institutional work, attending to epistemics experientially by beginning in apory makes it possible to go on to interfere in ontological happenings, and effect ontological shifts in our concepts as the knowns we work with and through. It is possible to do this knowingly if we suspend our habitual ways of beginning empirical inquiry, and commence instead by cultivating an ethos of respectful, careful epistemic incommensuration in learning to relax in apory. Different ontological entities *can be knowingly happened* in situations as knowns in collective knowledge making and doing, and in this way futures different than pasts can be generated.

Encounters that generate epistemic apory involve many participants – knowers and non-knowers. To engage the epistemic experiencing of multiversal relationality requires two moves of knowing participants in the encounter. First, a decomposing step of *not* knowing as they ordinarily would, as a modern thinker or otherwise. Second, it requires participants to compose what emerges in the encounter (Verran 2018: 25). The first requirement is expression of epistemic bad will, it involves cultivating a feeling of canny attentiveness to one's own habits of knowing. The itch, always present, to propose one's own common-sense must be systematically rejected, so as to think difference. Knowingly exercising epistemic bad will, a knower becomes able to both recognise the demands of their knowledge habits, and to refuse to implement them. In doing this they can acquire a capacity to attend to what emerges in the here and now of the epistemic space opened in the encounter. This is the stage for the practice of the second requirement, enactment of epistemic good faith. This second step expresses epistemic commitment to articulate interpretation within the conditions that constitute the here and now of the encounter itself. Acknowledging that, ontologically speaking, participants emerge self-different than what they were as knowers, while remaining aware of what their back-then-there knowing selves were. When difference is done together, none of the heterogeneous knowing participants becomes the other, yet they do not remain only what they were either. Another such telling of this approach has been composed by colleagues Blaser and de la Cadena (2018: 11) in their helpful explicating of my telling of practices involved in doing this with respect to the encounter of developing an innovative school mathematics curriculum with my Yolngu Aboriginal colleagues in the 1980s and 1990s (Verran 2018).

In beginning expression of epistemic good faith, the re-composing stage, six epistemic questions can provide guidance (Raasch/Lippert 2020). These are questions traditionally asked of epistemics, but of course asking these questions is merely an organising device, the fantasy of answering any one in anything more than a partial and vague way, in actually enacting answers, should not be entertained – wordy discourse is not a valued outcome of this sort of knowledge doing and making.

In any recomposing, axiological and teleological questions are important: asking ›Why and for whom might knowledge, generated in any re-composing, be significant and valuable?‹, and ›What purposes might be served by knowledge generated in recomposing?‹, and perhaps more important ›Whose purposes are these?‹ Answers to methodological and epistemological questions might also need attention. ›How to tell how this knowledge is generated?‹ and ›How to be certain enough it is knowledge?‹ But most significant of all in generating knowledge for futures different than pasts are ontological questions. ›What is known here?‹ and ›How are knowers configured?‹. These are the questions that for the most part have guided my use of this approach, but a younger generation of researchers following this approach is focussing on others. They focus more on questions of whose epistemic purposes and values, and how particular epistemic interests might be pursued (Spencer 2019; Smolka 2020; Smolka/Fisher/Hausstein 2021).

The experience of apory featured in each of my four visits to the *Unvergleichlich. Kunst aus Afrika im Bode-Museum/Beyond Compare. Art from Africa in the Bode-Museum* exhibition. Having surveyed the whole early on, I spent my time in different rooms. I chose specific rooms to train myself in what, following Wittgenstein I name as a particular ›thinking-seeing‹ or ›knowing-looking‹, selecting displays I felt connected to. These became my co-participants in beginning the process of working my way out of the experience of epistemic apory the exhibition wrought with me. What I offer in the next section is a decomposing, a story of finding words to negotiate passage out of uncomfortable experiences that I had in the museum. In this paper I do not offer recomposition on the basis of this carefully assembled experiential story data; interpretation of the unusual experience of this Bode exhibition I strove to contrive, is not part of this paper. That is not my purpose in this article, and in any case, it is not work for me, or any other person to do alone. That, I hope, is the work that collectives will do in making museum futures different than pasts.

A Story of Encounters with Bode's *Beyond Compare* Displays

Like all visitors to the *Beyond Compare* exhibition on each of my four visits, my experience begins with the display situated on its threshold. Along with my critical response to the explicit, wordy curatorial framing, I also recognize the curators know more than they are saying, or perhaps more than they know they know. Having worked with epistemic, in particular ontological, disconcertment for many years, in coming upon this display I feel a vivid delight in the juxtaposition: visual similarities connect – color, size, human body shape and even posture. But these similarities, material-semiotic superficialities in the meaning-making context of art, lie within an overall profound incommensurability. As art, each figure actively repels the other, yet it is difficult to discern where those tense mutually repellent forces arise, let alone discern their form. For me the display generates a moment of wonder: I feel that here indeed I am experiencing something that truly goes beyond compare. This sense of a form of cosmological concertation, a moment of commensuration, arrives reliably with each visit; it disconcerts me. I feel sure that I am not the only looker who experiences delight, and assume the location of this display signals that. This in part leads me to suspect the curators do know how to know differently.

In this moment of wonder, initially I feel keenly a lack of training in reading works of either European or African art. Yet I am emboldened by the systematic training in engaging with cosmology that I received over many years from my Yolngu Aboriginal Australian senior colleagues. From the very first, they generously offered tuition which invariably proceeded through art forms. My reading of and about the work of French philosopher Henri Bergson also heartens me. In Bergson, art is the answer in philosophy not the question; he argues that analytic possibilities arise in extension and expansion of disciplined training by an intuition grounded in that disciplined thinking (Guerlac 2017: 42; Jancsry 2019: 76). But what fortifies me most in this new venture, is that I know I know how to cultivate ontic experience of the exhibition, wordless experiencing, albeit within a particular language world. Long ago I learned from some helpful Nigerian children, bilingual in Yorba and English, that the ontic is not only knowingly habitable, but also that one's navigation within it happens in particular language worlds, albeit wordlessly, and further, that such navigation might be spoken of (Verran 2007). For me the ontic has become but one aspect of the fractalizing interface of multiversal relationality.

All four of my visits to the exhibition leave me uncomfortably disconcerted. My first visit is given over to surveying the exhibition, subsequent visits focus on particular rooms. In visits two and three I focus on the paired displays in rooms 108 and 208 respectively. I choose these in large part because I have travelled to Benin and Ashanti, the areas the African works in those two rooms hail from. Visiting the lively workshops of artists that could still be found there in the late twentieth century, I purchased small tourist art pieces as mementos of my visits. I have never visited Italy or Belgium, the places of origin of the European companion pieces of these African sculptures, here I can only trust I absorbed enough in my school history of art lessons, and in experiencing the gothic in Christian church architecture. On visit four the room of interest is 209, and in this visit I explicitly experiment with the form of my attention, in part in response to feeling I have made no headway in negotiating my way out of the apory the exhibition provokes.

In room 108, the *Beyond Compare* display features two wooden figures, ›dolls‹ is the word that comes to mind; both smallish yet still human baby-sized. One is pinkish, round and invitingly cuddly from fourteenth century Perugia, the other all head and arms with a face that demands attention, from nineteenth century Asante. I am drawn to each through feeling a sense of connection to the women for whom these figures mattered, whom I learn about from the notes provided (Sears 2017). But no moment of commensuration arises between the two as works of art. I come away from the display with a sense of failure and disconcertment. I have no idea how to begin to think these two partially together as art, while respecting their profound difference as expressions of disparate cosmologies. A similar sense of failure is complicated by feelings of disgust and horror as I take my leave of the display in room 208. The display »Portrait Heads« has a sixteenth century bronze memorial head of an Oba of Benin stolen by an unknown British soldier during a brutal collective act of British imperial perfidy; and a wooden, fifteenth century sculpture, a relic or, perhaps, a reliquary, a life-like portrait of the head of the Biblical figure John the Baptist, seemingly still in the act of dying. In the case of the first object, I find it almost impossible to separate the art work from the story of its journey from Benin to Berlin. In the second, the gory sculptural detail of a European type head on a plate seems to exactly capture the horror of the story of the perfidy of Herod and imperial Rome. Again, while recognising that each figure perhaps brilliantly expresses a particular cosmology, no matter that I struggle for a thinking-seeing, or a knowing-looking, I admit failure; the stories get in my way. I know not how to look partially in this situation, no partially commensurable lively forms are see-able by me.

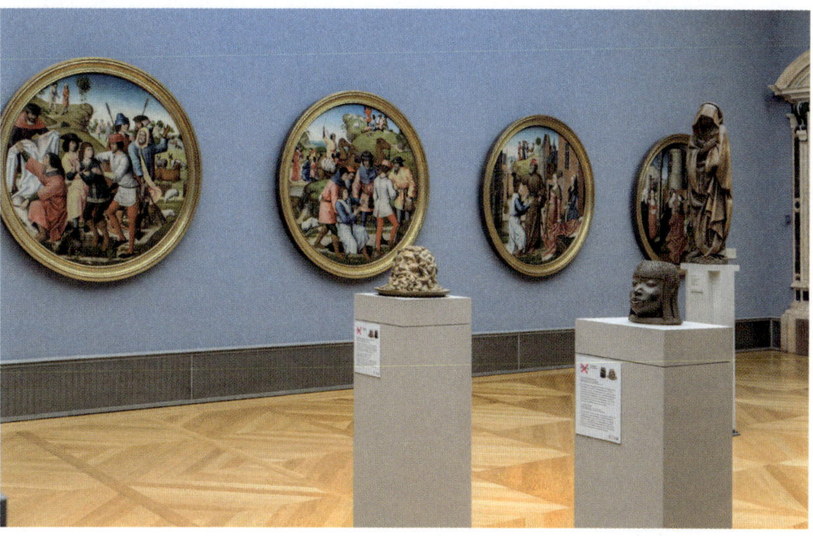

Fig. 4: The stories of John the Baptist and the Oba of Benin dominate. Staatliche Museen zu Berlin–Preußischer Kulturbesitz. Skulpturensammlung und Museum für Byzantinische Kunst. Photo: Wolfgang Gülcker, Berlin.

On my fourth and final visit to the exhibition in August 2019, I find the *Beyond Compare* exhibition displays are being dismantled. Fortunately, the displays on the second floor remain untouched, so the experiment in experiencing I have been planning is still feasible. I am headed for gallery 209, a display space that I know well, having lingered in it on previous visits. There, in the center of the room is a pair of objects that feature in the exhibition's advertising. The Bwiti figure made in the nineteenth century within the Bwiti community of the Kota or Kélé people in the Republic of Congo or in Gabon, one of that pair, seems to be the darling of the exhibition. The companion piece in the display, a reliquary bust of a bishop made in Brussels in 1520, seems to be merely a foil. On previous visits I had observed that visitors often lingered in the room of this display.

My experiment in thinking-seeing is designed so that I might experience the room both in its parts and in its wholeness, and also engage the art objects both in their individuality and in their being items displayed together. As I enter the gallery, I begin by confining my attention to objects in the room's periphery. In addition to the *Beyond Compare* object pair, this gallery is designed to display gothic-era art objects depicting Christian religious iconography. It contains a total of twenty-three art pieces, mostly delicate wood sculptures. As I make my way around the walls, it seems to me that the objects compete, each subject matter proclaiming itself as the most pious, each piece aiming for a realistic expression of Christian religious piety. For the most part, female piety is on display here: St. Ursula arraigned Christ-like on a cross, or protecting supplicants in the folds of her cloak; clusters of women tending the lolling dead body of the Christ; beautiful young European women playing with the baby Christ-figure; clusters of women reading out of books. Male piety is featured in just three displays. In two of these we see men reading off scrolls, and in the third a large figure of archangel Michael is slaying a writhing devil.

After photographing each of these accompanying objects with my phone, I retreat to a far corner, drawing a reprimand from the security guard as I make to lean back against the wall. My aim with this uncharacteristic gallery behavior is to try to experience ›the room‹. In contrast to my previous viewing of the ›resident‹ objects, from this position I want to bring the display of the whole of the room into focus, vague though this must be. Now the *Beyond Compare* pair are in the picture; I am facing the diminutive Bwiti figure. Watching other people enter the room, I see that the Bwiti figure draws a visitor's eye. Placed at the room's center, it changes the room; it conducts and concerts its companion art objects. Forms wrought in many different times and places by unknown knowing-doing human hands, in the ways human hands have in making art, sing in concert.

The dissonance I have previously experienced in the implicit competition for attention (God's?) in the gothic-era Christian objects turns to a calm around the Bwiti figure. It seems quiet and still in comparison to those around it. A tenderness emanates from its smooth bronze colored metallic surface. Shifting my gallery-gaze to include the reliquary bishop, the pair present a simultaneously both *›yon‹*, beyond each other, and yet *›par‹*, each other's equal. I muse that perhaps *this seeing* is specifically what the exhibition title refers to; what it indexes. Then, focusing solely on the bishop, the bust suddenly seems tawdry; the banality of its mimetic, realistic representation of some actual bishop, has me almost laughing out loud, but I am aware of the rather aged, hovering guard keeping me squarely in his sights.

My experiment in knowing-looking over, I retreat to the bookshop and a cup of tea. As I browse through the exhibition catalogue, I feel the inevitable sadness of goodbyes. These objects, many no doubt stolen from the African places in which they first came to life, or at very least exchanged in conditions where power was distributed very unevenly, will not be in this museum space next time I visit – coming to life, calling out or not, to the objects that surround them. I cheer myself with the thought that at least some of the art works might in the next few years, make their way back to their places of origin.

Museums Cultivating a New Epistemic Demeanour

My reading of the displays of the *Beyond Compare* exhibition refused to begin by assuming all objects in the displays *necessarily are* objects in the common sense of the modern

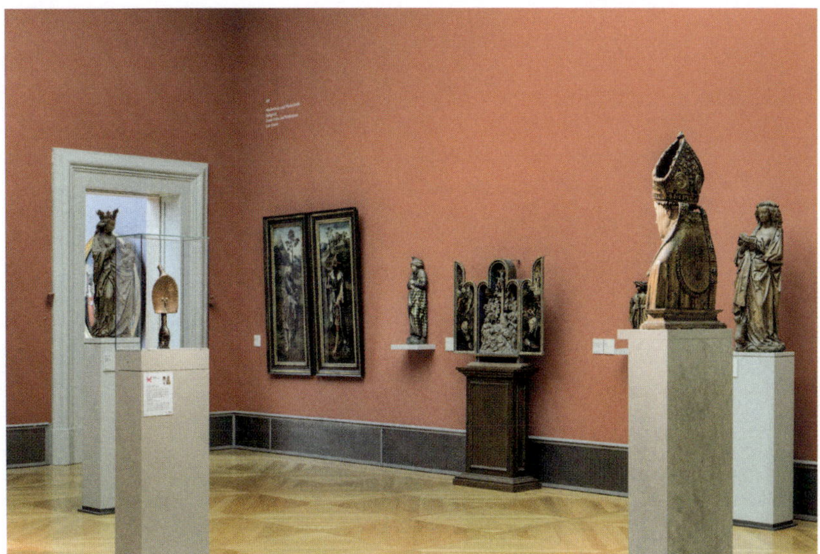

Fig. 5: The diminutive Bwiti Figure lights up the room. Staatliche Museen zu Berlin–Preußischer Kulturbesitz. Skulpturensammlung und Museum für Byzantinische Kunst. Photo: Wolfgang Gülcker, Berlin.

spacetime cosmology. I refused to focus on the entities I met as ›real lumps of matter set in spacetime‹ expressing various cultural and social qualities by which the objects might be compared and contrasted. I chose instead to cultivate experiential apory, to experience epistemic emptiness when confronted with the manifestations that were museum displays. I mobilised an alternative epistemic demeanour as I faced the challenge of engaging these manifestations in unknowing, attempting to offer opportunity for the manifestations themselves to announce their own terms. And indeed, that is what happened. I found I could learn how to look knowingly so that terms of manifestation of the entities in *that singular situation*, could be read, and the displays known in a non-modern way. As I learned to do this in passing my days amongst the displays, I discerned signs that the curators who had designed this exhibition had indeed already learned to engage with the artworks in the ways I was laboriously contriving. This of course, is not a surprising finding to arise from my experiment.

I propose the cosmology of my reading as a *translating* cosmology. I do NOT propose my reading, afforded as it is within a radically minimalist, partial modern cosmology, as a substantive cosmology. It is salient to epistemics, only albeit a politically inflected epistemics. Importantly, ontologically speaking it is utterly promiscuous; it can connect to any and all other readings which, in their manifold differences are necessarily cosmological. This translating cosmology, better proposed as an experiential methodology, proposes only a partial, limited and ephemeral commensurability which can nevertheless be reliably experienced. Such ontic experience reading artworks as icons fraught with difference, is enough to become a solid basis for politico-epistemic negotiation. Its explicit acknowledgement is crucial in allowing curatorial analyses and interpretations that begin in an incommensuration that opens up, rather than a posited commensuration that seals off.

Literature

ABRAMSON, Allen/HOLBRAAD, Martin (2014): »Introduction: The Cosmological Frame in Anthropology«. In: *Framing Cosmologies: The Anthropology of Worlds,* ed. by id., Manchester: Manchester University Press, 1–28.

BACKER, Malcolm (1996): »Bode and Museum Display: The Arrangement of the Kaiser-Friedrich-Museum and the South Kensington Response«. In: *Jahrbuch der Berliner Museen* Vol. 38, Beiheft: *›Kennerschaft‹. Kolloquium zum 150sten Geburtstag von Wilhelm von Bode,* 143–153.

BARAD, Karen (2007): *Meeting the Universe Halfway: Quantum Physics and the Entanglement of Matter and Meaning,* Durham: Duke University Press.

BLASER, Mario/DE LA CADENA, Marisol (2018): »Pluriverse. Proposal for a World of Many Worlds«. In: *A World of Many Worlds,* ed. by id., Durham: Duke University Press, 1–28.

CHRISTIE, Michael/VERRAN, Helen, (2013): »Digital Lives in Postcolonial Aboriginal Australia«, *Journal of Material Culture* 18, 299–317.

CHAPUIS, Julien/FINE, Jonathan/IVANOV, Paola (Eds.) (2017): *Beyond Compare: Art from Africa in the Bode Museum,* Berlin: Staatliche Museen zu Berlin.

EISLER, Colin (1996): »Bode's Burden. Berlin's Museum as an Imperial Institution«. In: *Jahrbuch der Berliner Museen,* Vol. 38, Beiheft: *›Kennerschaft‹. Kolloquium zum 150sten Geburtstag von Wilhelm von Bode,* 23–32.

FOCILLON, Henri (1992): *The Life of Forms in Art,* trans. by Charles B. Hogan/George Kubler, New York: Zone Books.

GUERLAC, Suzanne (2017): *Thinking in Time: An Introduction to Henri Bergson,* Ithaca: Cornell University Press.

JANCSRY, Jonathan (2019): »The Future as an Undefined and Open Time: A Bergsonian Approach«. In: *Axiomathes* 29, 61–80.

MACGREGOR, Neil (2006): »A Cache of Civilisations«. In: *Financial Times Magazine* 36, 36–37.

MAPLES, Amanda (2020): »African Restitution in a North American Context: A Debate, A Summary, and A Challenge«. In: *African Arts* 53: 4, 10–15.

RAASCH, Josefine/LIPPERT, Ingmar (2020): »Pioneers in Ontology in Science and Technology Studies: Helen Verran«. In: *Sage Research Methods Foundations,* doi.org/9781529750478 (30.06.21).

SEARS, Andrew (2017): »Representation and Embodiment«. In: *Beyond Compare: Art from Africa in the Bode Museum,* ed. by Julien Chapuis/Jonathan Fine/Paola Ivanov, Berlin: Staatliche Museen zu Berlin, 156–159.

SMOLKA, Marieke (2020): »Generative Critique in Interdisciplinary Collaborations: From Critique in and of the Neurosciences to Socio-Technical Integration Research as a Practice of Critique in R(R)I«. In: *Nanoethics* 14, 1–19.

SMOLKA, Marieke/FISHER, Erik/ HAUSSTEIN, Alexandra (2021): »From Affect to Action: Choices in Attending to Disconcertment in Interdisciplinary Collaborations«. In: *Science, Technology, & Human Values,* https://doi.org/10.1177/0162243920974088 (30.06.21).

SPENCER, Michaela (2019): »State-funded Services Delivery as Cosmopolitical Work. Opportunities for Postdevelopment in Practice in Northern Australia? «. In: *Postdevelopment in Practice,* ed. by Elise Klein/Carlos Morreo, London: Routledge, 203–216.

Uzoigwe, Godfrey N. (1984): »Reflections on the Berlin West Africa Conference, 1884–1885«. In: *Journal of the Historical Society of Nigeria* 12: 3&4, 9–22.

Verran, Helen (2001): *Science and an African Logic*, Chicago: University of Chicago Press.

Verran, Helen (2007): »Metaphysics and Learning«. In: *Journal of Learning Inquiry* 1, 31–39.

Verran, Helen (2008): »Science and the Dreaming«. In: Issues Magazine 82, http://www.issuesmagazine.com.au/article/issue-march-2008/science-and-dreaming.html (30.06.21).

Verran, Helen (2014): »Working with Those Who Think Otherwise«. In: *Common Knowledge*, 20: 3, 527–539.

Verran, Helen (2018): »Politics of Working Cosmologies Together While Keeping Them Separate«. In: *A World of Many Worlds*, ed. by Marisol de la Cadena/Mario Blaser, Duke University Press, 112–130.

Verran, Helen (2021a): »Writing an Ethnographic Story in Working toward Responsibly Unearthing Ontological Troubles«. In: *Experimenting with Ethnography: A Companion to Analysis*, ed. by Andrea Ballestero/Brit Ross Winthereik, Duke University Press, 235–244.

Verran, Helen (2021b): »Ontics«. In: Technologies in Practice (TiP) Lexicon, ed. by James Maguire/Brit Ross Winthereik, https://tip.itu.dk/category/tip-lexicon/ (30.06.21).

Verran, Helen (in preparation): »Knowing Ontological Happening. Towards a Decolonial Ethnographic Museum«. Submitted.

Wiredu, Kwasi (1996): *Cultural Universals and Particulars. An African Perspective*, Bloomington: Indiana University Press.

Wittgenstein, Ludwig (1958): *Philosophical Investigations*, trans. by Gertrude E.M. Anscombe, Oxford: Basil Blackwell.

Table of figures

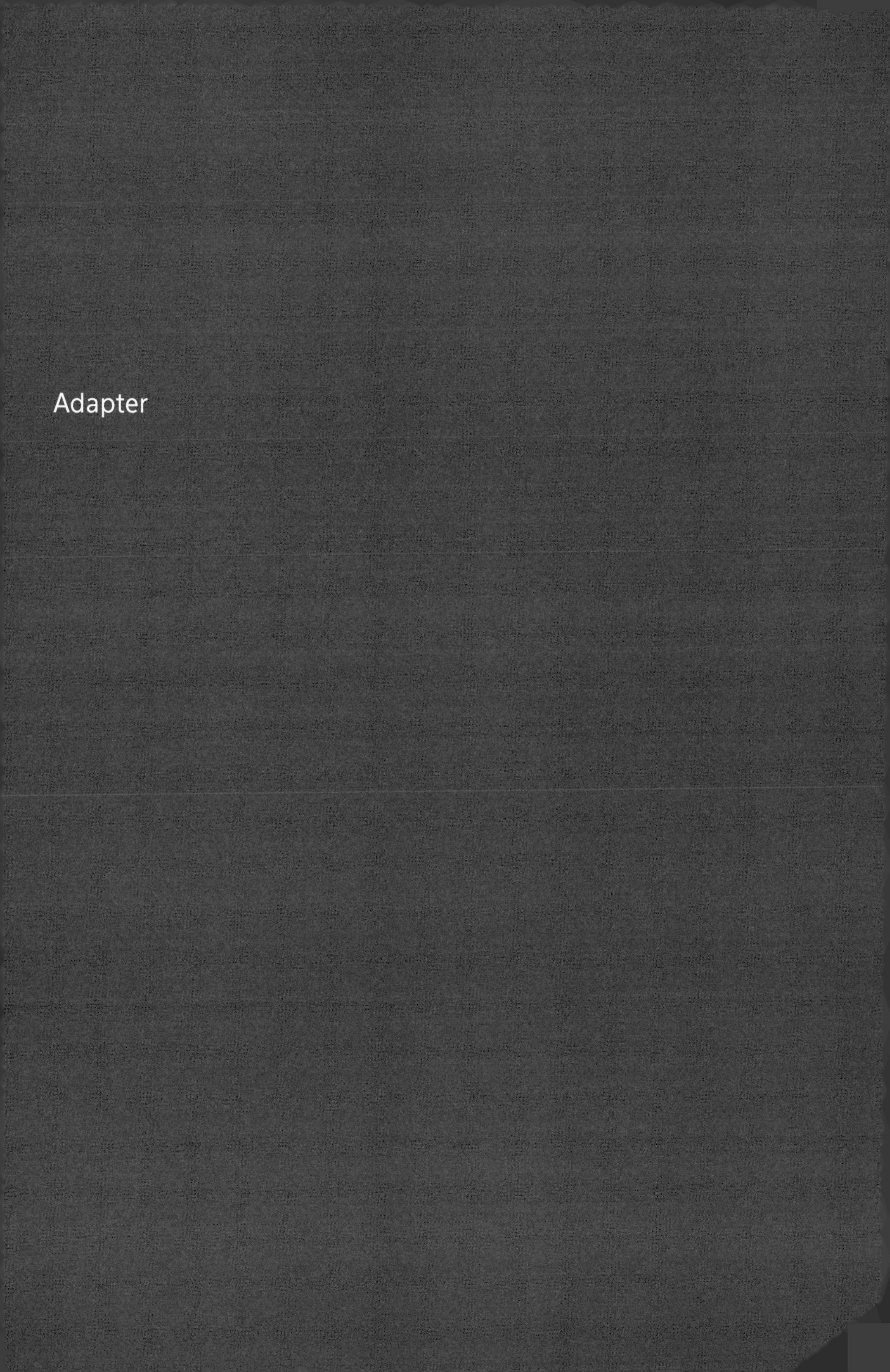
Adapter

Evidence and Fiction: An Untimely Alliance with the Photography Archive of Margot Dias and Jorge Dias

Catarina Simão

The work of the Portuguese ethnologist António Jorge Dias (Porto, 31 July 1907 – Lisbon, 1973) and his wife and collaborator Margot Dias (Nuremberg, 4 June 1908 – Oeiras, 2003), a German national, important also for its sheer volume, produced a very abundant quantity of archival materials. Nevertheless, Portuguese anthropology's history has assessed the work of Jorge Dias essentially on the basis of his intellectual and ideological output.[1] In this particular framework, Dias' work marks the paradigm shift within the Portuguese anthropology from the dominance of anthropobiology towards a particular branch of culturalism. His influence emerged at the end of the first half of the 20th century, in the last period of the Portuguese colonial era. Margot Dias, a professional pianist who moved her focus to ethnography and ethnomusicology, mainly worked as part of Jorge Dias' expedition team, in particular the expeditions to Mozambique and Angola, where she pioneered using film and sound recordings. After the death of her husband, she carried on as guardian of his legacy and devoted herself to continuing the work she had begun with him. Although the publication of her film records on DVD has recently highlighted her contribution to Portuguese visual anthropology,[2] their fieldwork has been little studied and explored. Their documentation consists of various media (journals, photography, film, and sound recordings) and can mainly be found in Portugal at the National Museum of Ethnology in Lisbon, an institution to which Jorge Dias contributed during its foundation in 1965 (at the time it was called the Overseas Ethnology Museum). In some cases, these materials are centralised and meticulously organised, while in other instances they are scattered or have shortcomings in terms of access and organisation.

1 Jorge Dias had a degree in Germanic Philology from the University of Coimbra. He did his lectureship between 1938 and 1947 at the universities of Rostock, Munich, Berlin, Santiago de Compostela, and Madrid. From his experience at German universities he absorbed and developed the anthropological disciplines that resulted, in March 1944, in his doctorate at the University of Munich in the area of philosophy, as well as *Volkskunde*.

2 The ethnographic films of Margot Dias have been edited on DVD in a co-edition of the Cinemateca Portuguesa-Museu do Cinema/National Museum of Ethnology of Lisbon (Costa/Da Costa 2016).

urn:nbn:de:hbz:6:3-zfk-2021-42015

This visual essay will focus on a selected group of images, which originated from an anthropological mission to the Makondes between 1957 and 1961 that Jorge Dias headed. This mission happened within the scope of the Mission of Portuguese Overseas Ethnic Minority Studies (Missão de Estudos das Minorias Étnicas do Ultramar Português) as an activity of the Overseas Research Council (Junta de Investigações do Ultramar). Directly subordinated to the Ministry of the Colonies/Overseas, the entity's main function was to coordinate the scientific studies, that were to be undertaken in colonial territories under Portuguese rule. Beyond the objectives proper to applied anthropology, the creation of those missions was linked to the attempt to diagnose and correct potential threats to Portuguese sovereignty coming from local movements in those territories, but also from those coming from neighbouring countries. In this respect, special attention was given to the study of the Makondes in the region of the Mueda plateau, because it is situated close to the Tanzanian border, on the territory of modern-day Cabo Delgado Province in the North of Mozambique.

This essay not only focuses on the Dias' photographic collection, but also regards it as an original creative act, thus permitting an intentional distancing from its subsequent disciplinary and scientific uses. The metaphorical choice of words for the title emphasises this same intention: to allow the research to go in and out of the central object, like in a dialogue with a living, complex, and incomplete figure. In my artistic research,[3] this translates into using an intertextuality between historical periods and disciplinary fields, while also approaching and relating diverse documents, be they objects, photographs, film or architecture. Beyond the concrete work that underlies the research – like searching for ›lost‹ parts of collections, reconstituting never-published books, and telling invisible micro-histories – I intend to displace the archive's nature out of its pretended neutrality in representation, in order to allow thinking the photographic inventory medium retroactively anew as a fostering technology for concepts such as ›authenticity‹ and ›coloniality‹.

3 It was only possible to work with these documents thanks to the availability and courtesy of the following people and entities (in the order in which they appear in the essay): João Pedro George, from the National Museum of Ethnology in Lisbon, Harry G. West, Ruy Guerra, Bernhard Guttsche, and Grassi Museum für Völkerkunde zu Leipzig.

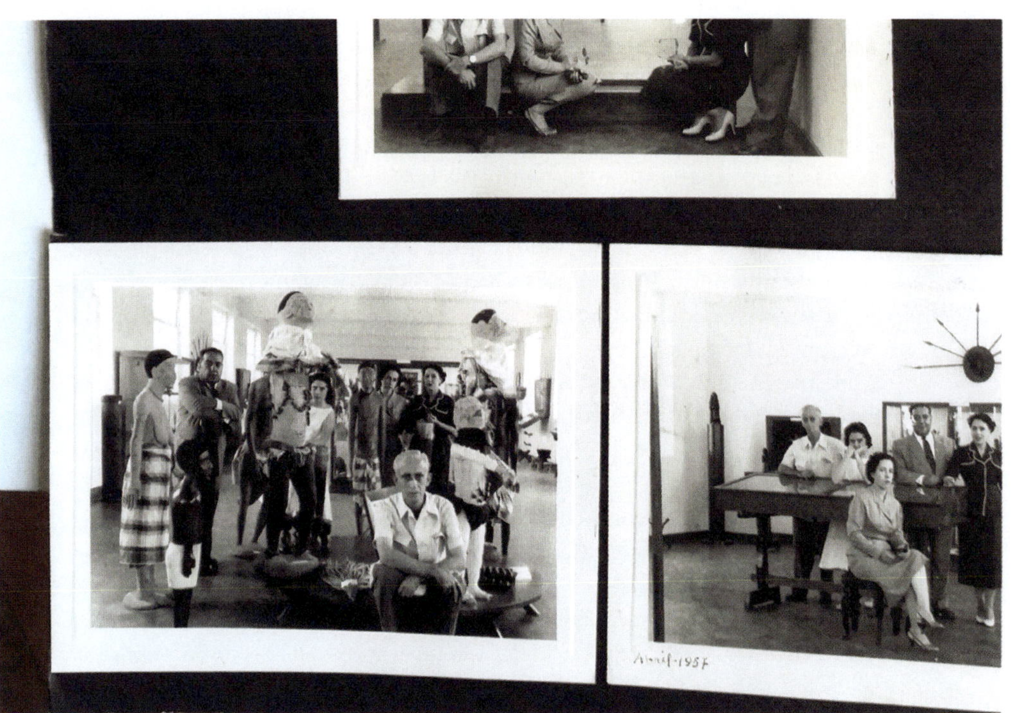

Fig. 1: NAMPULA

Fig. 1: *Inauguration of the Regional Museum of Nampula, Mozambique, 1956; black and white photograph, 10×7cm. Family album. Private Archive, Avellar George / Adelino Pereira Soares de Castro, Lisbon. Courtesy J.P.G.*

Central exhibition; a Makonde collection was part of the first set of objects incorporated into the Nampula Museum collection. Manuel de Avellar George and Adelino Pereira Soares de Castro (photo) were two of the main names associated with the Museum from the time it was created in 1956 until at least 1962.

In March 2018, I visited the National Museum of Ethnology in the city of Nampula, in northern Mozambique, and met the current director Mr. Kulyumba and his team. At the time, I showed them on my mobile phone a series of five black and white pictures. The team managing the Museum was not familiar with these photographs, despite having been taken sixty years ago at exactly the same place where we met. In one of the photographs, I helped identify the first two curators of the museum when it was inaugurated in 1956 under the name Commander Eugénio Ferreira de Almeida Regional Museum. In the image, the two curators were photographed with their families, standing in curious poses, camouflaged among sets of life-size wooden human figures that displayed ›ethnic scarification‹, *Mapiko* masks mounted on mannequins (or sculptures?), and other artefacts associated with initiation rites. At my request, one of the museum staff went and brought similar items from different sites in the building, until he had finally gathered a small set of objects that he recognised in the photograph, setting them out before me so that I could photograph them. This staff member thereby carried out the sequence of procedures that a photograph in a museum generates by acting as an index of the object. We are familiar with the fact that photographs are used in a museum to reference and catalogue its collection. However, this access system, which organises and reports documents in relation to each other, does not seem to exist in the same manner throughout the world. From the early years of its activities, citing a lack of resources, the Nampula Museum was gradually abandoned and finally closed. With the decolonisation process (1974–75), a part of the collection was taken by the colonisers, who returned *en masse* to Portugal with whatever they could carry in their baggage[4] (see Vicente/George 2021). I was not wrong in presupposing that these photographic documents would not be recognised by the current staff of the Nampula Museum. I quickly accepted the idea that the broken link between the Museum and its archive was the result of the violent rupture between Portugal and its colonial space.

From another angle, it may in fact be easier to disown an object when it cannot assume the appearance of a memory, for the lack of evidence of its representation, omission of traces of its material and symbolic permanence. Further research led me to consider a new stigmatizing factor that, associated with the nature of the historic disturbance, would contribute to portraying the Museum of Nampula as a ghost museum.

4 Scholars have recreated the history of the documentation of the Nampula Museum (a mix of family and museum archives) and the way it arrived intact in Lisbon a few years before Mozambique's independence.

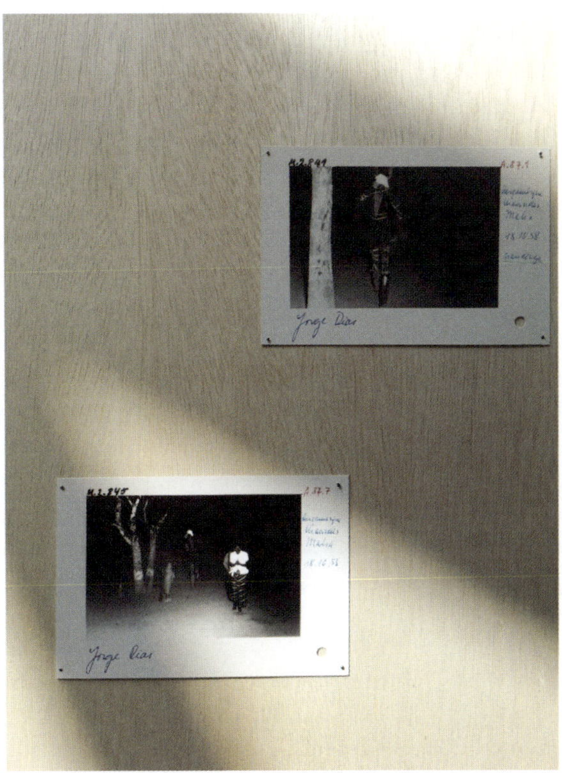

Fig. 2: JOHANNESBURG

Fig. 2: *Photo:* Ethnographically Intimate *Exhibition (partial). Witswatersrand University Museum of Anthropology, 10 & 11 May 2019, Johannesburg. Foto: Catarina Simão.*

In May 2019, I collaborated with the Witswatersrand University Museum of Anthropology, where, along with the academic Caio Simões Araújo and the Museum director George Mahashe, I co-organised a workshop entitled *Critical Entanglements: Colonialism, Anthropology and the Visual Arts.*[5] This workshop focused on the year 1959 in order to reflect on the museum's and university's pedagogical and political framework. In that year, the Portuguese ethnologist Jorge Dias was invited to present a series of lectures, while his anthropological study on the Makondes in northern Mozambique was still in progress. At the same time, the political struggles for independence in Congo and Tanganyika were having a stronger impact on the northern region of Mozambique. The prospect of major political change was a constant concern for the team of ethnologists on this mission. Proto-nationalist movements were organised in exile or clandestinely within the country. The Portuguese Secret Information Service intensified arrests and recruited informants in the villages among the Makonde population, especially along the border with Tanganyika. In 1959, Professor Jorge Dias received an invitation from the Department of Portuguese Studies at Wits University, which was funded by Ernest Oppenheimer, the renowned South African magnate involved in the diamond trade. The six public lectures were entitled *Portuguese Contribution to Cultural Anthropology*, and his lecture *The Makonde People of Portuguese East Africa* was an especially noteworthy part of the series. In 1961, these lectures resulted in a publication by the University, in which the chapters were organised according to the themes examined in each lecture. This alignment clearly reflected the series of concerns set out by Jorge Dias (1961a) in that context.[6] On the one hand, the exceptional nature of the Portuguese case in the history of Africa and the process of African colonisation and, on the other hand, the advances made in anthropological studies of the Makondes in colonial northern Mozambique and in the province of Cabo Delgado.

Monograph

As part of Jorge Dias' anthropological mission, a four-volume monograph (Dias 1964; Dias/Dias 1964; Dias/Dias 1970; Guerreiro 1966), entitled *Os Macondes de Moçambique* (1964–1970), was published and had an enormous impact as it circulated the results of their anthropological study on the social and cultural life of the Makonde. However,

5 The workshop *Critical Entanglements: Colonialism, Anthropology and the Visual Arts* and the exhibition *Ethnographically Intimate* were organised jointly with Dr. Caio Simões Araújo, a postdoc researcher at CISA, and the director of the Museum of Anthropology, George Mahashe, the South African artist and academic. The events were held on 10–11 May 2019, at the Wits University Museum of Anthropology.

6 Jorge Dias (1961a): *Portuguese Contribution to Cultural Anthropology*. Contents: 1) A Historic Introduction to Portuguese Anthropology; 2) The Makonde People: History, Environment and Economy; 3) The Makonde People: Social Life; 4) Portugal: Land and People; 5) Community Studies in Portugal; 6) The Portuguese Abroad.

there was no indication of the disruptive effect of the Portuguese colonial occupation. In contrast, the problems and tensions among the Makonde population were described in Jorge Dias' Mission Reports from 1957, 1958, and 1959. These reports were prepared at the request of the Ministry for Overseas Affairs and remained entirely confidential for many years. Being smuggled to Mozambique through networks sympathetic to the anticolonial movements[7] – and thus inaccessible to Portuguese researchers – these reports already informed the political elite and the first generation of post-independence Mozambican historians, contributing (somewhat ironically) to a reversal of the constraints of the colonial legacy.

Ethnographically Intimate, 2019

Alongside the workshop at the Wits Museum a selection of representative documentations, produced by Jorge Dias' mission to Mozambique, were displayed in the atrium of the workroom. It was arranged in a way that the audience could critically approach the visual and materials that described the presence of the anthropological team among the Makonde. This installation was insightfully called *Ethnographically Intimate*. I contributed to the exhibit with a piece made from reproductions of photograph file cards that I obtained from the National Museum of Ethnology in Lisbon (MNEL). I selected a series of file cards from the complete collection of photographs that were taken by Dias' team during the expedition to northern Mozambique. The photographic collection was organised in one of the museum's filling cabinets in the year of the team's expedition to Mozambique (1957–1959 and 1961).[8] Of a total of 25 selected cards, I identified three specific sets for the exhibition *Ethnographically Intimate*:

(1) Micro-sequences: This set consisted of small reports prepared in Makonde villages using successive records to accompany the unfolding of a given ritual. The selection included Makonde initiation rites. The reason given in the monograph for omitting glaring aspects of change in favour of a timeless and traditional description of the Makonde people also ended up orienting the selection of ethnographic photographs toward static choices with singular descriptions. In contrast to the criterion used for the monograph, I was interested in the photographs that could not avoid the risk of a direct comparison with reality. Here, I appreciated the virtues of amateurism while taking the photographs, which inadvertently captured members of the Portuguese administration and the Western bodies and clothes of the ethnologists themselves, within the context of scenes of ›anthropological interest‹. These photographs were considered ›unsuitable‹, because they represented subjectivity, sensuality, fascination, fear, and intimacy.

7 Although it is difficult to determine a precise date, according to Professor Yussuf Adam (UEM) the confidential reports Jorge Dias prepared appeared at the Centre for African Studies and the Mozambique Institute for Scientific Research through Aquino de Bragança.

8 The 4th year of the mission only continued in 1961. The Ministry for Overseas Affairs did not authorise the 1960 campaign, for fear of the political turmoil that ended up in the incident that became known as the *Mueda Massacre*, which took place in the town of Mueda, on 16 June 1960.

(2) Micro-occurrences: I used the term *micro-occurrences* to describe clues that were not evident at first glance but which emerged due to the regular and methodical organisation of the files. The captions themselves, along with succinct comments, favour an objective appreciation of the images, while the gestures captured therein are clearly of another nature.

(3) Micro-absences: This photograph stands out from the set presumably because it shows a space that is not associated with the environment of the villages. This is a photograph that depicts the interior of the residence of the Portuguese Administrator of Mozambique Island and focuses on the ebony wood figure of a ›Makondised‹ saint that was on exhibition. The natural correlation established by this photograph is with the monograph volume that was never published – and which became known as *the 5th volume*. This was initially envisaged by Jorge Dias and Margot Dias to examine exclusively the theme of the Makonde wood sculpture. The task of compiling documentation continued, since Margot Dias paid constant attention to this theme (as is evident in several of her published articles), but the 5th book of the monograph was never concluded. Very little is known about what happened in 1973 after Jorge Dias died and Margot Dias continued trying to resolve the challenges that this volume raised for her and for the collaborators, she invited to assist her. I began my presentation during the workshop with this photograph to mark the shift of my research away from the disciplinary history associated with this archive.

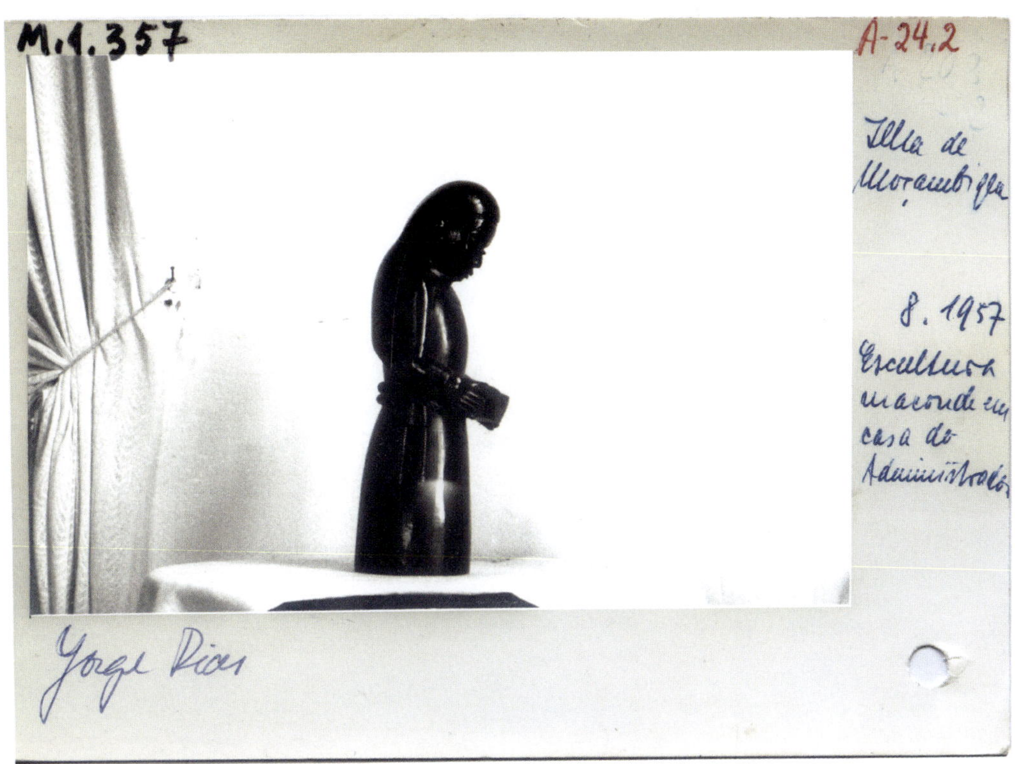
M.1.357
A-24.2
Ilha de Moçambique
8.1957
Escultura maconde em casa do Administrador
Jorge Dias

Fig. 3: *Photograph card: Mozambique Island; 8.1957. Makonde sculpture at the administrator's residence. Jorge Dias. (14.7×10.6cm). Photograph collection, Jorge Dias/Margot Dias archives. National Museum of Ethnology in Lisbon.*

»Makond-ised« saint in a hall at the residence of the Portuguese Administrator of Mozambique Island, 1957.

The photograph card shows a wooden female figure captioned »Makonde sculpture«. While, on the one hand, it reflects the private space of a residence (with European curtains), it also shows a totally different type of intimate aspect: the intimacy between the team of anthropologists and the Portuguese colonial administration. Close ties with the administration were essential to be able to carry out fieldwork. Not only was this collaboration unavoidable, but it was also necessary for the logistics of anthropological expeditions, such as hiring a team of local assistants (drivers, interpreters, etc.), organising accommodation, vehicles, and other activities. In his (unpublished) Mission Reports, Jorge Dias criticised the brutal and uncultured way the Portuguese administration treated the indigenous population. Jorge Dias' criticism was fuelled by a genuine belief in the theory of the exceptional nature of Portuguese »Lusotropicalism« in Africa, capable of promoting a harmonious fusion of allegedly »superior/inferior« cultures, as long as the »stronger group« is able to skilfully conduct »its assimilationist action« (Dias 1961b). In her field work notebook, Margot Dias showed herself to be more emotional than her husband and did not hide her irritation with the fact that European cultural practices tended to distort the population's ›traditional culture‹. The commissioning of ebony sculptures, such as the one in the photograph, was part of the instrumentalization of the population by the Catholic religion.

grafia ou uma passagem e diziam-me "Era assim, compreende?".

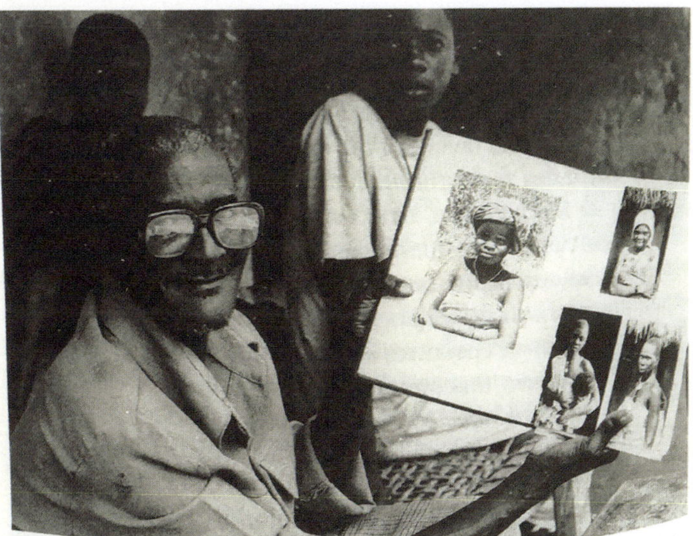

"Rafael Mwakala segurando *Os Macondes de Moçambique*, aberto numa página em que figura uma fotografia de sua mulher e criança (página do lado direito, imagem no canto esquerdo inferior da página)"
Foto: Museu Nacional de Etnologia

Com ... ciar cada vez

Fig. 4: *Image reproduced in a book: Rafael Mwakala holding Os Macondes de Moçambique, open at a page with a photograph of his wife and child (right hand page, image at the lower left corner of the page). Photo: National Museum of Ethnology in Lisbon. (West 2006: 150)*
Courtesy Harry G. West.

Rafael Mwakala in 1991, showing the monograph by Jorge and Margot Dias. Harry G. West. Photo taken from his 2004 article »Inverting the Camel's Hump: Jorge Dias, His Wife, Their Interpreter, and I« In Significant Others: Interpersonal and Professional Commitments in Anthropology. (ed.) R. Handler. Madison: The University of Wisconsin Press. – here in the Portuguese version of 2006.

Between 1991 and 2005, the anthropologist Harry G. West carried out anthropological research on the effects of colonialism, war, and social reconstruction in the same district as Jorge Dias studied the Makonde in the late 50s. In an article published in 2004, West analysed Jorge Dias as the anthropologist who had preceded him by studying the same region of northern Mozambique on the eve of the Mozambique liberation war (1964–1974). The article described his meeting with Rafael Mwakala, the interpreter who accompanied Jorge Dias (he was his favourite interpreter) during an expedition he headed 30 years before. According to Mwakala, he was recruited expressly by Jorge Dias – who had not been satisfied with the level of his other interpreters' Portuguese – at the Catholic mission where he lived, a few kilometres from the town of Mueda. In the photo, Mwakala can be seen smiling, holding the monograph *Os Macondes de Moçambique*, open at the page where his wife and baby appeared as objects of study in the book. Mwakala himself could not be included as an object in this monograph. He did not count as one of the ›traditional‹ Makonde. From the perspective of Dias' team, he had been changed by the school and by the church, and he did not have the traditional physical markings on his body, the »scarification that would have identified him with his ethnic group«. However, they valued his intelligence and his proficient Portuguese and in Dias' eyes, this made it possible for him to successfully carry out all tasks, which involved translating from the Shimakonde language to Portuguese, and vice versa. This fact was greatly appreciated by the team, since they did not speak any of the local languages. However, this was not the reason for the criticism that West voiced in his article.

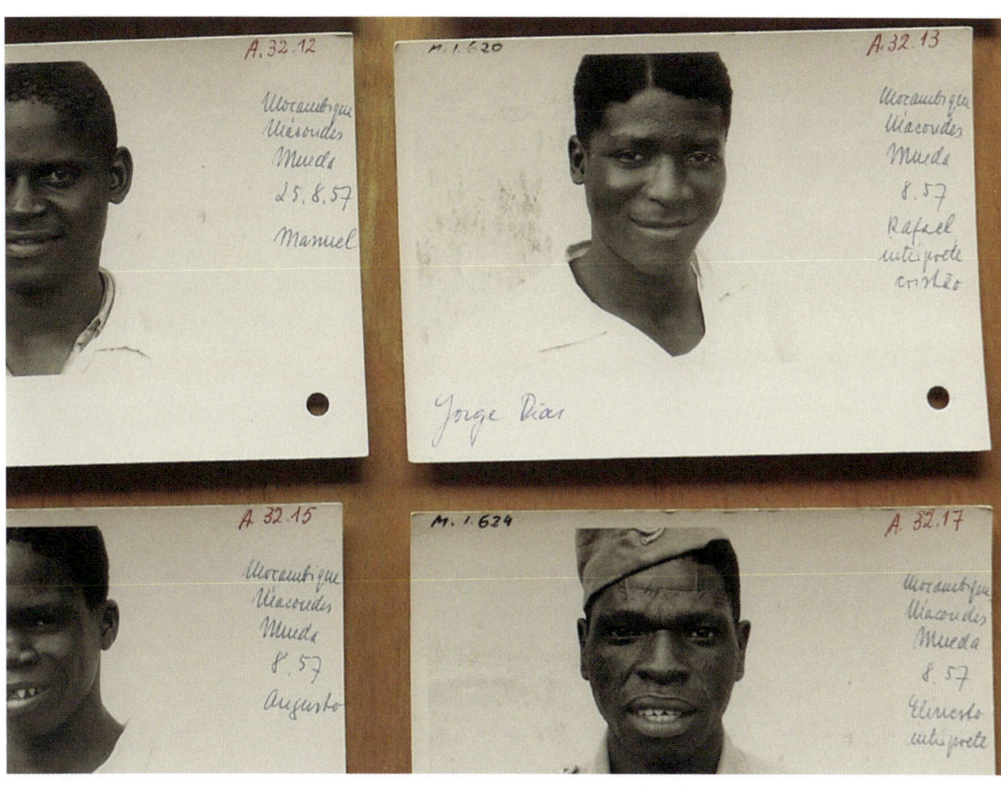
A.32.12
Mueda
25.8.57
Manuel
M.1.620
A.32.13
Mueda
8.57
Rafael
Jorge Dias
A.32.15
Mueda
8.57
Augusto
M.1.624
A.32.17
Mueda
8.57

Fig. 5: *4 photograph cards. Upper right corner: Mozambique, Makondes, Mueda. 8.57. Rafael, Christian interpreter. Jorge Dias. (14.7×10.6cm). Photograph collection, Jorge Dias/Margot Dias archives. National Museum of Ethnology in Lisbon.*

----

4 photograph cards. Upper right corner: Rafael Mwakala shown in 1957, as a member of the »staff«.

The meeting between Rafael Mwakala and Harry West enabled the latter to ascertain the anthropologists' impact on the Makonde community that they were visiting. He argues that, while the images printed in the monograph were proof of their ›traditional‹ and unchanged culture, their impact created a confused suspension of memory, affecting their identity. One of the revelations made by Mwakala West talks about, is about his own life at the time of the expedition. Rafael had been secretly involved in a proto-nationalist movement (MANU). From 1963 onward, he was even one of the first recruits to be sent to Algeria for military training by the newly-formed FRELIMO,[9] which was created by merging three smaller movements (one of which was the MANU). West emphasises, that this radical aspect of Rafael's life history is particularly useful to demonstrate what Dias and his colleagues were unable to envisage or at least failed to describe in their ethnographic work on the life of the Makonde people.

9 FRELIMO stands for Mozambique Liberation Front and was created in 1962 in Dar es Salaam as the result of the merger of the three main anti-colonial movements that since ever since the 1950s had been organizing acts of resistance against the presence of the Portuguese in Mozambique.

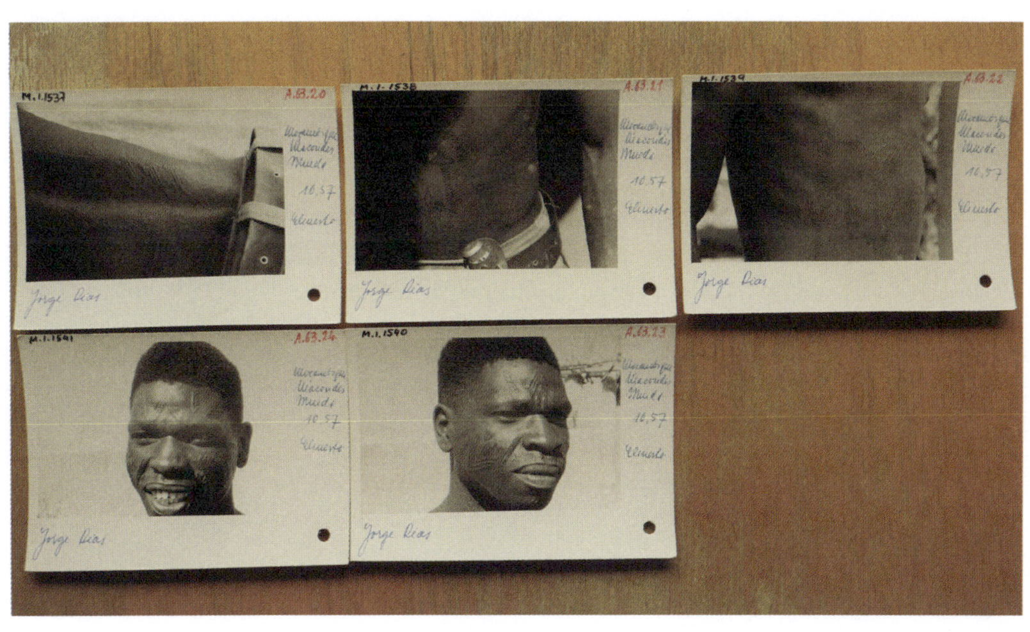
M.I.1537
A.63.20
10.57
Jorge Dias
M.I.1538
A.63.21
10.57
Jorge Dias
M.I.1539
A.63.22
10.57
Jorge Dias
M.I.1541
A.63.24
10.57
Jorge Dias
M.I.1540
A.63.23
10.57
Jorge Dias

Fig. 6: *5 photograph cards: Mozambique, Makondes, Mueda. 10.57. Elinesto Jorge Dias. (14.7×10.6cm). Photograph collection, Jorge Dias/Margot Dias archives. National Museum of Ethnology in Lisbon.*

----

5 photograph cards: Details of »Elinesto's« body in 1957; scarification on the lower back, the abdomen and face; dental mutilation.

In this set of photographs, Elinesto reveals his skin (shown without sepoy uniform) to show five specific parts of his body. Unlike in the case of Rafael Mwakala, the tattooed body of Sepoy Elinesto qualified him to be a ›traditional‹ subject. Photographs of Elinesto appear in volume I of the monograph *Os Macondes de Moçambique – Aspectos históricos e económicos* (54) and in volume II, *Cultura Material* (14). The overlapping of Elinesto's different functions – object of study, interpreter, and simultaneously a sepoy – sheds light on a certain procedure that originated in the colonial Portuguese administration. The administrator would choose from among the more qualified and ›trustworthy‹ individuals who worked for the local administration, indicating those who could serve as assistants for the anthropological team's work. This group of local assistants would take the anthropologists to situations in villages in the region that were of interest to their studies. Generally, these villages corresponded to their own communities. Thus, the set of interpreters chosen by the Portuguese administration would end up determining the circuit of villages and the situations of interest recorded by the scientific team. The team of anthropologists could have been aware, or not, of the functional importance of the indigenous informers' role as interface in their ethnographic work. However, the interpretation that this ›interface‹ had for the community of the villages was obvious. The community knew the psychological profile of the Makonde people working for the ›whites‹, who were forced to defend the interests of the colonizers and reject their own.

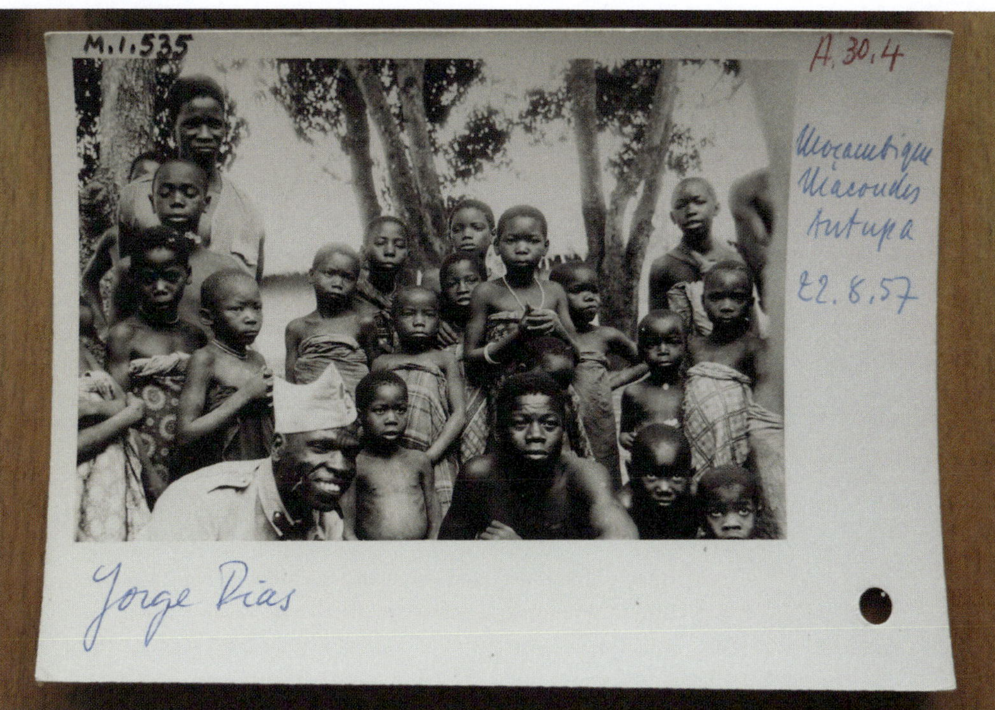

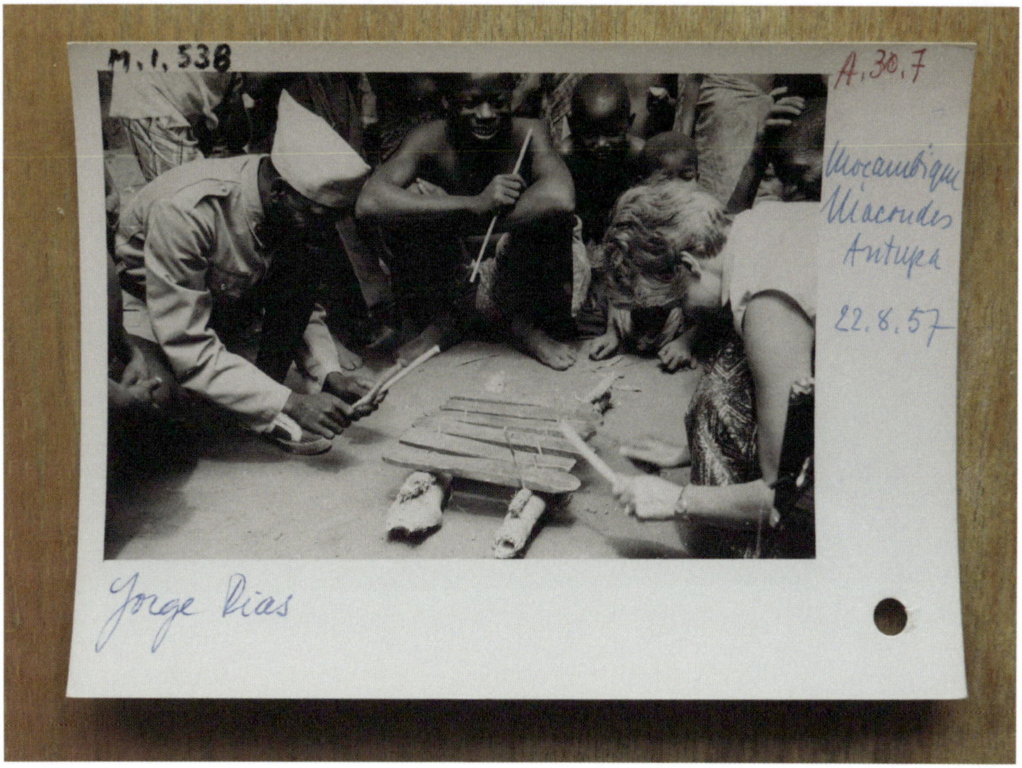

M.1.538
A.30.7
Moçambique
Macondes
Antupa
22.8.57
Jorge Dias

Fig. 7 and 8: *2 photograph cards: Mozambique, Makondes, Antupa. 22.8.57. Jorge Dias. (14.7×10.6cm). Photograph collection, Jorge Dias/Margot Dias archives. National Museum of Ethnology in Lisbon.*

----

2 photograph cards: Elinesto in his sepoy uniform in 1957; during an audio recording, Elinesto and Margot Dias simultaneously played a percussion instrument, surrounded by children and some adults from the village.

In the archives of the Portuguese Secret Police (PIDE) in Lisbon, Elinesto is described as a cruel, obedient soldier and he was therefore highly appreciated by the Portuguese administration of Mueda village. He was a ›good sepoy‹ and his name was always suggested whenever the Portuguese administration considered it ›necessary‹ to carry out harsh punishments against other Makonde. His name also appears in the documentation linked to events that sparked an incident of colonial violence on 16 June 1960 at the administrative post in Mueda. In Mozambique's history, this incident became known as the Mueda Massacre. The term was strategically coined by FRELIMO during the armed struggle (1964–1974), which converted this event into a strong weapon of counter-propaganda at a time when Portugal was still promoting the narrative, that their colonizing actions were exceptionally mild – which the »Lusotropical« vision that Jorge Dias defended helped to cement. In 1959, Elinesto was summoned by the Mueda administration to escort the famous Makonde proto-nationalist Faustino Vanomba on his return to Tanzania. Indeed, Faustino Vanomba had come from Dar es Salaam to negotiate the return of the Makonde he was representing, who had immigrated to Tanganyika to escape the oppressive rules imposed by the Portuguese. They were making claims to regain power over their land in Mozambique, as the political changes for independence in Tanzania no longer ensured work and livelihood in that country, but at the same time exhibited a model of successful peaceful negotiation that leads to a radical power shift. According to the official PIDE dispatch, and demonstrating a complete antinomy with the political changes going on in the neighbouring country, Elinesto was to take steps *en route* to discourage Vanomba from returning to Mueda with such demands for independence (though he did nevertheless return, placing the two Makonde once again in conflict, as will be seen in the next chapter).

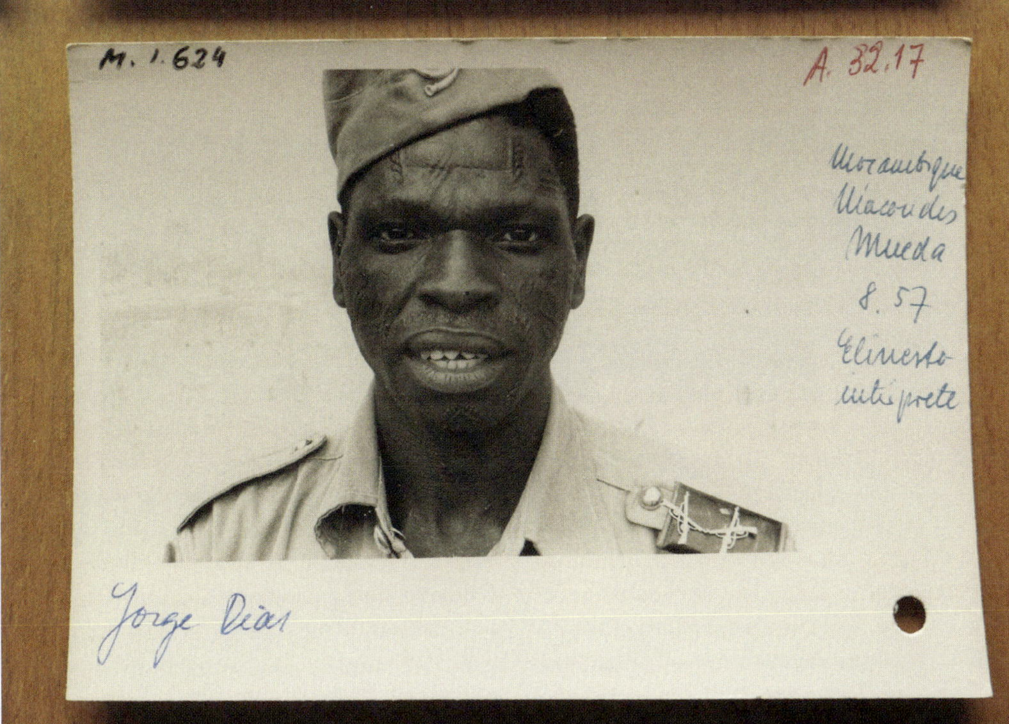
M. 1.624
A. 32.17
Moçambique
Mueda
8.57
Jorge Dias

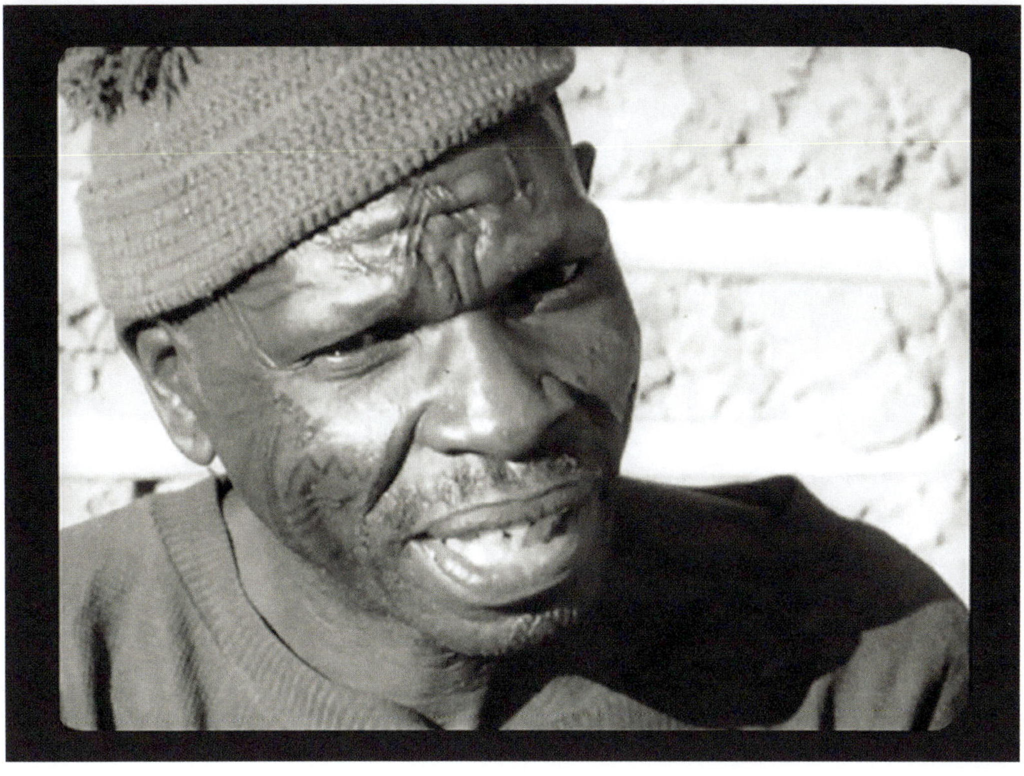

Fig. 9 und 10: *1 photograph card: Mozambique, Makondes, Mueda.8.57. Elinesto, interpreter. Jorge Dias. (14.7×10.6cm).*
1 screenshot (distribution copy): Mueda, Memória e Massacre, Ruy Guerra, 1979–1980 (INC, Mozambique). INAC (Maputo)/Arsenal – Institute for Film and Video Art – Berlin. Courtesy Ruy Guerra.
----
1 photograph card: Elinesto in his sepoy uniform in 1957.
1 screenshot: Ernesto Tchipakalia in 1978, during one of the sequences of the film in which he appears: »I shot too. If they died, I can't say, because they were all on top of each other. People died that day. A lot of people.«

The film *Mueda, Memória e Massacre*, by Ruy Guerra, enshrines the legend of the Mueda Massacre as a national event. According to the official FRELIMO narrative, this was the watershed moment, the point of no return, which legitimised the use of weapons and the armed struggle to achieve independence. In 1978, Ernesto – who was no longer called Elinesto – was interviewed for the film as a witness of the massacre that occurred due to successive political demands and adverse attempts by the Makonde proto-nationalists to negotiate with the Portuguese administration. In the film, Elinesto introduces himself humbly: »My name is Ernesto Tchipakalia and I used to be a sepoy for the Administration of Mueda«. Subtly evasive, Ernesto Tchipakalia's testimony is a mixture of a voluntary confession about his involvement in the massacre as well as his equally ambiguous conversion to the cause of independence, in which he »also killed… I don't know if they died« and that »many people died«. Considering Ernesto's/Elinesto's psychology, his reappearance in official images, once the country became independent, could hardly have been accidental. In this aspect, his involvement in the 1979 film is similar to his role in 1957 during Jorge Dias' and Margot Dias' expedition. He already knew this role of obeying the authority in power and defending its interests and had embodied it so diligently. Of the testimonies the film compiled to narrate the history of the massacre, only two among them were from the side of the ›aggressor‹. But in the final (censored) version, only Ernesto/Elinesto appears in the film. The other testimony that of the erstwhile colonial administrator, was removed. Responsible for this was Garcia Soares, the Portuguese administrator responsible for the administrative post at the time of the Mueda Massacre. Soares spoke openly about the fact, that the incident had been adulterated by FRELIMO propaganda. Unlike the description the former administrator gave for the film, Ernesto/Elinesto is consistent with the official version of the massacre, in which, supposedly, 600 Mozambicans were killed by Portuguese soldiers. The claim, that Ernesto's/Elinesto's reappearance in official images was not accidental, is reinforced by the complete invisibility of Rafael Mwakala in the history of the struggle for liberation. According to Harry West, after Mozambique achieved independence Rafael left the FRELIMO to join the enemy movement RENAMO[10] once

10 RENAMO stands for Mozambican National Resistance. It was a political organisation in Mozambique, that was initially sponsored by Rhodesian intelligence. Created in 1975, RENAMO was part of the anti-communist movement in opposition to the ruling FRELIMO party. The movement had its roots in a group of anti-FRELIMO dissidents who emerged immediately before and shortly after Mozambican independence.

he saw that his value was not being recognised within the FRELIMO movement. The character of Ernesto/Elinesto can also be connected to TaTac Mandussi, the character of the administrator's faithful sepoy in the film. It is said, that TaTac Mandussi was hung by his own people in a ›popular trial‹ for publicly claiming that the black people would not be capable of governing the country after independence. During that time, Ernesto/Elinesto remained silent and was therefore spared.

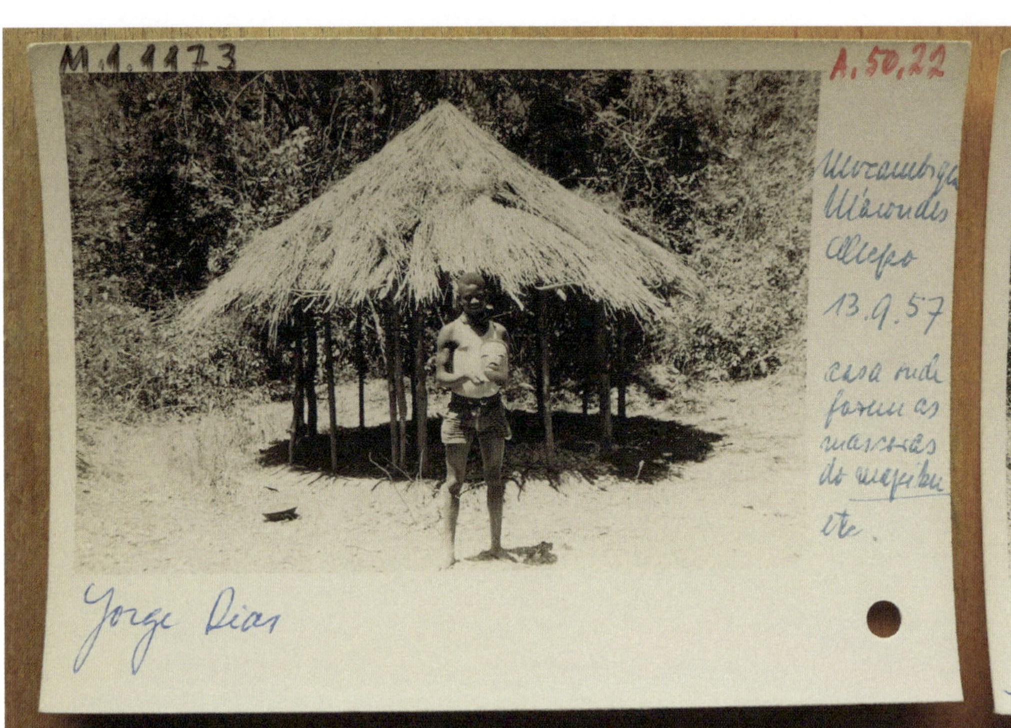

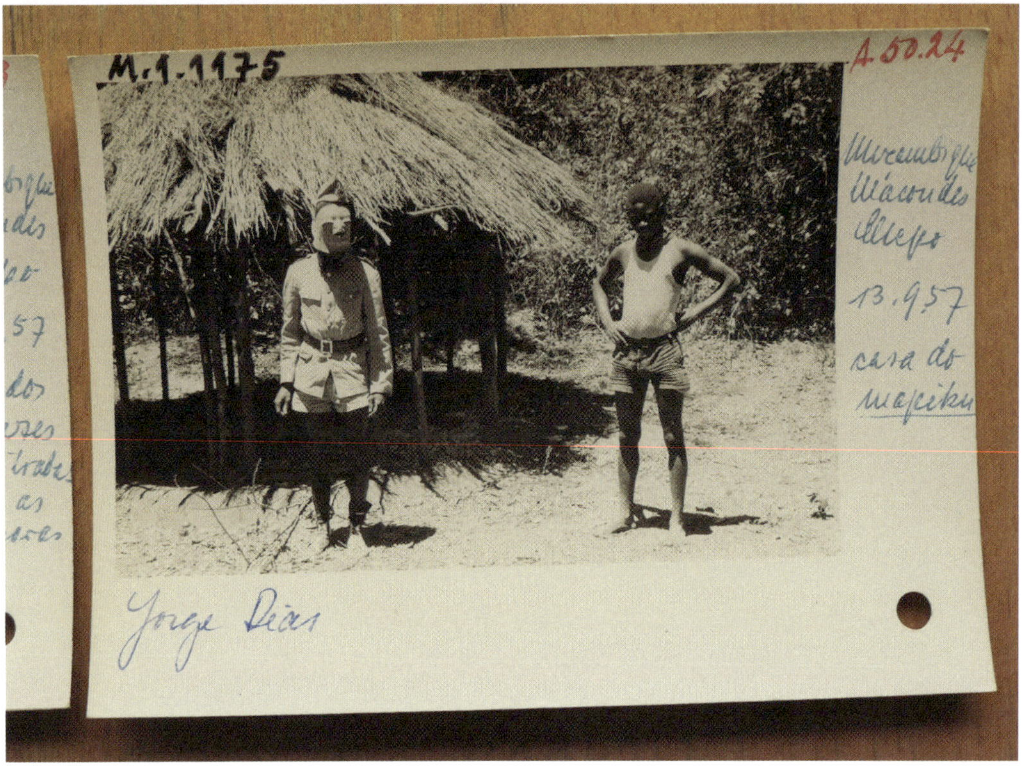

M.1.1175
A.50.24
Moçambique
Macondes
13.9.57
casa do mapiko
Jorge Dias

Fig. 11 and 12: *Composition of 2 photograph cards. Casa do Mapiku Jorge Dias. (14.7×10.6cm). Photograph collection, Jorge Dias/Margot Dias archives. National Museum of Ethnology in Lisbon.*

Composition of 2 photograph cards. Elinesto (Ernesto Nengo Tchipakalia) poses for a photograph with a Mapiku mask on his head. His sepoy bonnet, which identifies him, is placed on top of the helmet-like mask.

The card system of Jorge Dias' and Margot Dias' photograph collection plays an important role in the consolidation of their scientific narrative and in the perception of a heterogeneous unity. However, other ›possible‹ portraits and other characters can be extracted from the way the cards were organised. For this approach, it is necessary to work on a counter-factual basis, following the clues of micro-occurrences, such as, for example, the paradox contained in Ernesto Tchipakalia's baptismal name. Ernesto, a Portuguese name, contains the sound of the r that is common in the Portuguese language (and which does not exist in Shimakonde). This means that in 1957, Ernesto pronounced his own name in a form that was adapted to his own language, substituting the sound of the r with an l. Later on in my research, I accidentally learned that he was more commonly known as Nengo among the Makonde. After independence, he stayed in Mueda until his death in the early 2000s. Those who knew him say, that he was a great supporter of the FRELIMO commemoration of the 16th of June, volunteering eagerly every year to speak publicly about his ›conversion‹ after defending the Portuguese on the day of the Massacre.

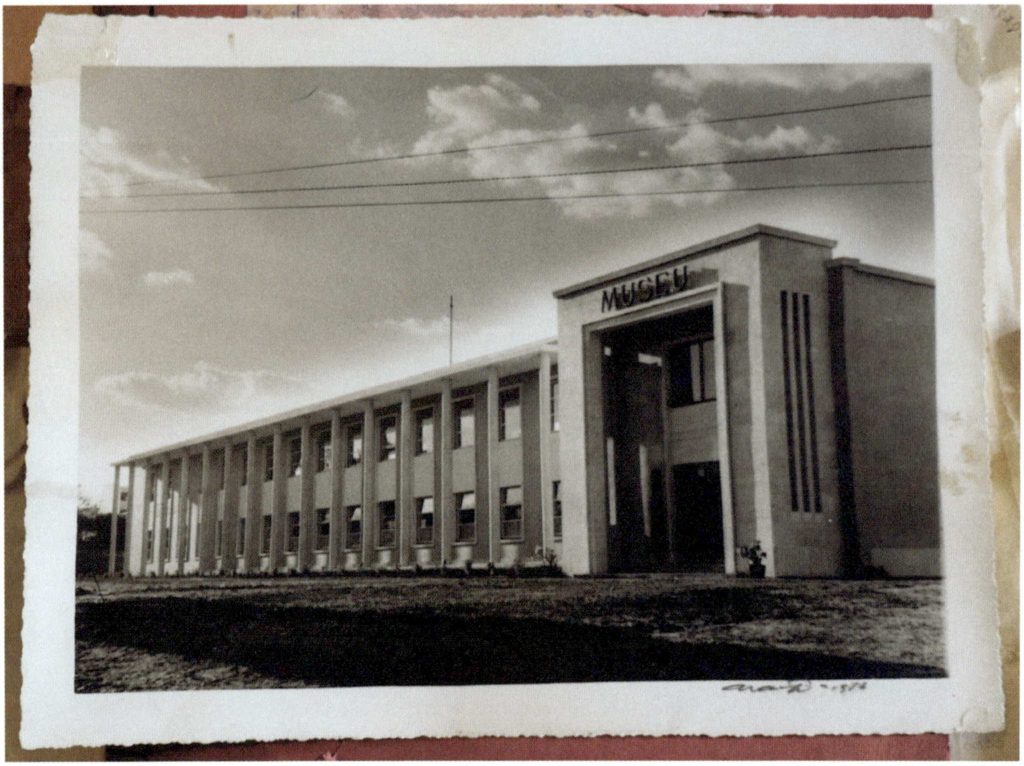

MUSEU

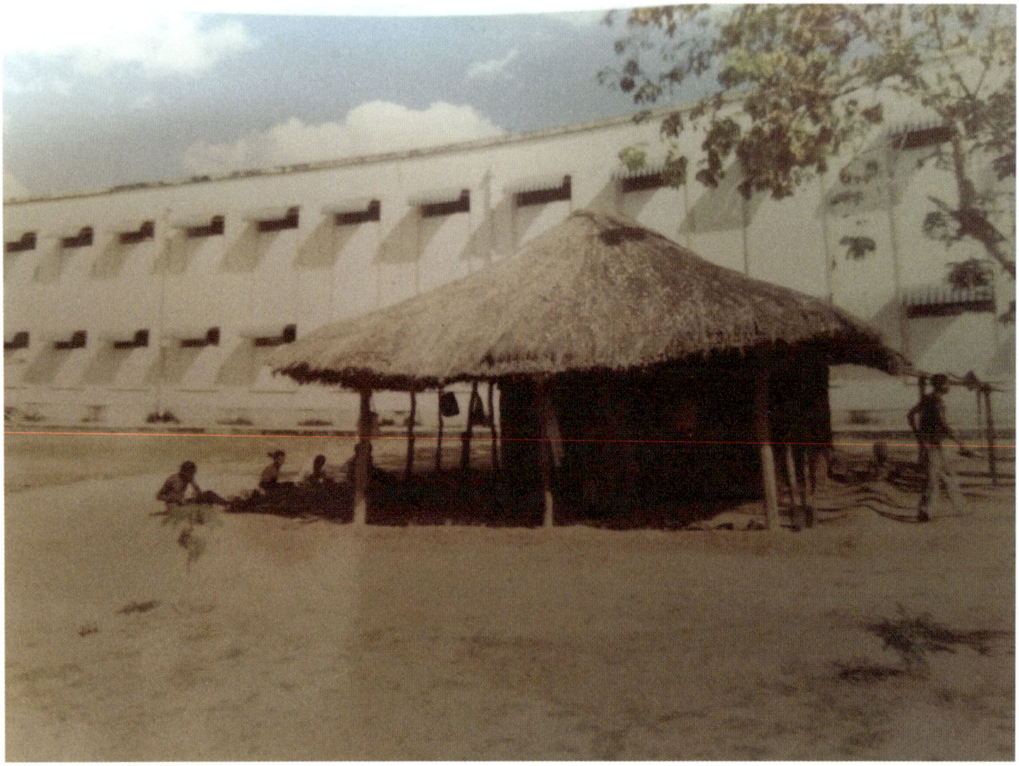

Fig. 13 and 14: *Black and white photograph: Nampula Museum, 1956. Family album. Adelino Pereira/Avellar George archives, Lisbon. Courtesy João Pedro George.*
Colour photograph: Thatched hut of Makonde sculptors (1986) built behind the Nampula Museum. Private album of a former GDR worker in Mozambique. Courtesy Bernhard Guttsche.

---

2 photographs: Front (1956) and rear (1986) of the Nampula Museum, Mozambique. In 1986, the thatched huts built at the back of the Museum hosted Makonde sculptors who came from Cabo Delgado to produce objects for the exhibitions. Paradoxically, the installation of the thatched huts recreated the ambience of the museum during the colonial period (as described in documents from the period). Even today, after visiting the exhibition, the public can leave by the rear door and see the Makonde sculptors work in thatched huts and temporary structures and can purchase items and souvenirs from them.

Nampula is the capital city of the province of the same name that is situated on the Mozambique coast and immediately south of the modern Cabo Delgado province. In colonial times, the Nampula Museum had an important collection of *Makonde* artefacts. This collection is a result of the ›administrative‹ acquisition of objects from villages in Cabo Delgado and also consists of pieces provided by staff and administrators in that region. Responding to an appeal for contributions, staff and administrators made personal donations to the Museum's collection. In the collection of ebony Makonde sculptures, many had been bought to decorate their homes – such as the figure of the Makond-ised saint in the first photograph card. As for the exterior, a composite architecture similarly mirrored the spectrum of the colonial inventory. The opposition and resistance to the colonial system were absent, they would be controlled by co-opting ›assimilated‹ individuals into ›white‹ civilisation. However, it was necessary to imagine the members of the ›pre-assimilated‹ culture, since they were being modified by the ›superior‹ European culture. In light of the evidence of change, the fiction of ›tradition‹ was supported by museographic and scientific tools (even if amateur). The dissociation of the bodies and the objects took root. The Makonde sculptors' work was catalogued and studied inside the museum's building, while in the square behind the museum, the workers of this ›local culture‹ were made to correspond to an ethnographic context that was suitable for their ›cultural cycle‹.

Margot and Jorge Dias visited the Nampula Museum in 1958 with a mixture of interest and disquiet. In 1961, in order to compile material for the fifth volume of *Os Macondes de Moçambique*, they commissioned a professional photographic inventory from the Mozambique Institute for Scientific Research in Lourenço Marques. The request consisted of surveying collections of Makonde art in Mozambican museums, resulting in 4 boxes of photographs, where 225 photographs corresponded to the collection at the Nampula Museum and 37 corresponded to the ethnographic section of the Museum of Natural History situated in Lourenço Marques, which is today Maputo, the capital city of Mozambique. Nowadays, these 4 boxes of photographs are located at the Museum of Ethnology in Leipzig, Germany.

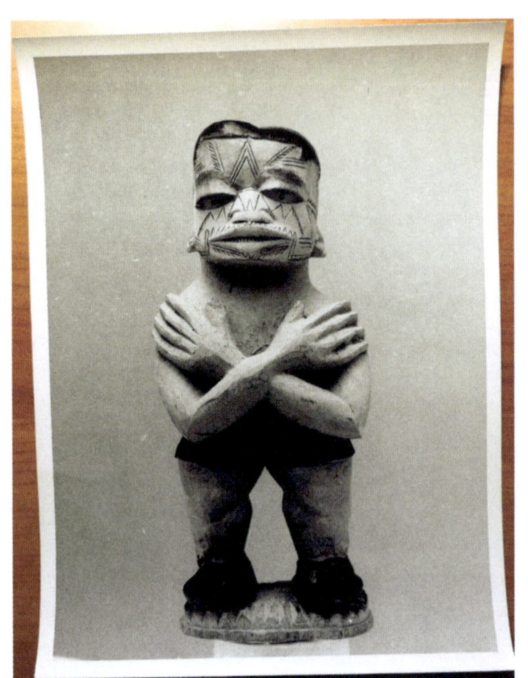
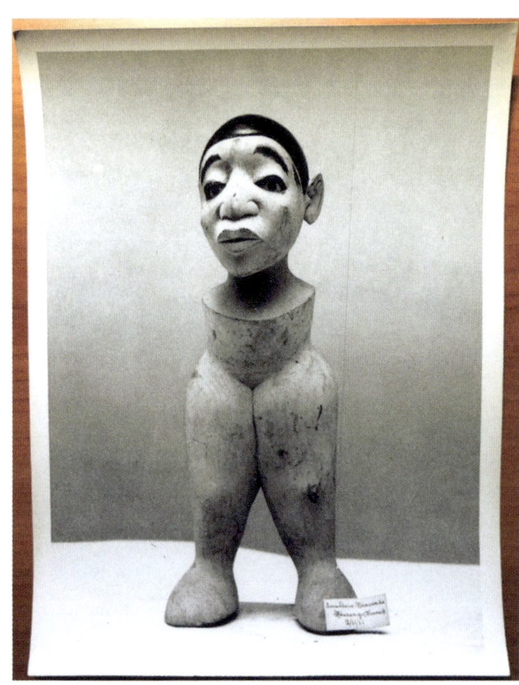
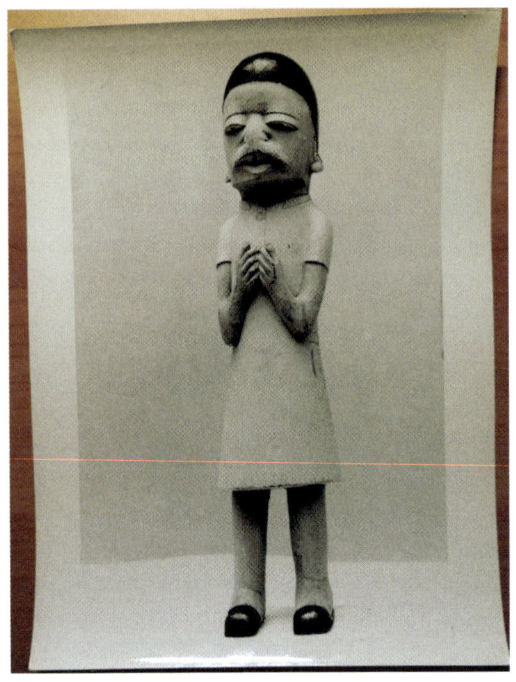
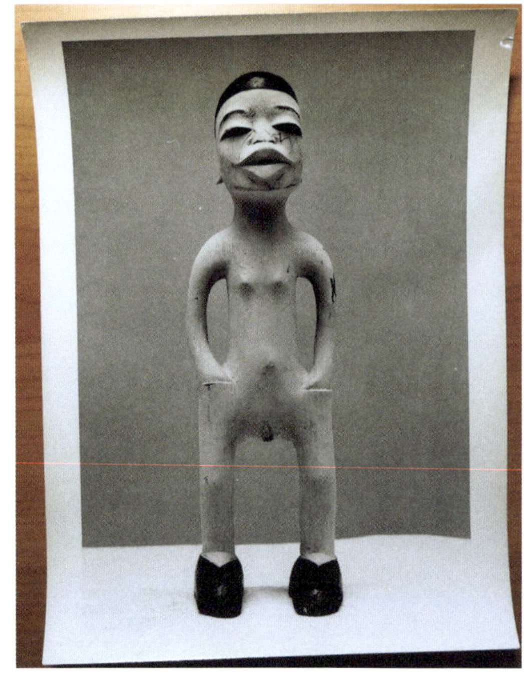

Fig. 15–18; 19–22; 23–24: LEIPZIG

Fig. 15–18; 19–22, 23–24: *Selection of photographs: Makonde sculpture, from the collection of the Nampula Regional Museum of Ethnology, 1961. Photographs credited to Manoel Manarte (Head of the Photographic Department of Mozambique Institute for Scientific Research), 18×24 cm. Nampula, Mozambique. Grassi Museum für Völkerkunde zu Leipzig.*

Photographs from the collection that Margot Dias gave to Giselher Blesse, in 1991. Unknown photographer (Mozambique Institute for Scientific Research), Leipzig (2019) – recently, it was possible to prove that these photographs were taken by an ›African‹ and ›assimilated‹ photographer working for this Institute.

The indices in the search engines of public libraries in Germany constantly bring up the prefix *Ost* in publications associated with the word Mozambique: *Ost*, German for east, as in *Ostafrika* and *Ostdeutschland*. In early 2018, my research work during my artistic residence at the Grassi Museum of Ethnology in Leipzig,[11] concerned the relations between Mozambique and the former GDR. One of my inquiries was, whether historical materialism has had an application in exhibitions, particularly those that made use of the museum's colonial collections. In 1977, Giselher Blesse, the curator responsible for the East Africa and South Africa collections at the Leipzig Museum, prepared his first exhibition, bringing together contemporary art from Mozambique and Makonde objects from the museum's colonial collection. The exhibition was called *Mosambik: Kunst und Handwerk einer jungen Volksrepublik* [*Mozambique: Arts and Crafts of a young Peoples' Republic*]. When I interviewed him, Blesse affirmed that the theoretical justification for the exhibition was a key question that needed to be resolved. One operated within the notions of base and superstructure, using an adaptation of the German *Kulturkreislehre* (especially the variant of Hermann Baumann). Within this theoretical alignment, the exhibition narrated the ›culture and way of life‹, interrelating religion and society. At the Leipzig Museum, I found the reference to the 4 boxes with the photographs of the Makonde art from Mozambique. The black and white photographs showed a sequence of Makonde art figures that brilliantly caricatured the ›white‹ Portuguese colonisers.

11 The residency at the Grassi Museum took place during 2018 and was hosted by director Nanette Snoep. This residency was part of the project Exodus Seasons #4, organised by curator Marta Jecu.

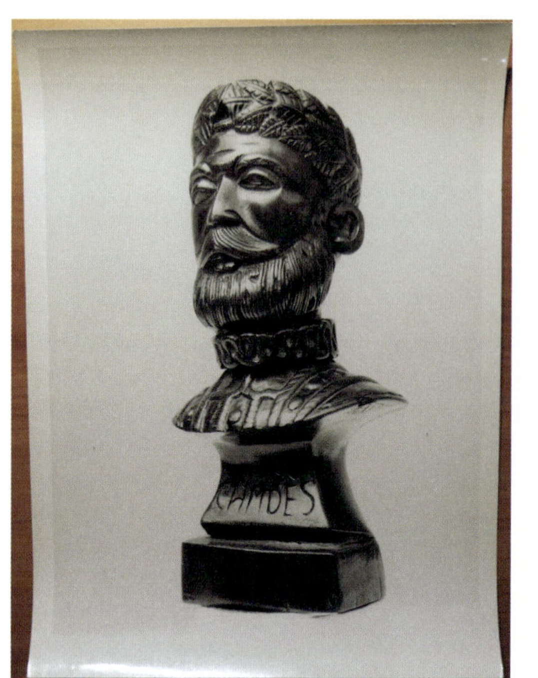
CAMÕES

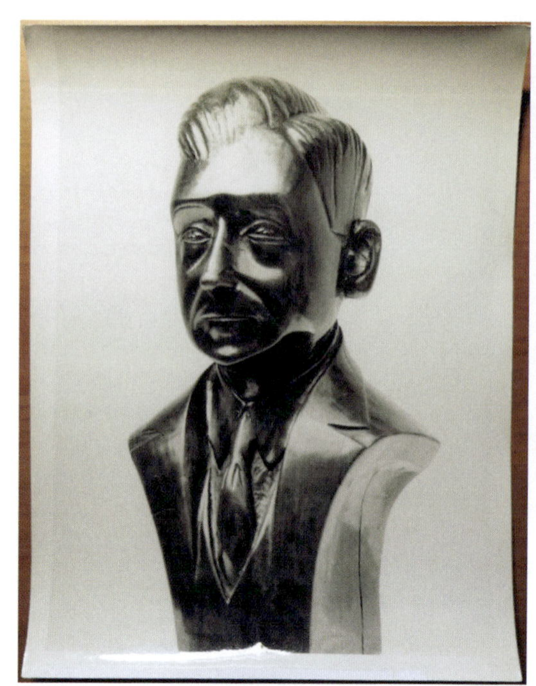

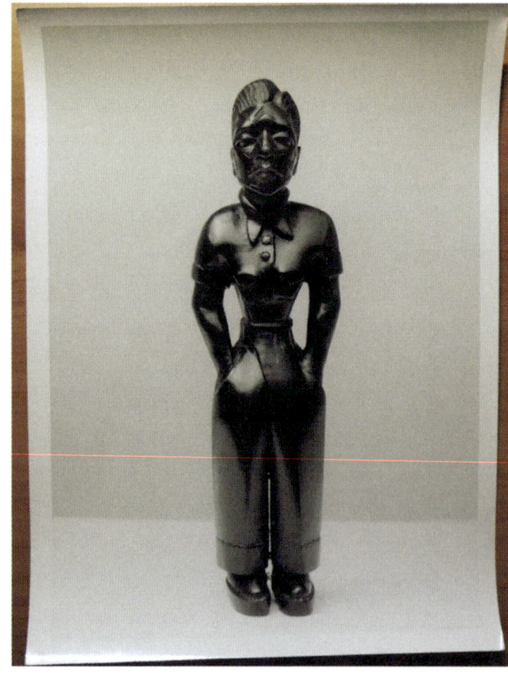

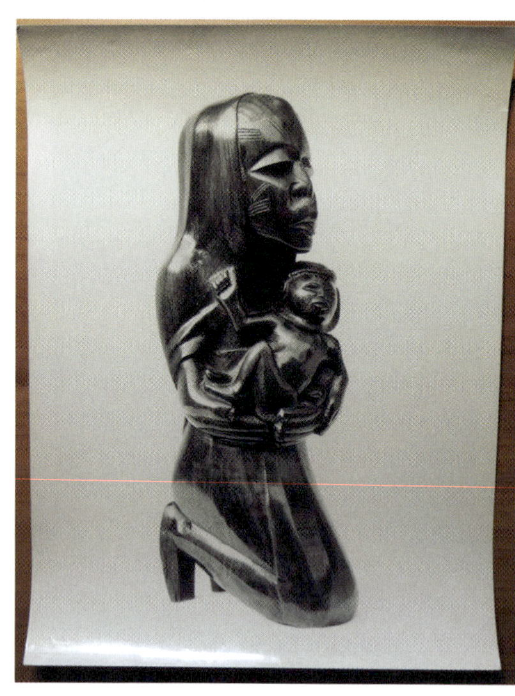

In addition to the caricature, other pieces were faithful ebony wood representations of figures from Portuguese history and literature, such as Salazar[12] and Luís Vaz de Camões.[13] Yet others showed Makonde figures incorporating signs, gestures, and attire from the colonising culture. In 1991, after the political transformation of Germany, Giselher Blesse came to Lisbon to meet Margot Dias, with whom he had corresponded years before. While preparing the 5th volume, Margot Dias asked the Leipzig Museum for information on the Makonde masks and sculptures in the collection of the German anthropologist Karl Weule – who had also once been the director of that Museum. This collection originated from his expedition to southern Tanzania in 1906, when this region was still a German protectorate. As for the 4 boxes with photographs of Makonde sculptures from Mozambique, they were of little use to Margot Dias, since they could not be categorized as either ›traditional‹ art nor as so-called ›modern‹ Makonde art. Blesse was interested in precisely this phase of the transformation of Makonde art that was linked to religious and social phenomena toward so-called modern art, even if it was disconnected from these representations (see Branco/Simão 2021). The project for the 5th volume would not have included these photographs – unless Blesse were to pursue the project. The boxes were given to him and, in his turn, Blesse donated them to the Leipzig Museum. Generically considered to be ›commissioned art‹, the disconcerting critical expression of some of these pieces, the sarcasm, and the humour offer resistance to the strict cataloguing of this collection. The Makonde collection at the Nampula Museum could have been challenging the colonists from the heart of their power apparatus (the museum) – in any case, it demonstrates a paradoxical repertoire of coloniality that is fundamentally rooted in a perception of itself.

12 Antônio de Oliveira Salazar (1889–1970) was a prominent figure of the Portuguese colonial-fascist dictatorship, he dominated Portuguese politics for more than 40 years.

13 Luís Vaz de Camões (Lisbon, c., 1524 – Lisbon, 1579 or 1580) was a portuguese poet. He is considered one of the main authors of classical Portuguese literature and the mythical narrator of Portugal in its »expansionista awakening«.

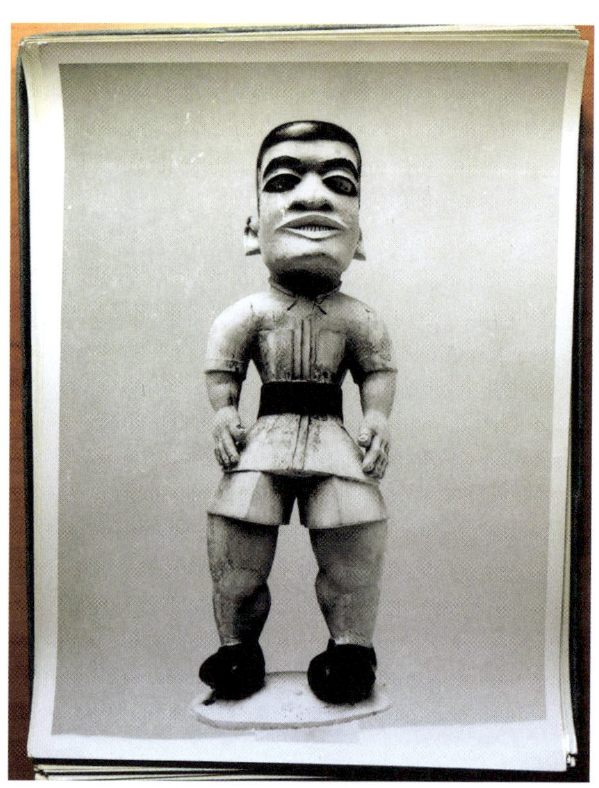

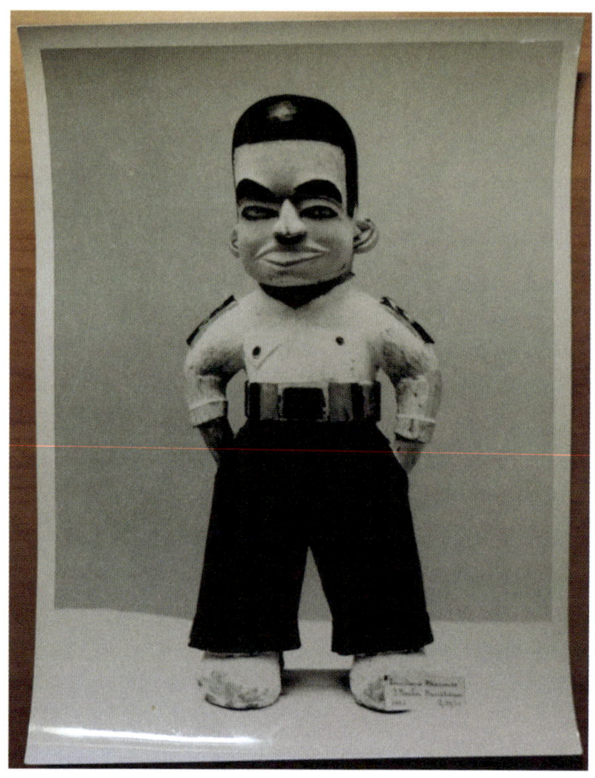

Defunct Context

With regard to the exhibition and the workshop held at the Witswatersrand University Museum of Anthropology, I was essentially interested in presenting an ›evolution‹ of the representations – as opposed to the year 1959 – in ways of viewing objects and in the system that they are a part of, irrespective of whether it related to works of art, human remains, or archive documents.

This was facilitated by one attribute in particular, which was provided by the environment of the Wits Museum itself: the fact that this museum had been divested of its ethnographic collection. Effectively, the anthropology museum today is engaged in a programme of debates on the »defunct context«, a term coined by its director, George Mahashe, to announce the museum in the absence of »artefacts of the Bantu peoples«, which had once filled its halls and display cabinets. The concrete experience of this museum without objects provided a real safe environment, in which to examine the work of Jorge Dias. Free from the effect of this tutelary weight (as well as the authority of the archives), these photographic materials were taken much closer to the *strata,* from which the subjects in this photographic collection originated.

My presentation was hosted as part of a defunct metaphor that served to approach the post-representational question of museological contexts. In the final part of my presentation, I showed the set of black and white photographs, that I had recovered through my research at the Leipzig Museum and which represented the Makonde collection at the Nampula Museum in 1961. Surprisingly, the audience at the workshop reacted to these photographs with loud guffaws. The force and beauty of this reaction strengthened my resolve to pursue this research, in order to show these images at an opportune moment to an audience in Portugal. This happened a few months later, on 14 June 2019 in Porto, in the context of the *Reframing the Archive* workshop, organised by the Archivo Platform. This event was held in a building that had once been the prison and court of appeals in Porto, which is currently the Portuguese Centre for Photography. As I suspected, presenting the photographs to a Portuguese audience did not elicit even a smile, but only resulted in a deep and uncomfortable silence.

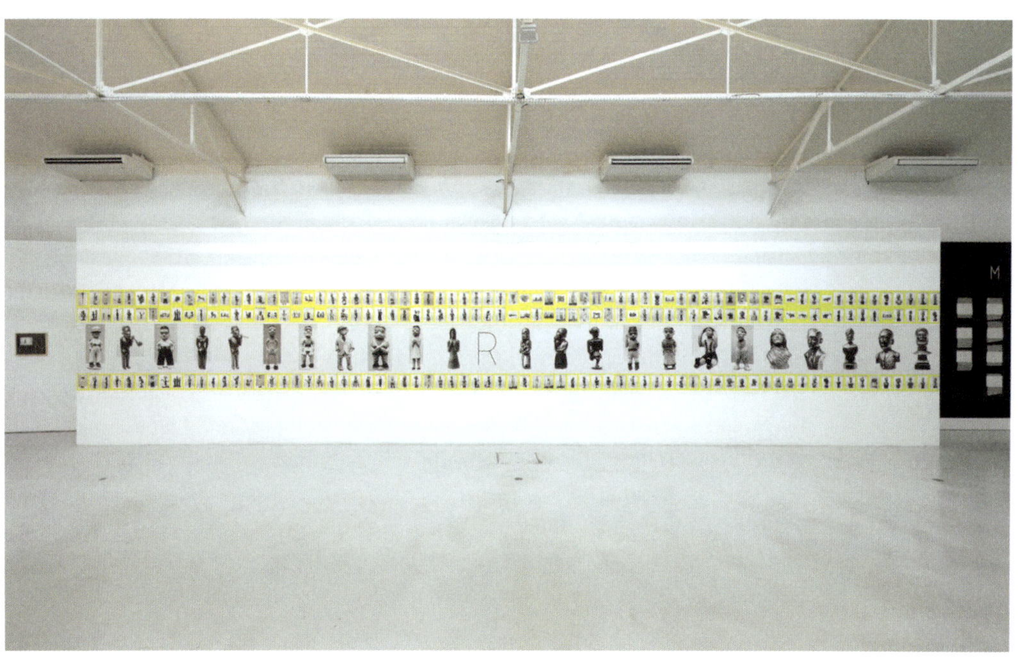

Fig. 25: LISBON

Fig. 25: *Mirror-wall. Catarina Simão, R-Humor Exhibition 2020. Galerias Avenida da ndia, Lisbon Municipal Galleries. Photograph: João Neves.*

On 26 January 2020, an exhibition was inaugurated at the Galeria Avenida da Índia – an avenue with a colonial name – that brought together a significant part of my artistic work linked to the Mozambique archives. With the portmanteau *R-Humor*, which I chose as the title, the exhibition heralded a specific way of inventorying the 26 pieces that comprised the display. This decade-long approach to my work was the result of a reflection on the challenges that I faced working with archives at different forms of incompleteness. The exhibition urged one to reimagine archives through the forms of absence therein: deferred strategies, temporary restrictions and public secrets, such as rumour or humour, as unsuspected proof of the clairvoyance of reality. Using a device that I called the mirror-wall, the exhibition consisted of a central piece made up of a composition of blown-up photographs depicting the old collection of Makonde art at the Nampula Museum. Facing this mirror-wall, the *R-Humor* exhibition juxtaposed excerpts from the Mozambican film *Mueda, Memória e Massacre (1979–80)*, by Ruy Guerra, where the representation of the ›Other‹ entails an equally paradoxical affectation. In the case of this film by Ruy Guerra, Mozambican actors play the role of the ›whites‹, very often ridiculing them and causing guffaws amid the audience. There is no distancing among an oppressed population, because colonisers penetrate their lives and offer no respite, thus representation takes place in another way, by means of incorporation, by means of a change, an appropriation that is transformed. This exhibition did not present the conclusions of any research. On the contrary, it was a hybrid space, even if partially representative, but open to a procedural dimension. The archive was no longer used to represent, becoming a moment of practising the tradition of representing, with its particularities, since it chose a suspended programme. Equally in suspense was its final determination, as an artistic or political practice – it is the context to which the production is linked, that dictates the assimilation, or not, of one form by the other.

Translation from Portuguese: Roopanjali Roy.

Literature

Branco, Jorge Freitas/Simão, Catarina (2021): »About the 4 Photo Boxes of Margot Dias – Interview to Giselher Blesse«. In: *Direito à Informação/Right to Information*, ed. by Catarina Simão, Lisbon: Galerias Municipais/EGEAC, 68–82.

Costa, Catarina Alves/Da Costa, Paulo Ferreira (2016): *Margot Dias: Ethnographic Films 1958–1961*, Lisbon: Cinemateca Portuguesa-Museu do Cinema/National Museum of Ethnology of Lisbon.

Dias, Jorge (1961a): *Portuguese Contribution to Cultural Anthropology*, Johannesburg: Witwatersrand University Press.

Dias, Jorge (1961b): »Conflitos de Cultura«. In: *Estudos de Ciências Políticas e Sociais* 51, Lisbon: Separata de Colóquios sobre Problemas Humanos nas Regiões Tropicais, 109–125.

DIAS, Jorge (1964): *Os Macondes de Moçambique. Aspectos Históricos e Económicos, vol. I*, Lisbon: Junta de Investigações do Ultramar.

DIAS, Jorge/DIAS, Margot (1964): *Os Macondes de Moçambique. Cultura Material, vol. II*, Lisbon: Junta de Investigações do Ultramar.

DIAS, Jorge/DIAS, Margot (1970): *Os Macondes de Moçambique. Vida Social e Ritual, vol. III*, Lisbon: Junta de Investigações do Ultramar.

GUERREIRO, Manuel Viegas (1966): *Os Macondes de Moçambique. Sabedoria, Língua, Literatura e Jogos, vol. IV*, Lisbon: Junta de Investigações do Ultramar.

VICENTE, Filipa/GEORGE, João Pedro (2021): »Family Colonialism: The Nampula Museum Archive«. In: *Direito à Informação/Right to Information*, Catarina Simão, Lisbon: Galerias Municipais/EGEAC, 84–101.

WEST, Harry (2006): »Invertendo a Bossa do Camelo. Jorge Dias, a sua Mulher, o Intérprete e Eu«. In: *Portugal Não é um País Pequeno. Contar o »Império« na Pós-Colonialidade*, ed. by Manuela Ribeiro Sanches (org.), Lisbon: Livros Cotovia, 141–190.

Table of figures

Fig. 1: Inauguration of the Regional Museum of Nampula, Mozambique, 1956; black and white photograph, 10×7cm. Family album. Private Archive, Avellar George / Adelino Pereira Soares de Castro, Lisbon. Courtesy J.P.G.

Fig. 2: Photo: Ethnographically Intimate Exhibition (partial). Witswatersrand University Museum of Anthropology, 10 & 11 May 2019, Johannesburg. Foto: Catarina Simão.

Fig. 3: Photograph card: Mozambique Island; 8.1957. Makonde sculpture at the administrator's residence. Jorge Dias. (14.7×10.6cm). Photograph collection, Jorge Dias/Margot Dias archives. National Museum of Ethnology in Lisbon.

Fig. 4: Image reproduced in a book: Rafael Mwakala holding Os Macondes de Moçambique, open at a page with a photograph of his wife and child (right hand page, image at the lower left corner of the page). Photo: National Museum of Ethnology in Lisbon. (West 2006: 150) Courtesy Harry G. West.

Fig. 5: 4 photograph cards. Upper right corner: Mozambique, Makondes, Mueda. 8.57. Rafael, Christian interpreter. Jorge Dias. (14.7×10.6cm). Photograph collection, Jorge Dias/Margot Dias archives. National Museum of Ethnology in Lisbon.

Fig. 6: 5 photograph cards: Mozambique, Makondes, Mueda. 10.57. Elinesto Jorge Dias. (14.7×10.6cm). Photograph collection, Jorge Dias/Margot Dias archives. National Museum of Ethnology in Lisbon.

Fig. 7 and 8: 2 photograph cards: Mozambique, Makondes, Antupa. 22.8.57. Jorge Dias. (14.7×10.6cm). Photograph collection, Jorge Dias/Margot Dias archives. National Museum of Ethnology in Lisbon.

Fig. 9 and 10: 1 photograph card: Mozambique, Makondes, Mueda.8.57. Elinesto, interpreter. Jorge Dias. (14.7×10.6cm); 1 screenshot (distribution copy): Mueda, Memória e Massacre, Ruy Guerra, 1979–1980 (INC, Mozambique). INAC (Maputo)/Arsenal – Institute for Film and Video Art – Berlin. Courtesy Ruy Guerra.

Fig. 11 and 12: Composition of 2 photograph cards. Casa do Mapiku, Jorge Dias. (14.7×10.6cm). Photograph collection, Jorge Dias/Margot Dias archives. National Museum of Ethnology in Lisbon.

Fig. 13 and 14: Black and white photograph: Nampula Museum, 1956. Family album. Adelino Pereira/Avellar George archives, Lisbon. Courtesy João Pedro George. Colour photograph: Thatched hut of Makonde sculptors (1986) built behind the Nampula Museum. Private album of a former GDR worker in Mozambique. Courtesy Bernhard Guttsche.

Fig. 15–18; 19–22; 23–24: Selection of photographs: Makonde sculpture, from the collection of the Nampula Regional Museum of Ethnology, 1961. Photographs credited to Manoel Manarte (Head of the Photographic Department of Mozambique Institute for Scientific Research), 18×24 cm. Nampula, Mozambique. Grassi Museum für Völkerkunde zu Leipzig.

Fig. 25: Mirror-wall. Catarina Simão, R-Humor Exhibition 2020. Galerias Avenida da Índia, Lisbon Municipal Galleries. Photograph: João Neves.

Debate

Introduction: Discussing »Tacit Racism«

Michi Knecht and Martin Zillinger

Two years after the murder of George Floyd by a police officer in Minneapolis, and sixteen years after Oury Jalloh was abused by police in Dessau and then burned to death in police custody under circumstances that are still not clear, at a moment in time, in which the state of research with regard to systematic racist violence in the police has large gaps, especially in Germany (Hunold and Wegner 2020, KOP – Kampagne für Opfer rassistisch motivierter Polizeigewalt 2021) what can cultural and social sciences do? What is their task in the midst of intensified societal polarization, one of the salient features of which is the rise of both recurring and new forms of racism as well as the struggle and protest against many forms of group-based misanthropy? In a time of proliferation of openly displayed, shamelessly exhibited and publicly performed acts of racism in the streets, in parliaments and educational institutions, in old and new media, what methodological and analytical possibilities can the humanities and social sciences muster to make the scope of the problem visible and contribute to change? Why, in other words, do we turn towards more hidden, unconscious, or tacit practices of racism and why should that be helpful in a moment, in which the debate in Germany about the necessity of empirical social science research on systematic police violence has not yet been won (at least not at the federal level) and in which social and cultural scientists like Didier Fassin in France are commissioned by victims of police violence to conduct ethnographic counter-investigations? It is in the context of these and related questions that we invited Anne Rawls and Waverly Duck to contribute an essay to this debate section and introduce the argument of their book *Tacit Racism*, published just a few months before we started to prepare this issue. *Tacit Racism is Institutionalized in Interaction in the US: What about Elsewhere?* invites readers and fellow commentators to explore how racism is co-produced in interaction. It therefore advances an argument that tries to complement existing research in, for example, Critical Race Theory by asking »how the inequalities that have been documented […] in the large scale economic and social relations […] and the differences revealed by research on intersectionality, translate into interactional practices« (in this volume, p. 214). The authors thus direct our attention to aspects of our daily lives where we might least expect to find racism at work – in the very micro-practices by which we co-produce our social worlds. Those are situated practices, and they are likely to differ between societies. The authors challenge us to think about how racism is encoded in the everyday social expectations in societies other than the U.S. with its particular history of racism, labour exploitation and inequalities.

In recent years, diverse forms of racism, antisemitism and other forms of systematic discrimination and neo-colonial orderings have taken centre stage in public debates in Europe. In Germany, pioneering work of authors such as Annita Kalpaka and Nora Räthzel (1986), Mark Terkessidis (1998, 2004, 2019), Erol Yildiz

urn:nbn:de:hbz:6:3-zfk-2021-42021

(1999, 2014), Pipo Bui (2004), Paul Mecheril (2007), Serdal Güler (2009), Ilka Eickhoff (2010) and Annita Kalpaka, Nora Räthzel and Klaus Weber (2017) have helped paving the way for a new generation of public intellectuals raising their voices on racism (Amjahid 2017, 2021; Hasters 2019, 2020; Kelly 2021) and demanding a public debate on long standing forms of discrimination. Scholars like Arndt (2005), El-Tayeb (2001, 2016), Foroutan (2019), El Mafaalani (2021) have helped to establish the crucial importance of these topics for social and cultural theory, as much as for a functioning democratic society.

In hindsight, it can only be called a major scandal in the history of European and North American *Geistes- und Sozialwissenschaften* (humanities and social sciences) that, for too long, majority thinkers have treated the suppression of minority scholarship and racism as side issues (for an analysis of the situation in American Anthropology see Allen and Jobson 2016). They have thus contributed to »trivialize the centrality of the problem... and allowed it to fester«, as Waverly Duck and Anne Rawls argue in their contribution (see p. 211 in this volume). They remind us that the marginalization of voices that have tried to do otherwise has contributed to upholding the illusion that racism is not a problem within the workings of democratic, Western societies and, by extension, within their universities (in this volume, p. 211). The need to address racism and to decolonize academia applies to all disciplines, and even though the topic has gained some ground in recent years, the difficulty scholars continue to face when trying to build a career on this topic bears witness to this history of continuous neglect and rejection. Moreover, a short survey of the diversity of students' and university teachers' bodies, for example in German universities, makes it poignantly clear that the trivialization of the topic has had far reaching consequences for universities and the societies they are meant to serve. Students, who are continuously exposed to racism at the university, have started to form associations and organize workshops to counter racism. Whoever attends one of these self-help forums (often instigated by AStAs at universities and independent student organizations) cannot but fall silent in view of the painful reports of BPOC-students recounting their experiences with teachers, administrators and fellow students. The pain, tears and fears, that the very institution that is meant to produce and protect a community of learning, inflicts on the young people who strive for knowledge and education are not only shameful, but testify to systematic and endemic forms of exclusion. It is one of the unsettling arguments of Duck's and Rawls' article that such forms of exclusion are normalized or even naturalized, when they are either primarily rendered as problems of individual mind-sets (and thus located at the level of individuals), or somehow ascribed to the workings of structures and institutions (and thus at least partly out of reach).

In their paper, Waverly Duck and Anne Rawls propose to revisit forms of everyday racism, not at the margins of societies but in their midst – directing their empirically detailed attention to routines, tacit expectations and systemic, and often unconscious, patterns of racist interaction. It is a privilege of White people and a structural feature of racialized societies that such patterns are often little commented upon in diverse publics and equally little reflected upon in the everyday lives of many Whites (Cakaya and Mepschen 2019). Waverly Duck and Anne Rawls explore how systemic racism is »institutionalized in taken-for-granted practices of interaction«, in what they call »interaction orders of race« . Both have been working together on this for many years. Their perspective is primarily sociological, more specifically: ethnomethodological. One of the crucial features of ethnomethodological research is to foreground practice to all other elements in a given situation or social setting. In many ways this is counter-intuitive, since most social and anthropological theories continue to invoke structures and institutions to explain social orders (and thus, for example, how a regime of White supremacy is enacted) or actions and actors with their intentions and identities to explain practices (and thus, for example, racist discrimination). Following Garfinkel, the authors turn this taken-for-granted model of the social world on its head and zoom in on the modes in which structures, actions and intentions are co-constituted in interaction. For this purpose they lead us into the ethnomethodological world of micro-studies and sequential analyses.

Inspired by W.E.B. Du Bois' concept of »double consciousness« (which, as Meyer remarks, must also be understood as »double membership«) and Harold Garfinkel's ethnomethodology Rawls and Duck carve out what they call »grammars of interaction« (see the responses by Jean Beaman and Christian Meyer). These racist grammars of interaction are empirically investigated in three diagnostically rich situations of interaction, partly under laboratory conditions and partly on the basis of filmed visual sources which are later analyzed: situations of ›first contact‹ in everyday life, of systematic devaluation of *Black* people in professional roles, and a hard-to-bear scene of an interaction between *White* police officers and a *Black* civilian. (We need to issue a trigger warning at this point: The description of this interaction does not entail physical violence but may nevertheless have retraumatizing effects in some circumstances.)

There is, of course, a thoroughly extensive body of research, for example on the phenomenology of racism (reports and auto-ethnographies from the perspectives and experiences of those repeatedly affected by racism in everyday life) as well as on everyday racism (Essed 1990) as a systematic and structural problem anchored in the centre of social reproduction, representational strategies, and forms of interaction. Notably institutionalized forms of everyday racism have been widely researched (see only as examples Fassin 2016 and 2021; Heinemann and Mecheril 2017; Hunold and Wegner 2020, Jäger 1992, Terkessidis 2004, Wacquant 1997). Schools, labour markets, educational systems, housing and the media have been studied in terms of how they not only absorb and transmit racist and racializing discourses, but also in terms of how they independently produce discrimination and disadvantage. In the case of our own working environment, i.e. German universities, empirical educational research has shown that the system of higher education in Germany has particularly exclusive effects – referring to a variety of discriminations and disadvantages, for example on the basis of class/stratum, immigration, language or religious affiliation.

So what is missing or should be renewed with regard to the current state of research? It is evident that even after years of cultural and social studies research, pressing questions and research findings about everyday racism remain outside the canon of our disciplines and are still underrepresented. Equally, they are still underrepresented in the centre of cultural and social theory. Waverly Duck and Anne Rawls themselves argue that much of the research on everyday racisms is still caught up in the old dichotomy of individual versus structure. To put it more succinctly: Much research on everyday racism in their perspective has either examined opinions, attitudes, prejudices, and psychological mindsets on the side of the individual or structures – discourses, laws, constitutions, markets, sciences, and institutions – understood as external factors of influence that often seem out of reach for everyday actors.

In contrast, with their interactionist and ethnomethodological research program focusing on empirical details in micro-situations and their theoretical concept of interactional expectations, Anne Rawls and Waverly Duck have developed interesting tools to overcome this dichotomy. Most commentators confirm and reinforce this argument and see the bringing together of fine-grained qualitative empirical data with a program of analysis that focuses on »racialization in action« (Meyer, in this volume, p. 244) as a particularly innovative and relevant step in their contribution.

Our own impetus for why we curated this debate can be summarized in three points.

First, we wanted to re-examine what Duck and Rawls refer to as »tacit« more explicitly as situated in the current polarized and politicized debates about racism and anti-racism. »Tacit« is translated in German either as *stillschweigend* (which refers to the Latin verb *tacere, schweigen, to keep silent*, as the word root of the term Anne Rawls and Waverly Duck use both in the title the essay published here and in their book) or as *implizit*. We wanted to discuss how implicitly racist expectations embedded in everyday interactions change in the context of an explicit debate about racism. Is this really still about »unconscious« racism, an ›interaction order of Race‹ only subliminally known by Whites? Or can Michael Polanyi's reflections on »tacit knowledge« help us to interpret the orders of racist expectations and embodied everyday knowledge as more active appropriations and more controversial, if implicit, decisions. Polanyi sees tacit knowledge, like every form of knowledge, as including an »appraisal«, a »personal coefficient, which shapes all factual knowledge« (Polanyi 1962:17). One of the strengths of Polanyi's thinking on »tacit knowledge« certainly lies in his rejection of dualistic distinctions between theoretical and practical, objectified and subjective, and between tacit and explicit knowledge. For him, all knowledge practices are »skillful actions« (Polanyi and Prosch 1975: 44). Following Polanyi, we were interested in discussing the proximal notion of »tacit« in the context of racially patterned expectations and to see what can be learned about »tacit« racism as an active blocking of knowledge, as a racist attitude appropriated in the context of socially distributed and widely available alternatives (see Ann Stoler's plea for shifting the discourse about »amnesia« in the context of ›unremembered‹ or ›forgotten‹ colonialism to »aphasia«, a distinctly more salient and complex language disorder to analyse (Stoler 2011; see Beaman in this issue).

Second, we thought it productive to ask how Waverly Duck's and Anne Rawls' research with its focus on the United States would be received and discussed in European contexts and what modifications, extensions, or alternative research designs it might prompt. This question is taken up by our commentators in a variety of ways and it is interesting to read how they address national or supranational differences in the everyday orders of tacit racism. Given the diverse transnational or global interconnections of lifestyles, social movements, political forms, and discourses of all kinds, forms of comparison operating under the assumption that their units of comparison are disconnected and discrete increasingly turn obsolete. Any attempt for comparison or clearly cut juxtapositions seems to be at loss in the face of traveling concepts and entangled lifestyles, the globalization of social movements and the proliferation of international social media and political networks. Movements such as Black Lives Matter translated into different social and national settings and the concepts and forms of political resistance traveling with them have empowered minorities to articulate their anger and their demands. However, how racist interaction orders are globally intertwined and intermingled is usually little addressed (but see Beaman in this issue). This perhaps indicates a research desideratum of its own. The entanglements of orders have long been evident in everyday life; however, empirical studies on such entanglements are, to our knowledge, largely lacking.

Third, and perhaps most crucially, we wanted to explore the scope or extent to which updated ethnomethodological approaches and a practice-theoretical orientation towards everyday forms of »racialization in action« (Meyer, in this volume) might be well equipped to anchor everyday racisms more firmly at the centre of social consciousness. Casting ›Race‹ not as a pre-empirically existing category, but instead making the processes of its production visible in situ and in process (see Balkenhol and Schramm 2019), as ›Race‹ in practice or interaction, contains a hope. Being identified as practice theorists ourselves, we tend to see value in the description of racist everyday (inter)actions as emergent and in permanent need of doing / undoing. The leeway in »doing racism« (Balkenhol and Schramm 2019) might include active disregard of existing anti-racist or at least less racist alternatives (Meyer, in this volume).

Not all of the esteemed colleagues we invited to this debate shared the concerns that are raised by Rawls and Duck, and some of their scepticism was mirrored by the anger we encountered when we discussed their text in different settings. After all, practice theory is not a theory of action. The »interactional expectations« examined in the text go beyond individual intention. They are so deeply ingrained into social lives and the ways how social worlds are reproduced in ordinary interactions that they are difficult to avoid. Those who belong to the *White* majority may not even recognize racism when it manifests. This kind of tacit racism that readers encounter in the text, is outrageous, it hurts.

But the detailed analyses of racialized interactions in everyday life might also promote an awareness of possibilities for change, or even more: the need for change. In other words: there is potential for enlightenment. Rawls' and Duck's descriptions of micro-interactions, which, of course, are made from a specific positionality indicating different, often antagonistic social positions, intend to amplify societies' potential for making inconspicuous racisms conscious and known, alongside the explicit racist violence that is so visible. If it is true that, with a radicalized theory of practice, the capacity for social reflection is expanded, then there is also hope for change. With their plea for a ›White double consciousness‹ the two authors turn their analysis into a manifesto. Making visible what is hidden enables you to put yourself into the place of the other. What is needed, therefore, is more research on these mundane interaction orders that constitute everyday life, within and without the universities.

The multi-voiced and lively dialogue that has emerged in the debate that follows is inspiring and provides numerous indications of how the research approach of Anne Rawls and Waverly Duck (which they explicitly reflect as specifically US-American) invites further thinking, indeed: more than we could have hoped for. So, for example, when Jean Beaman points to the analytical potential for theorizing global racisms, which, starting from Du Bois, is already inherent in the observations and indications of Duck and Rawls, but should be explored more systematically and comprehensively in the future. When Martijn de Koning takes up the ball and discusses tacit racism on the basis of his own empirical research on racialization and anti-Muslim racism in the Netherlands (in this volume, p. 234). When Giolo Fele locates the sly and persistent forms of tacit racism (more clearly than Rawls and Duck can address it here themselves) in the context of a specific theory of modernity less based on shared expectations than on conflicting negotiations. When Christian Meyer, in turn, continues to spin this thread and points to the importance of empirical investigations that address precisely not the noiseless consummation, but the ruptures and breaches of racist expectation orders in everyday live. Such research will be able to make visible and delineate alternatives more thoroughly and explore the production of racializing and racist orders of interaction as compromised and/or opportunistic acts of choice. Last but not least, Levent Tezcan, from a German perspective, argues for paying attention to the multiplicity and dynamics of figuration processes in (post)migration societies. In doing so, he is concerned with a recognition of both the malleability and the multiformity of »systemic and tacit« racist interaction. We would like to thank our admired commentators very much for their excellent contributions, all of which open up future research strategies.

The transnational Black Lives Matter Movement (Williams 2015) marks and combats structural racism and institutional discrimination as forms of everyday racisms. Current everyday, ›tacit‹ racism in its many forms has not only been handed down, but is also publicly reinvented and partly re-normalized. The social and cultural sciences are undoubtedly called upon to publicly counter these developments. In our opinion, this implies an extension of scientific responsibility from texts, ideas, knowledge and research programs to include universities as the institutions we work in as well as the social and political contexts in which we are embedded. We hope that the debate on tacit racism initiated by Waverly Duck and Anne Rawls will have some power to support this.

Tacit Racism is Institutionalized in Interaction in the US: What about Elsewhere?[1]

Anne Warfield Rawls and Waverly Duck

We were asked to write a summary of our book *Tacit Racism* (Rawls/Duck 2020) to stimulate discussion of our research approach in Europe. In doing so we confront several challenges. First, a summary leaves out details, which is problematic because our argument rests on detailed analysis of social interaction. Summarizing the relationship between our argument and prior theory and research on Race, including the Black American and minority scholarship from which it takes inspiration, is also complicated.[2] Our research is unique. But there are important relationships and we address these below (see also Rawls/Whitehead/Duck 2020). That Europe and the US have different histories of Race and colonization, and that the discussion in Europe is in a ›post-colonial‹ phase, is another challenge. There is no corresponding ›colonial‹ phase of relations between Races in the US. The whole country began as a former colony.[3] Black Americans were not colonized by White Americans, nor were they ever ›immigrants‹ in the European sense. The language and literature of post-colonialism do not fit.[4] Furthermore, the idea of Race is itself problematic. As we discuss it, Race is an American invention, a social construction as W.E.B. Du Bois argued, with no basis in biology. Du Bois also argued that while Race is the most significant category dividing the

1 Die deutsche Übersetzung ist unter https://doi.org/10.25819/ubsi/10116 frei zugänglich.
The German translation is openly accessible at https://doi.org/10.25819/ubsi/10116.

2 We capitalize Race and other exclusionary category terms as a possibly irritating reminder that Race is a social fact and not a biological fact in all our publications. Although the social fact status of Race has been acknowledged since Du Bois introduced the idea – there are still too many who consider Race a natural distinction. From there it is easy talk about how natural it is for people to be afraid of differences. What differences? Our answer is that the differences that scare people – the ones that ›count‹ – are socially constructed differences, not natural differences.

3 In our book we do discuss the possibility that White Americans are suffering from a colonial mentality that dates from the 1600's. But it is quite evident that Black Americans are not.

4 However, recent immigrants to the US from former European colonies in Africa, the Caribbean and elsewhere, have brought the post-colonial mentality to the US, creating problems in the Black American community that we discuss in our book.

US population, it is also the primary unifier within the Black community. The experience of racism that Du Bois called »double consciousness« gives Black Americans insight into racism and democracy that White Americans lack. While aspects of that insight may have been exported along with the concept of Race, it has no European counterpart.

Tacit Racism is a book about how systemic racism in the US has become institutionalized in the taken-for-granted practices of everyday interaction – in what we call ›interaction orders of Race‹ – such that ordinary people are constantly doing racist things without being aware of it. Most discussions of Race and racism have focused either on individual prejudice or on formally institutionalized racism in legal and other formal organizations. This centers the discussion on ›racists‹ rather than ›racism‹ and on formal processes rather than interaction (e.g., the currently popular terms ›micro-aggression‹ and ›implicit bias‹ both focus on individual behavior). We hope to change this narrative by refocusing the discussion on the systemic racism embedded in social interaction. Our research is unique in treating interactional expectations as ›structures of racism‹ that are ›institutionalized‹ at the level of social interaction. Acting on these structures produces racist outcomes – *in what people do* – regardless of individual intent or awareness.

We expect that something similar is happening in Europe, as immigrants seeking to join new societies confront the cultural biases coded into the interactional expectations and social categories of the countries they now live in, and we invite researchers from around the world to join us in documenting this problem. However, we caution that the conceptions of Race and the tacit structures of interaction involved will not be the same across countries (or even regions).

In our book, we consider these issues in the context of a Black/White binary racial category system that developed in the early North American colonies in the late 1600s and persists today as an American tradition. We do not use the term tradition to refer to differences between societies, but rather to refer to differences within the US that are shaped by the 400-year domination of Black Americans by White Americans, and the resulting privileges that some 60% of White voters in the 2020 presidential election still claimed as their right. These traditions date from slavery, and the racial domination they encode still grounds US economy and society.

Suppression of minority scholarship is also an American tradition. The marginalization of pioneering research on Race and slavery contributed by Black and Jewish scholars, and the trend toward individualism and positivism in research and theory aligned with White ideals that silenced their voices, contribute to the invisibility of racism (Rawls/Duck 2019). Racism and a Race-based system of labor control and oppression sit at the foundation of US society. Treating Race as a side issue, of relevance only to minorities, has trivialized the centrality of the problem, hidden it from view, and allowed it to fester. In the US, those who cling to tradition and resist change are clinging to racist domination and White supremacy whether they realize it or not.

Misunderstandings of what Race is are also problematic. Race is a social category with no biological basis, a point made originally by Du Bois (1940). Until recently, his position was ignored, and Race treated as a natural scientific category. Societies generate the social categories members use to organize themselves and their experiences. As such, Race varies against the history and social organization of any given society or country. How Race categories developed to force Africans to labor as slaves for the benefit of their English owners in the early colonies (which we discuss below) shaped not only the development of conceptions of Race, but how tacit racism is embedded in the interactional expectations of Black and White Americans today.[5]

Our studies of how tacit racism has become institutionalized in interaction orders are situated within this exclusively American background. While most approaches to racism treat it either as a psychological effect of prejudice and hate, or as an aspect of formal structures, we argue that focusing on individuals and formal structures has had the effect of hiding dimensions of racism that are socially institutionalized in interaction, thus helping to perpetuate it.[6]

The solution we offer is to expose the interactional practices of systemic racism, as they are institutionalized in the daily practices of Americans, while calling attention to the Black and minority scholars whose insights we build on (including key Jewish scholars), and the innovative research practices they developed (ethnomethodology and conversation analysis EM/CA). We hope to produce awareness among majority thinkers of how racism shapes literally everything. Du Bois called the Black American awareness of racism »double consciousness«. In homage to him we call the awareness we hope our research will produce »White double consciousness«.

Our approach involves the claim that some phenomena popularly referred to as ›micro‹ and considered a matter of individual attitudes (›micro-aggressions‹ and/or ›implicit bias‹) actually involve structures of interactional expectation that are constitutive of self, social objects and meaning. There are no social selves/identities without society. The popular psychologizing of social action, and the treatment of actors and social objects/meanings as existing independent from interaction – has been an obstacle to getting this point across. The interaction that creates these objects happens *between* people – through seeable, hearable sounds and motions that occur in time and space that cannot be reduced to ideas and intentions. As social structures, interaction orders do not vary with the beliefs and attitudes of individuals, but rather involve structures of shared interactional expectation used by individuals to *make* meaning, self and social objects.

In using the term ›structures‹, we do not mean either ›macro‹ or ›micro‹ structures. We refer to the structure of interaction orders; sets of expectations that are constitutive of the objects and meanings they produce; something like the rules of a game. The argument parallels Chomsky and Wittgenstein who proposed grammars of syntax and »language games« respectively. Our approach expands the idea to grammars of action or culture (an idea first proposed by Garfinkel and Sacks; see Garfinkel [1967]2020 and Rawls 2019a, Rawls/Turowetz 2019).

Garfinkel (1963) proposed a set of reciprocity conditions – »trust conditions« – as a requirement for »orienting« these rules cooperatively. Working with Garfinkel, Sacks proposed that the rules for a speech exchange system could be identified empirically (Sacks 1962). We recognize Garfinkel and Sacks as pioneers with insights into the processes of exclusion that originated in their own experiences as Jewish minorities (Garfinkel [1947]2012; 1956). For Garfinkel these experiences took place in the American ›deep south‹ (North Carolina, Tennessee, Georgia, Texas, Mississippi) in the 1930's and 1940's where he was not considered White (Rawls/Whitehead/Duck 2020; Rawls forthcoming a).

5 When ›scientific‹ racism emerged in England and at the beginning of the Twentieth century it elaborated on earlier conceptions of Race that had originated in the US colonies.

6 Getting people focused away from individual ›good intentions‹ toward how society is structured is necessary. If the overall structure is fundamentally racist and exclusionary, then good intentions, no matter how good they make us feel about ourselves, will perpetuate systemic racism (as in Mannheim's ([1929]1936) example of how a person who gives money to a beggar is actually supporting the economic system that makes beggars out of people in the first place).

The ›trust conditions‹– constitutive conditions of reciprocity in interaction – which Garfinkel (1963) proposed, are roughly that participants must use the same definition of the situation, orient the same expectations or rules, extend benefit of the doubt to others, assume other participants are competent until they show they are not, confirm competent presentational work by others, and assume that others are doing the same and assuming the same of them. All of this occurs at an unconscious level of taken-for-granted, and thus largely hidden, practices.

Given these conditions, participants can orient shared rules in an infinite number of ways and innovate endlessly. But, for actions to be mutually understood they must be recognizable as ›moves‹ that orient the constitutive expectations of a particular game, or social/cultural practice. As Garfinkel ([1967]2020) argued, taking the other persons' pieces off the board in chess, or putting your mark outside the lines in tic-tac-toe, is not »playing the game« and people cannot play it with you if you do it. The same is true for the interaction orders of everyday life.

The interactional expectations we identify with tacit racism are institutionalized structures in this sense. They are expectations – constitutive grammars of interaction – that belong to a situation of social action such that they are ›constitutive‹ of *the recognizability of an action as action* of a particular sort (greetings, introductions, confirmations, instructions, etc.), for people who share those expectations. When actions do not meet the constitutive expectations of others, those others cannot recognize what has been done, or said. They will typically be troubled by this, and assign motive/blame to the individual who has done the unexpected thing. We find that this happens often between Races in the US because systemic inequality has led to the development of clashing interaction order expectations for Black and White Americans (Rawls/Duck 2020; Duck 2015; Duck 2016).

Failures at the level of interaction order are consequential not only because they result in loss of meaning, but because in violating ›trust conditions‹ they impact judgments of the competence of participants, their motivation and their trustworthiness, reducing the general willingness of people to try interacting again. Discovering and analyzing troubles at this level of interaction order requires detailed ethnographic observation supported by audio/video data, an interactional approach to self and identity, and an approach to meaning that does not focus on concepts, or comprehensive symbolic systems, but rather on how social categories are created and used *in-situ*, and on the ›order properties‹ of the ›sequences‹ of social action that people tacitly orient in making sense together.[7]

In what follows we offer some historical and theoretical background for our approach and then discuss three of our findings in the context of the historical oppression of Black labor in the US and the insights of Black and minority scholars about those conditions. First, we find that there are Race differences in interaction order expectations about what should be said and done when Americans first meet one another, in what we call »introductory sequences«; Second, we find that high status Black Americans experience frequent failures by others to recognize their legitimate identities, which we call »fractured reflections« of their presentations of self; and, third, we document a Black American practice we call »submissive civility«, a conception inspired by Du Bois' argument that the Black American value of submission to the good of the whole is a valuable democratic practice that could offset the undemocratic

7 »Order properties« is being used in both a literal and a technical sense here. Sequences have order properties such that whether something said or done comes first or send, for instance, has implications for what it means (Sacks/Schegloff/Jefferson 1974).

›White strong man ‹ ideal.[8] We analyze this practice through a Black/White Police/Citizen encounter that was video-recorded. Overall, we argue that Black Americans are not only the democratic heart of the US, but that they are consistently punished by the majority for their democratic behavior.

Background for our Conception of Interaction Orders of Race

Our conception of ›interaction orders of Race‹ builds on groundbreaking early work on Race and inequality by Harold Garfinkel (1940; [1942]1949; [1942]2012), in combination with Erving Goffman's conception of interaction orders (joined later by Harvey Sacks' examination of how Race categories are used in conversation). The research is also informed by W.E.B. Du Bois' (1903) foundational writings on Race, and Eric Williams' (1944) pioneering analysis of slavery and capitalism. Our theoretical formulation began in the 1970's (in consultation with Garfinkel) and continued through the 1980's with an initial focus on narratives about slavery (Rawls 1983; 1987; 1989; 1990). After 1987 the empirical research on Race differences in social interaction began. The intent has been to make interactional aspects of Race and inequality that ordinarily remain hidden and taken-for-granted visible. This has been done through an EM/CA inspired analysis of interaction and its expectations as revealed by troubles in interaction and narratives about those troubles. This approach – *to make the hidden visible* by focusing on problems and accounts – is the essence of Garfinkel's studies of ethno-methods in social interaction, which we treat as a method for producing a kind of ›double consciousness‹ about social practices.

While Du Bois is not generally thought of as a social interactionist, we argue that his work provides a starting point for analyzing racism in interaction, and for conceptualizing the Black American worldview and social expectations that developed in opposition to that racism (Rawls 2000). Our approach also acknowledges the contributions of approaches to Race and ›implicit bias‹ developed in Critical Race Theory (Bell 1973; Crenshaw/Gotanda/Peller/Thomas 1995, Delgado/Stefancic 1995), and the groundbreaking conception of ›intersectionality‹ developed in Black Feminist Thought (Crenshaw 1989; Spillers 1987; Hill-Collins 1990). However, our research focus is different and has independent origins. Whereas Critical Race Theory and Black Feminist Thought focus on experiential and structural implications of Race, gender and inequality, we explore how those inequalities have become institutionalized in the interactional structures of everyday social interaction – in typically unnoticed ways – such that interaction orders vary by Race identity and positioning in American society.

This dimension of racism in interaction has been largely overlooked by other approaches. The question we ask is how the inequalities that have been documented by Critical Race Theorists in the large-scale economic and social relations that characterize the separate worlds of Black and White Americans, and the differences in awareness of the relationship between individual selves and the larger community revealed by research on intersectionality, translate into interactional practices – into clashing ›interaction orders of Race‹. In doing so, we reprise a largely neglected interactional side of Du Bois' argument and connect it to Garfinkel's research.

8 ›Submissive civility‹ can be difficult for White people to understand. From a White perspective it has negative connotations of both ›femininity‹ and ›submission‹. But, why should anyone think it is inferior to be feminine? Or, why should anyone think that considering the good of the whole before one's own self-interest is either weak or negative? Black Americans do not think that being democratic and treating people as equals makes a man feminine. White men aggressively refusing to save American lives in the name of their own personal freedom during the COVID-19 pandemic gave us all an important illustration of this point.

While Du Bois (1903: 134) did not address the issue of interactional differences in detail, he did include communicative issues in his consideration of ›double consciousness‹, arguing that there are four levels of »race contact«: the first level is physical proximity, the second concerns economic relations, and the third, political relations. The fourth level, which he calls »less tangible«, involves interaction and conversation. Indeed, his own first experience of racial inequality is described in the context of a schoolroom interaction. It is this fourth level which we take up. According to Du Bois, this interactional level of Race contact consists of:

»[t]he interchange of ideas through conversation and conference, through periodicals and libraries, and, above all, the gradual formation for each community of that curious tertium quid which we call public opinion. Closely allied with this come the various forms of social contact in everyday life« (Du Bois 1903: 135).

Du Bois' treatment of interaction as an essential form of Race contact includes the role that daily interactional practices play in the formation of individual self-consciousness, in the achievement of mutual intelligibility, the creation of narratives, rumors, stereotypes, and finally, in the interplay between those institutional structures that result from, and then place constraints on, differences in communicative practices. Du Bois says:

»It is, in fine, the atmosphere of the land, the thought and feeling, the thousand and one little actions which go to make up life. In any community or nation it is these little things which are most elusive to the grasp and yet most essential to any clear conception of the group life taken as a whole« (Du Bois 1903: 147).

While interaction is essential, its »elusive« workings, he says, are *curiously invisible*. This, for Du Bois, »is peculiarly true of the South«. Describing interactions in the south during the first Jim Crow period, Du Bois (1903: 148) emphasizes the subtlety of the forces at work, which are so unobtrusive, he says, that »the casual observer visiting the South sees at first little of this«. People are quite literally living in different socially constructed worlds. Du Bois (1903: 148) says that the visitor: »realizes at last that silently, resistlessly, the world about flows by him in two great streams; they ripple on in the same sunshine, they approach and mingle their waters in seeming carelessness, then they divide and flow wide apart«. Between these two worlds, according to Du Bois, there are almost no points of intimate or intellectual contact:

»Now if one notices carefully one will see that between these two worlds, despite much physical contact and daily intermingling, there is almost no community of intellectual life or point of transference where the thoughts and feelings of one race can come into direct contact and sympathy with thoughts and feelings of the other« (Du Bois 1903: 149).

The lack of close contact that began during reconstruction is different from the close daily contact that occurred between Races in the south before the Civil War, and Du Bois dates the separation between Races to the Reconstruction period. C. Van Woodward (1955), in his famous book *The Strange Career of Jim Crow*, insists that racial segregation was an invention of the Jim Crow period, and not part of »southern tradition« as those who have resisted civil rights for Black Americans claim. Jim Crow, and its modern iteration in mass incarceration (Alexander 2011) and the *Chokehold* (Butler 2017), have effectively created and sustained two separate worlds, blocking Black Americans from participation in the White world, while requiring the pretense that their submission to Jim Crow is voluntary, and that they are full participants.

In his first publication, Garfinkel (1940) made the hidden, taken-for-granted character of this complicity the central feature of his approach, pointing out how the tacit social structures of Jim Crow broke down when two Black bus riders made them explicit by refusing to participate in their own humiliation. Making racism explicit undermines the polite surface veneer behind which it hides, which is one reason why the prospect of Black equality is such a fearful thing to those still wedded to traditional Jim Cow assumptions and practices.

The problem, as Du Bois eloquently develops it, includes the idea that not being able to achieve mutual reciprocity and equality with a group of others, particularly through close daily contact, is damaging to the development of both self and mutual understanding.

>»In a world where it means so much to take a man by the hand and sit beside him, to look frankly into his eyes and feel his heart beating with red blood; in a world where a social cigar or a cup of tea together means more than legislative halls and magazine articles and speeches, one can imagine the consequences of the almost utter absence of such social amenities between estranged races, whose separation extends even to parks and street-cars« (Du Bois 1903: 150).

While Black and White Americans may occupy the same physical space, we rarely occupy the same interactional space. Because interactional expectations developed separately for 160 years, displays of social behavior by members of one Race can look deviant to members of the other. Interaction orders demand compliance with expected use, which is constitutive of the social production of self, social objects and meaning (Goffman 1959; 1961; 1963; Rawls 1987; 1989). Actions within a practice can constitute recognizable social identities and objects that cannot exist without it: But only when they orient expectations in recognizable ways. Because the expectations of the two interaction orders are not the same, White and Black Americans often violate each other's expectations and the resulting judgments of incompetence have a moral tone.

Black Americans experience an added difficulty: as selves who must interact in two conflicting interaction orders, they are held to two conflicting sets of demands. In order to recognizably construct practices in one interaction order, they often must violate the expectations of the other. These conflicting interactional requirements confront the African American self in American society on a daily basis. A degree of social/moral tension greater than the challenge of having one's role or identity differentially shaped and valued from situation to situation is involved. White Americans tend to be unaware of this. In spite of their lack of awareness, however, White academics have been confident in dismissing the insights of Black scholars.

The Invention of Race in the US

The argument, as we make it, is grounded in a Race-based labor system designed by an English colonial empire in the 1600s that shaped the US economy, politics, law and social structure, and persisted across 400 years to become institutionalized in contemporary interaction. Race was invented to support the system of colonial labor in the American colonies when it confronted a sudden scarcity of unfree English/Irish labor (due to the start of industrialization in England around 1660), just as unfree African labor became plentiful (after the treaty of Westminster gave England access to the African slave trade in 1654). This, according to Theodore Allen (1994; 1997), gave birth to the modern idea of Race and explains why English colonies in North America developed a Black/White Race binary while Spanish and Portuguese colonies did not. It has little to do with the colonizing culture and everything to do with labor control issues.

Before this, Race categories were not used in the colonies, or anywhere else in the world. Previous references were to color, physical description, religion, nationality and culture. So, in an important sense *the birth of the modern conception of Race occurred in the US because early plantation owners needed their newly freed English/Irish laborers to begin suppressing their former African workmates*, with whom they had previously been allied. The new category ›White‹ was used to encourage that suppression, a development that became so popular that White Americans are now, according to Jonathan Metzl (2019), *Dying of Whiteness*.[9]

Social categories, and expectations about their use, constrain possible identities and situate people in a status quo. New uses of categories can create a new status quo, or challenge an old one. That the US American Black/White binary developed to serve the purpose of suppressing Black laborers is a moral loading that is inherent in the categories. A person who says they are »proud to be White« invokes that moral loading whether they intend to or not. ›Whiteness‹ has meaning only against that binary. Being »proud to be Black« has very different moral loading.[10]

In considering how and why this Race category system has persisted over four centuries and through the development of science, industry, and an allegedly ›free‹ labor system (that continues to suppress Black workers), we invoke Durkheim's ([1893]1933) distinction between consensus-based social forms that are organized on the basis of traditional beliefs and categories (that resist change), and dynamic practice-based social forms that can self-regulate without consensus in contexts of diversity and specialization. This is not a distinction between the US and other societies. Rather, we distinguish between places/situations within the US that cling to traditions based on slavery and Jim Crow segregation, and others, where people have begun to embrace new forms of self-regulating practice-based science, technology and occupations. The latter have multiplied in cities and on the coasts, where populations are more diverse, and specialized occupations have concentrated. In places where resistance to racial equality is strongest, the diverse populations and specialized occupations that generate self-regulating practices have not developed to the same degree, leaving those places dependent on consensus.[11]

This leaves the US divided between two forms of society with conflicting moral and organizational requirements. Often referred to as a »culture war« we treat it as a conflict between two ways of even having a culture/society (Rawls 2021). Traditional consensus-based societies and businesses not only tolerate inequality, they can thrive on hierarchies within and boundaries between themselves and others. However, in diverse specialized societies and occupations/sciences, where self-regulating practices predominate and experts are essential, the reciprocity requirements of practices – the ›trust conditions‹ – require equality/justice within the practice (Rawls 2019b). While people may adopt a *belief* in justice, unless they do the hard work of rooting out injustice, residual consensus will remain embedded in new

9 Metzl (2019) documents how the mythology of Whiteness encourages White Americans to support the interests of the rich in ways that lower their own quality of life and health; increases the proliferation of guns and gun violence (including high rates of suicide among White men), defund schools in an effort to hurt minority students, cut taxes for the rich in ways that strip infrastructure budgets, cut social services and vote against affordable health care.

10 In every country there will be ordinary words that have such moral loadings that need to be explored.

11 It is a sad fact today that tax surpluses from Blue states need to be given to Red states to make up their budget deficits, while the voters in Red states complain that their tax dollars are supporting Black Americans in big cities, and vote to cut their taxes even more. Red states are not supporting Blue states. Red states continue cutting their own social services because they believe this. It is a vicious cycle supported by false beliefs. If Blue states refused to support them most Red states would immediately go bankrupt.

self-regulating orders of practice – such that a belief in justice exists alongside tacit forms of injustice that contradict the social requirements of those practices and keep them from working for all people. This is why a failure to root out the racist foundations of US social structure have been so devastating.

Some places/situations openly embrace a tradition of racism. Others reject that tradition in principle, but because it is so deeply embedded, have not yet been able to reject it in practice. Consequently, while parts of the US that still rely on traditional consensus are more overtly racist, in more diverse and educated communities lingering injustices have become tacit, and tacit racism has become the predominate form perpetuating racism in those places.

Durkheim's classic ([1893]1933) explanation of this clash between traditional consensus and self-regulation is one of the minority insights that have been lost because majority scholars insisted on misinterpreting him as a consensus theorist when he argued against the need for consensus in modernity. One reason White scholars might have missed the point of Durkheim's critique, is that in ordinary times they live in a world where most things accord with their beliefs and challenges their majority views are rare. It feels like consensus. By contrast, minority scholars and women confront constant challenges to the validity of even their own personal experiences, giving them an awareness that there is no consensus holding things together.

All societies have some consensus and some self-regulation. The difference is in the proportion. As societies develop a significant proportion of self-regulating practices, they often still retain enough residual consensus to prevent equality and justice from actualizing – even when people fervently *believe* in justice. This is problematic because self-regulation in diverse modern contexts requires more cooperation and flexibility than consensus permits. Without an explicit program of moral education, Durkheim (1925) feared that traditional injustices would remain entrenched and societies would take problematic abnormal forms.

The US currently finds itself such an ›abnormal form‹. We live in a type of society that requires justice in its scientific and technical practices and between members of a diverse population – but we are without actual justice – and we have not adopted a system of moral/civic education that could solve the problem. In fact, we have been retreating toward a consensus-based educational system that strengthens tradition and weakens self-regulation.

Once a society has diversified and become dependent on science and technology a strong traditional consensus is a problem. Forms of interaction that require equality cannot succeed between unequal categories of people. The illusion of fairness can be maintained for majority people (who can often manage to talk only to people in their category), while at the same time inequality prevents successful interaction across Race. Given this illusion, talk about racism rarely occurs in day-to-day interaction and when it does is problematic, which leads White people to avoid it (DiAngelo 2018). Thus, the majority have the illusion of justice, when the whole system is built on racism.

The excluded tend to be alone in being aware of this. When their voices are eliminated, as they have been, the illusion that there is no problem can be maintained. The theory and methods that support this illusion of fairness are hegemonic, and minority voices that criticize that hegemony (Du Bois; Durkheim; Williams; Garfinkel; Goffman; Sacks), have been marginalized by a combination of misinterpretation and outright suppression of their work. In challenging this hegemony, and arguing that an interactional approach that treats order as constitutive of meaning is necessary to document systemic racism, we build on Du Bois' insight that after reconstruction (after 1876) US society developed two separate streams that flow side-by-side with little contact, and that only the excluded, who develop »double consciousness«, are aware of this.

It is our position that in a diverse society riddled with systemic racism, and given an academic context that has excluded minority voices and suppressed studies of interaction, huge amounts of tacit racism can be present without majority people being aware of it. Consequently, when Black Americans describe their experiences with racism, most White Americans have not recognized what they are talking about and dismiss their claims. The extraordinary summer of 2020 witnessed a change as White Americans began waking up to the Trump administrations' overtly racist policies/actions (although only 4 in 10 rejected this racism at the polls). But unless we get a better grip on tacit aspects of the problem quickly – interest in it will fade once the more overt aspects of racism become less public – they are no longer so obvious to the majority.

Race Differences in Expectations about ›Introductory Sequences‹

When people meet each other for the first time they have basic expectations about what information should be shared and how it will be shared. Names are usually exchanged first, and colleagues at the same company might identify the part of the company they work in. But it turns out that beyond those basics, in the US the expectations vary so much by Race that ›introductory sequences‹ between Races are typically fraught with misunderstanding. In the early 1990s, narratives about »nosy White people« relayed by Black colleagues and students, alerted us to problems at the very beginning of interracial interactions in ›introductory sequences‹. White Americans were routinely asking for information that Black Americans considered private. This was concerning, as it would likely prevent friendships from developing even between Black and White people who wanted to form them. White people we talked to at the time had no idea what this narrative meant, while almost every Black person we asked recognized the narrative, laughed and then told us a story about their experiences with »nosy White people«.[12]

Garfinkel (2002) called this method of giving a story to get a story a »coathanger«: the story becomes a coathanger for the person you interview to hang their own matching story on. The selection of what story matches the one told by the researcher is done by the interviewee, which is a good exploratory method when a researcher is not a member of a practice. Once we understood more about the narratives, we realized they were evidence of a pervasive phenomenon that should be examined in detail. The challenge was that ›introductory sequences‹ between the same two people only happen once. We needed to be present at such meetings to collect data.

Also, because interaction order expectations are largely tacit, only coming to consciousness when they fail, we realized that the narratives we had collected were likely generated by *failures*, representing the imputing blame and motive phase of post interaction troubles. This left open the question of what success would look like if two Black speakers did not violate one another's expectations? Or, two White speakers?

We did manage to observe a few such introductions ethnographically. But they don't happen often and go by quickly. We decided to make them happen in a setting we controlled and asked for student volunteers. The challenge was to create a context in which ›introductory sequences‹ would occur as naturally as possible so that we could record them on video and analyze how they were organized across an actual interaction. We asked for student volunteers, got their permission to be interviewed on video-tape, and sat them together in a room and then left them to introduce themselves while they waited for us to

12 Waverly Duck, an undergraduate at the time, joined the team in 1996 and has been part of the work ever since.

return. We matched some students in same Race pairs and others in mixed Race pairs. However, we invited only female students, making all pairs female/female, to prevent gender differences from complicating the interactions.

The set-up was designed to allow for the introductory talk Black and White speakers prefer to occur without prompting.[13] We recorded many such sequences. While each is different in details, we were able to identify preferred characteristics of what we call the Black introductory type and the White introductory type that are constitutive of mutual understanding for those familiar with the expectations, while producing problems for those who are not. We also held dozens of large interracial focus groups, workshops and community meetings about these recordings during which we discussed our analysis and collected feedback.[14]

In the original paper (Rawls 2000) and in our book we reproduce transcripts of ›introductory sequences‹ accompanied by an in-depth turn-by-turn analysis of what the order properties involved reveal about Black and White interaction order preferences. We identify a typical White/White introductory sequence that proceeds by asking questions about category information like where a person lives, works, goes to school, their marital status, whether they have children etc. White Americans prefer to *ask and be asked* for this information, and do not generally volunteer information not asked for. Black speakers, by contrast, prefer not to be asked such status and category questions, and prefer to *volunteer* the information they do give. To say that these are preferences means that the occurrence or non-occurrence of asking for category information in the respective interaction orders is meaningful, and that assessments of moral character and mutual commitment are based on whether and how these expectations are fulfilled.

The big point here is that the implications of the same conversational ›move‹ are different in a Black introductory sequence than they are in a White introductory sequence. White speakers *should* ask category questions. If they *don't* it means something and is ›accountable‹ (they are held accountable for the lack). Black speakers *should not* ask. If they *do* it means something and is ›accountable‹. When White Americans talk to Black Americans, who do not answer and ask such questions, it can trigger narratives like »Black people are rude« and »they were holding back, I don't think they liked me«. White Americans are apt to feel that they tried their best to be friendly and were rejected. Sometimes they conclude that Black people did not like them because they are White – triggering the narrative that Black people are racist.

For Black Americans such category information is personal. It also quickly reveals social status – which Black Americans avoid – instead focusing on topics drawn from the immediate setting. We find that this does not vary by social class as many scholars expect. If anything, high status Black Americans are more scrupulous about reserving such information about themselves.

This clash explains the Black narrative »White people are nosy«. The Black American introductory sequence prefers to proceed on the basis of topics available in the local setting, while avoiding category identifiers that reveal social status and inequality. The emphasis is on what can be seen, heard, smelled, etc., in the immediate surroundings: on ›personhood‹ instead of social status identifiers. *The Black preference is the mirror opposite of the White preference.*

Avoiding categories leads to intimacy among African Americans, whereas it is treated as a way of

13 The videos of ›introductory sequences‹ were made for a 1994 project in which student volunteers participated (discussed in more detail in Rawls 2000; Rawls/Duck 2020).

14 The analysis went on for six years. The recordings were played in class, for focus groups and alumni groups and at public forums.

avoiding intimacy by White Americans. Maynard and Zimmerman (1984: 304f.), for instance, found that talk focused on the immediate setting seemed to function as a technique for avoiding intimacy and maintaining anonymity in conversations between White college students. By contrast, African Americans in our data report that talk focused on immediate surroundings is respectful of them as persons, and thus preferred. Furthermore, the quest for category identifiers by White participants is treated by Black Americans as devaluing their personhood.

Expectations about this are not the same in Europe, where the White American practice is often considered pushy and rude.

The differences can be both confusing and upsetting. Whereas the preferred White sequence has several clearly identifiable elements that usually come up (residence, job, education, marriage, children), there are no such identifiable elements of a preferred Black American introductory sequence because of its focus on the immediate setting. Avoiding the use of stereotypical identities and categories, participants are expected to talk about things in the setting, such as: »You in the class?« »What's this interview about?« »How you doing?« This preference preserves equality and dignity against the inequalities encountered by Black Americans daily in White American society.

In not relying on category identification as the foundation for building new relationships, Black Americans are engaging in a purer form of reciprocity that promotes equality by relying more exclusively on the self-organizing mutual exhibition of preferences and reciprocities face-to-face and move-by-move, and less on category information. Whereas the African American preference avoids information that would locate persons in a social hierarchy – where most Black Americans are at a disadvantage because of systemic racism – White ›introductory sequences‹ focus on category information that places people into status and role categories. As Goffman (1959) maintained, the meaning of words and actions depends on the *definition of the situation* and the *role* or *identity* a speaker has within that definition. *This gives status and stereotypes relevance* in ways that bring racial inequalities into interaction from the start. White speakers focus on getting information to settle such identity issues – without being aware of its relationship to systemic racism – while Black speakers work to minimize the relevance of stereotypes and unequally distributed identities: in the process neutralizing inequalities.

»Fractured Reflections« of High Status Black American Presentations of Self

400 years of systemic racism have created a White racial framing of American life (Feagin 2014). Living within this frame Americans – Black and White – learn not to expect to see Black men and women in high status locations and identities. It should be obvious that this racialized way of ›seeing‹ Black people would impact on their ability to perform high status identities. But the general belief seems to be that success can neutralize racism for high status Black Americans.

Our first observation of Fracturing occurred in 2003 when the authors witnessed a puzzling interaction in which a Black man who was confronted with a failure to recognize his competent performance of his high status identity refused to acknowledge that failure. After much discussion and the collection of additional instances, we realized that we had witnessed something important. As with our other findings, it took extensive discussion and observation to achieve an understanding of this phenomenon from both a White and a Black perspective.

Black men and women are constantly confronted by failures to recognize their high status identities (not only by White people). However, they often do not either recognize or repair these failures. Nor do they respond the way the literature on the internalization of negative self-image would predict (Fanon 1952).

Instead, they often refuse to acknowledge the legitimacy of those who denied them recognition. They were also talking to each other about these occurrences.

We found that this interaction order preference for refusing to acknowledge such failures, combined with systemic racialized expectations about status and identity was producing what we call »fractured reflections« of self-presentation, a type of interactional event we argue is frequently experienced by Black Americans (Rawls/Duck 2017). Approaches that assume a colonial, post-colonial model of Race expect a loss of self-esteem and/or attempts to repair presentation of self that were not occurring. Approaches that treat self and identity as given prior to interaction also miss the significance of this interactional event.

As with the ›introductory sequences‹ discussed in the prior section, our data collection focused on narratives about the Fracturing event. Like the experiences Du Bois drew on for his conception of ›double consciousness‹, ›fractured reflections‹ are a well-known ›experience‹ that high status Black men and women tell each other stories about. But they remain unknown to the White Americans who produce them by failing to recognize legitimate Black identities.

To get more detailed descriptions of the existence and contours of the phenomenon we recorded in-depth interviews with 38 high status Black men who were top executives, collecting and transcribing their narratives about Fracturing. We focused on Black men for two reasons: First, Black men are the targets of the most extreme stereotypes about violence and crime, which we had good reason to believe followed them into high status positions; Second, one of the authors is a Black man who had better access to men to discuss this sensitive topic. As with our earlier study of ›introductory sequences‹, which focused only on women, we decided to avoid confusing gender with Race by focusing only on men. All 38 of the high status Black men we interviewed recognized our narrative about a Fractured Reflection and told us stories about their own experiences with it. O ur original paper (Rawls/Duck 2017) reproduced transcripts of these narratives, and our analysis establishes that Fracturing occurs frequently, provides a description of how it occurs, and, takes up implications. Here we offer only a short description.

During any interaction, people are expected to present an identity they have a right to and that is appropriate to the situation they are in (Goffman 1959). A Black corporate Vice-President we call Robert giving his administrative assistant a task is an exercise of appropriate identity. There is an essential moment in the process when a presentation of identity/self has been made and it is the turn of Other(s) present to recognize, respond to, and ratify that presentation. The integrity, legitimacy, the very existence of the self *as presented*, depends on (and can be changed by) that response. In Robert's narrative, he describes how, when he asks his assistant to do something, she goes behind his back to ask other people (including the company President) if she should do what he says. This is a Fracturing event that Robert refuses to acknowledge to her – but it leads him not to trust, even though he believes that she wants him to succeed. He calls her actions »insubordinate«, interpreting her ›checking‹ as evidence that she does not think he is competent.

Fracturing occurs when the person presenting self, in this case Robert, is given back a reflection of their identity performance that is not recognizable to them (indicating that the Other did not recognize the appropriateness of their identity, or their competence in presenting it), and this happens not only once, but so often that over time they learn not to treat it as accurate feedback that they are doing something wrong.

Typically, we expect a presentation of self that is not confirmed to be repaired by the presenter. For Black Americans, however, there are so many situations in which, what Joe Feagin (2014) calls a »White racial frame«, prevents Others from recognizing their competent high status identities, that they learn to ignore the problem. Failures to recognize and ratify competent presentations of self, reported frequently by the high status Black men interviewed, threaten to strip them of the social identities they are entitled to, and the dignity, power, and authority associated with those identities. Not only is this an injustice in the conventional sense, it violates the »trust conditions« (Garfinkel 1963), and equality (Durkheim [1893]1933) necessary to make self and social objects together in societies where self-regulating practices predominate.

The ›Non-Recognition‹ of identity experienced by Black Americans (and White women in high status positions) threatens the process of sense and self-making, and led the Black men we studied to take the evasive action we call a »Null-Response«.[15] Because these men can retreat into their own Black interaction order to confirm their sense of self they are not destroyed by Non-Recognition. But it makes their jobs more difficult and they are constantly faced with inappropriate responses that test their creativity and ingenuity. While the high status Black Americans who have this experience are well aware of it, when it occurs, the White Americans who initiate the Fracturing typically do not understand why their Black friend or boss is doing a Null-Response, or how upsetting it is.

When Black Americans say they experience racism on the job *every day* this is one of the things they mean. There is no place in White American society where a Black American, however accomplished, can count on having their competence and qualifications recognized.

15 This lack of response is also familiar to the White female author as a preservation technique. But it is doubtful if many White women manage to use it with any consistency.

»Submissive Civility«: An Orientation of Black Masculinity to Oppression and Inequality

Du Bois (1890) argued that being submissive to the good of the whole is an important strength highly valued by Black Americans that is not valued enough by White Americans. He referred to the Black ideal in terms of a ›submissive man‹ who is submissive to the good of the whole, contrasting it with what he called the ›White strong man‹ ideal. Du Bois' offered Jefferson Davis, president of the confederacy during the Civil War, as an example of a ›strong man‹. Davis, who sacrificed the country to serve his own interest in continuing slavery was not orienting the good of the whole. Today Donald Trump represents the same willingness to sacrifice others. In the context of the 2020 presidential election, we offer Joe Biden as an example of a ›submissive man‹ who puts the good of the whole before his own interest. The ›strong man‹ ideal does not represent strength, but wanton self-interest. Similarly, in being submissive to the good of the whole the ›submissive man‹ is strong. The labels do not carry literal meaning.

A just social contract requires citizens to give up some things for the good of the whole. As Hobbes ([1651]1909) initially argued, it is the exchange of the full freedom of animals – to eat and be eaten – for the benefits of living in a society. Debates since Hobbes have mainly been over what a fair social contract would look like, not over the need for one. The question is why so many people revere the ›strong man‹ who takes whatever he can from the whole, while feeling that there is something less admirable in ›submission‹ to the good of the whole.

Given the existence of two such conflicting ideals, we expected that there would be empirical evidence of this in interaction that would be observable as clashes in interactional preferences. It also seemed likely that ›submissive civility‹ would lead to trouble in inter-racial interactions, when the actions of

Black men (in particular) in being ›submissive‹ were misunderstood by White Americans.

While writing up our research on ›fractured reflections‹ around 2015 we observed several interactional responses to racist violence and threat by Black men and women that exhibited a cooperative posture we thought could best be described in Du Bois' terms. After collecting ethnographic observations, we realized there might be recorded instances in archival video of Black/White police/citizen encounters that would facilitate a detailed sequential analysis.

In our original article (Rawls/Duck/Turowetz 2018) we introduced the interactional practice we call »submissive civility«, in the context of video data from a Black/White police-citizen encounter. We reproduced a partial transcript of a 16-minute video accompanied by a turn-by-turn CA analysis of the sequential structure of the interaction. The transcript is long and the analysis extensive. Here we summarize only one part of that analysis. The Black male citizen caught up in the encounter, in trying to establish his identity as a resident of the house and city neighborhood where the police approach him, adopts a submissive and cooperative posture. We argue that this is a preferred resource for Black Americans in situations where they are confronted by racialized domination and threat.[16] Because it clashes with the individualistic White American ideal, however, this preference for ›submissive civility‹, which relies on heightened-cooperation and formal respect, is often misunderstood by White Americans, *who tend to interpret social action as if White interactional preferences were the only legitimate expectations*. The two police officers wonder aloud why this Black man is being so cooperative and suggest that he is trying to hide something. That he is trying to show them everything so that they will not suspect him does not occur to them: It is not a practice they recognize.

While ›submissive civility‹ is a Black American preference with strong democratic virtues, the police in our data do not recognize either its preferred status, or its legitimacy. Instead, they treat this Black citizen's cooperation as grounds for suspicion and a pretext for arrest, enforcing White interaction order preferences as if they were legal requirements.

In a democratic society, *access* to situated identities – like ›neighborhood resident‹ – should be equally available by Race. Because of racial oppression and exclusion, however, African Americans are not expected to hold legitimate identities in many situations. When identity problems do occur, interaction order differences in how Black and White Americans try to resolve these problems can create additional misunderstandings.

›Submissive civility‹, is being smart, polite, and civil, going above and beyond what is required to avoid trouble.[17] For Black men, particularly in talking to White police officers, this can be challenging. We find several identity issues at work in the encounter that have particular relevance to how the event unfolds. The Black citizen resident (CR) could not get the officers to recognize him as a person who belongs at his mother's house: a common problem for Black men that is a Fractured Reflection of their identity. Instead, the officers orient a criminal/illegitimate identity from the beginning; a racial stereotype CR refuses to accept. There is a second identity issue working at a deeper level of reciprocity failure. The officers do not see the ›ordinary reasonableness‹ of CR's actions. If he does live here, and is waiting for his mom, his actions are *all* reasonable, and due to the public nature of the case *we know they were*. But the

16 Gabbidon (2007) has argued that Du Bois also laid the foundations for a sociological approach to criminology.

17 Fassin (2013: 93) found that Arab/Black youth adopt a similar submissive posture when confronted by the French police.

two White officers (PO2 and PO1) keep saying that the situation and his behavior are strange.

From the White male officer's (PO2) initial attempt at ›humor‹ (line 33), which makes fun of CR for trying to break into his mother's house, we see that from the officer's perspective this ›Black guy‹, was acting in a way he did not consider ›normal‹ from the beginning. But he can't arrest him without a reason: a pretext. Resisting is a preferred pretext (Bittner 1967; 1973; Chevigny 1969). However, CR will be ›submissively‹ civil, but he will not laugh at a joke that demeans his identity, and it is unreasonable to expect him to do so. While the opening ›joke‹ may (or may not) have been intended as an ›icebreaker‹, it positions CR as a deviant, and PO2 told the ›joke‹ and laughed at it (by himself) four times over the course of the incident. Regardless of the officer's initial intent, this is a serious failure of reciprocity (Jefferson 1979), indicating that PO2 is not engaged in mutuality with CR: He is being disrespectful, and not responsive to how CR feels about it.

Already, in the first seconds of the interaction the parties can be seen orienting two different definitions of the situation, a misalignment that continues. PO2 projects a ›humorous‹ conversational course that CR refuses to follow, instead interpreting the situation as serious. If PO2 had wanted to produce a problem in the interaction (so that he can accuse CR of resisting, which he later does), he has been effective. If he was hoping to communicate, then he has undercut his own purpose.

At line 33 PO2 indicates that it seems funny that he has accused a man of breaking into his mother's house and, that when the police get there, he is still sitting on the porch. As PO2 says several times over the course of the interaction, it is a very unlikely scenario. Nevertheless, he will continue to say this and laugh about it four separate times as he questions CR in front of his house. CR's responses display that the situation does not seem funny to him. It is in fact happening to him. He told the first officer who he was and she indicated that she was satisfied. But, after the two officers conferred at the police car, PO2 approached for the first time and opened with the ›joke‹ that CR treats as an accusation. CR's responses indicate that he treats the encounter as having immediately become much more serious.

#2: Greensboro Part Two: PO2 Body Cam time Code: 01:34

33 PO2: What are you doing breaking into your mom's house?
34 (0.6)
35 CR: I'm not breaking in here.
36 (0.2)
37 O2: Uh(h) heh huh heh
38 (1.4)
39 PO2: What's with the shovel?
40 (0.6)
41 CR: The shovel was here before.=I just picked it up off the yard when I got here sir.
42 (0.6)
43 PO2: Yeah they said you tried to open the garage door with it.
44 (0.5)
45 CR: No I didn't.=I want- all- this is what I did.=This is what I did.
46 (3.7) ((CR walks over to garage door and demonstrates))
47 CR: This is what I did.
48 (1.1)
49 CR: I got to make sure the dog wasn't in the- uh: garage. That's all I tried to do.
50 (1.4.)
51 CR: That's all I tried to do.
52 (0.7)
53 PO2: Alright.
54 (0.4)

After a pause in which CR does not respond to his laughter (line 38), PO2 asks another question hearable as an accusation, »What's with the shovel?« (line 39), and CR treats it as such. In asking for an account for the shovel, PO2 implies that CR's possession of it is problematic and requires justification. The female officer had introduced the shovel in the context of her description of the citizen call to the police. But, PO2 asks a direct question: »What's with the shovel?« (line 39). As Bolden and Robinson (2011: 96) observe, questions that solicit accounts and/or justifications embody »a type of suspension of ›trust conditions‹ (Garfinkel 1963) by claiming that [the speaker] cannot make ›typical‹ sense of the causes of, or motives for, the event«.

CR responds with an account of what he did with the shovel (line 41). PO2 follows this with a more explicit accusation – the third from CR's perspective: »Yeah they said you tried to open the garage door with it« (line 43). But, this time PO2 does so indirectly, reporting the speech of an absent third party, likely another reference to the citizen caller: »they said«. In response, CR makes an explicit denial, »No I didn't« (line 45), followed by *a physical reenactment* of »what I did« (line 46), during which he gets off the porch, walks to the garage, and then returns to the porch. The reenactment is accompanied by an account: »I got to make sure« (line 49), that refers to his concern about whether his dog is locked in the garage. CR's turn-final »That's all I tried to do« (line 49), which he repeats (line 51), is an extreme case formulation (Pomerantz 1986): *All* places a maximal boundary around his actions, and the intent behind them, as does his subsequent turn, »[t]hat's it. Nothin' more nothing less« (line 55).

We refer to this reenactment as a sequence of ›submissive civility‹ in the face of a series of what CR treats as accusations – all following an initial misalignment occasioned by PO2's ›joke‹. The reenactment is elaborate: going above and beyond what he is asked to avoid trouble.

In a democratic society, ›submissive civility‹ *should* be preferred. By contrast, the ›strong man‹ ideal aligns with the racist/sexist/classist ideology that those who can't ›pull themselves up by their own bootstraps‹, don't deserve voting rights, health care, food, shelter, or education; that those who are different weaken society; that government should let the strong do what they choose to the weak; and that White people ›have made the most important contributions‹ to the country and its culture. This undemocratic ideology equates contributions to society with the ›strong man‹; freedom with the unrestricted right to dominate others; and considers the weak and poor unimportant except insofar as they can be forced to make profits for the rich (Mayer 2016). It is important also to point out that in the US the so-called strong men at the top, who are said to have made it on their own, have always had others to pull their ›bootstraps‹ up for them: first through literal slave labor and now through forms of labor that pay so little that people can be forced to work under any conditions.

Du Bois offered submission to democratic principles as a counter-narrative to this hyper-individualistic ›American Dream‹, ›bootstraps‹, ›free market‹ ideology: positioning Black Americans as the democratic heart of the nation. They still are. For democracy to work, each individual must commit to the principle that equality and democracy are more important than any individual's self-interest: The modern civic person must be submissive before the principle of civil democratic publics, and the interests of the ›strong man‹ must bow before the general interest – or there is no democracy. In this regard, Du Bois proposed that *the Black American grasp of democracy is stronger than the White American grasp*, precisely because the Black American *experience of racial oppression*, and the development of a »double consciousness« about that oppression, creates a commitment to equality and democracy among Black Americans. We argue that ›submissive civility‹ exemplifies that commitment.

How will the Situation in Europe and Elsewhere Be Different?

One of the warnings to take from the US experience is that Race and exclusion can be efficiently exploited to support an anti-democratic agenda in ways that can seem reasonable on the surface. Every social group has some apparently reasonable complaints: They have been left out of the economy; they don't want their ›freedoms‹ impinged on; they don't want their taxes to support people they don't approve of; they don't want their way of life to change. Finding the systemic racism hidden behind these complaints requires a broad consideration of how the ›way of life‹ being defended and the freedoms being claimed not only originate in inequality, and in case of the US in slavery and segregation, but continue to be maintained by racial inequality: That ›our‹ traditions in the US have always meant White traditions that actively exclude minorities; that the people ›we don't approve of‹ are Black and Brown; that the reasons we don't approve of them involve false stereotypes that rationalize slavery and the suppression of Black civil rights; that White freedoms have never been available to Black Americans; that the wealth and privilege of White workers still comes at the expense of the mass incarceration and under-employment of Black and Brown workers, which is why they need social support; and, finally that the reason White people feel threatened by the prospect of racial equality is that it not only requires giving up those unfair and unearned traditions and privileges, but will also require finally acknowledging that the whole thing has been built on racism all along.

What had been invisible until recently is how false fronts backed by *Dark Money* (Mayer 2016) that funded the rise of a radical Right in the US had organized to exploit those ›reasonable‹ complaints. It turns out that powerful actors have infiltrated universities with false ›science‹ designed to convince White people that their real complaints were not about the poor jobs and bad pay they actually have, but about Black people and foreigners who they are told have taken their jobs. These false fronts push false stereotypes to hide the very real inequalities among White Americans that have been increasing year-by-year through legislation supported by the same dark money that has stripped American citizens of rights, social programs, education and jobs. The apparent reasonableness of these complaints has also been supported by ways of speaking publicly about racism through ›dog-whistles‹ (coded language) that can only be heard by those who are aware of the hidden racist positions (Anderson 2016; 2018; Haney-Lopez 2013).

Each country, or political/economic area, should expect to find that it has developed similar problems of its own – even if they are just beginning. But, in each country the process will work differently – and what it takes to make it visible and reveal those who are manipulating things behind the scenes – will be different in each case. It will require a focus on the details of interaction that can make what has been taken-for-granted visible.

In areas still organized by traditional consensus, Race and exclusion should be more obvious and overt than in diverse places where traditional consensus has begun to be replaced by self-regulating practices. This does not mean that there is less systemic racism in places with more diversity, however. In the latter, overt racism will likely have gone underground and become embedded in ordinary interactional practices as tacit racism. Because these diverse places have an even greater need for equality and reciprocity to support self-regulating practices – it is precisely here that racism can do the most damage.

Every colonial empire was structured differently in how it used racism and exclusion to support labor relations, and every country or area will have its own unique hidden dynamics. Sometimes the response to oppression by minorities will have taken the form of a »colonial mentality«, as described by Franz Fanon

(1952), in which the excluded emulate their colonizers and collude in their own suppression. This response was sometimes characteristic of the public responses of Black Americans in the Jim Crow South in the US before WWII (although according to Du Bois it never accurately conveyed their private response). In other cases, the response may have led to the development of alternate forms of identity and social solidarity – like the ones we found in Black and White interaction orders in the US – because assimilation was not either possible or desirable.

All of these issues will be filtered through a ›color‹ lens that sometimes operates more like the US binary, while in other cases – like Brazil, which has at least 23 ›color‹ distinctions – many categories developed. But, everywhere, social and identity expectations are assigned by color to some extent, although in varying ways. In Latinx culture the phrase »there is no Latinx without Black« has become a new way of acknowledging that all people who identify as Latinx have some African/native heritage that in the US binary is categorized as Black – even though many Latinx here identify as White.

Black communities in the US have openly and broadly embraced an awareness of Blackness as a positive status since at least the 1950s – and have typically rejected calls to assimilate since that time, insisting that there is something wrong with the majority culture that they do not want to emulate. Our findings document how these criticisms of majority expectations as dishonest, fake, individualistic, and disrespectful of personhood, manifest in the preferences of the Black American interaction order, which orient equality and democracy.

One of the advantages of the US binary, according to Du Bois, is ironically, that because it did not allow Black Americans to assimilate, it forced the best and brightest people with African ancestry to remain in the Black community to shape its ideals and fight for its freedom. It is not surprising that under these conditions the ideals of the Black American interaction order and its interactional preferences are more vibrant and democratic than the status-oriented preferences of the White interaction order and its ›White strong man‹ ideal.

The way social theory and research methods developed in each country, and how they have either supported the status quo and silenced minority voices or, promoted awareness, will also be different. Critical theory, which was developed in Germany in the 1930s by Jewish intellectuals on the basis of their experience of exclusion has been one important source of awareness. Du Bois, Garfinkel, Eric Williams, and more recently Critical Race Theory and Black Feminist Thought, have played a similar role in the US. But, in most countries such movements did not occur, and apart from some European universities in the 1960s and early 1970s Critical Theory did not become dominant anywhere The international thrust has rather been driven by developments in US sociology during WWII toward a type of statistical quantitative methodology that naively treats secondary data sets as facts in a way that supports majority White thinking (Rawls 2018).

No matter what the history of a country or area has been, every new disaster, natural or man-made, that produces refugees and/or asylum seekers will generate its own exclusionary dynamics and stigmatized categories of people. Some will create entirely new categories of Race and exclusion, but most will play out against an embedded historical background, and many of the dynamics should be similar. All will provide fodder for elites who strive to benefit from exploitation – and the processes will often become tacit and hidden.

Our work is intended to suggest a pathway for uncovering what has been hidden.

Responses

On Tacit Racism in France

Jean Beaman

In 1955's »Equal in Paris«, an essay in *Notes on a Native Son*, writer James Baldwin wrote of his experiences as an African-American living in Paris and the racism he witnessed and experienced:

> »It was quite clear to me that the Frenchmen in whose hands I found myself were no better or worse than their American counterparts. Certainly their uniforms frightened me quite as much, and their impersonality, and the threat, always very keenly felt by the poor, of violence, was as present in that Commissariat as it had ever been for me in any police station. And I had seen, for example, what Paris policemen could do to Arab peanut vendors. The only difference here was that I did not understand these people, did not know what techniques their cruelty took, did not know enough about their personalities to see danger coming, to ward it off, did not know on what ground to meet it. That evening in the Commissariat I was not a despised Black man. They would simply have laughed at me if I had behaved like one. For them, I was an American. And here it was they who had the advantage, for that word, *Américain*, gave them some idea, far from inaccurate, of what to expect from me« (Baldwin 1955: 106, emphasis in the original).

I thought of Baldwin's rich retelling of his encounter with Parisian policemen after being suspected of stealing a hotel bedsheet when reading both Rawls and Duck's essay, *Tacit Racism is Institutionalized in Interaction in the US: What about Elsewhere?*, and their recently published book, *Tacit Racism* (Rawls/Duck 2020). In this particular incident, Baldwin reflects upon both the racism facing France's racial and ethnic minorities, as well as the relative privileges associated with being an American in Paris. Here, Baldwin is not treated as a »despised Black man«, and therefore, to borrow Rawls and Duck's analysis, did not fit within particular expectations for interracial interactions in French society. His identity as simultaneously Black, yet American, violated particular rules of interaction in Paris.

In their essay, Rawls and Duck rightfully note how »racism shapes literally everything« (2020: 3). This is also true in the context of Europe, despite how many societies actively disavow the existence of Race and racism and relatedly relegate such issues outside of Europe.[18] Therefore part of how racism manifests itself is through the continual silencing of Race and racism as salient. It is particularly provocative to consider tacit racism and the related rules and structures of interaction in France, as it has long disavowed Race and racism as real and consequential. In what follows, I relate Rawls and Duck's illuminating analysis of the institutionalization of tacit racism to the French context. Specifically, I discuss the relevance of Du Boisian »double consciousness« for minorities in France; the role of colonialism in shaping France's racial grammar; and the state of academic and public discourse on racism in France and comparisons between France and the United States. While conceptions of Race and its tacit structures of interaction are contextual, it is also fruitful to consider how they compare and contrast across differently organized societies.

18 Here, I reference David Theo Goldberg's (2006) framework of racial Europeanization, in which Race is seen as a problem everywhere but in Europe.

W.E.B. Du Bois (1903) wrote of the »global color line«, or the relation of the darker to the lighter Races around the world. Therefore, his theorizing of Race and Blackness necessarily had a global component. His conception of ›double consciousness‹ relates to how Black Americans have a second-sight into racism and broader norms and rules of society that White Americans do not. Such a conception of minority consciousness, or the state of being a racialized minority in a society, is also relevant in France. In my own ethnographic research with adult children of Maghrébin, or North African, immigrants (Beaman 2017), I found that Maghrébin-origin individuals similarly had to be both conversant in French codes or ways of being and Maghrébin codes or ways of being, and in doing so, had insights on racism and post-colonialism in France that their White French counterparts lacked. As these individuals became upwardly-mobile compared to their migrant and working-class parents, they found themselves as part of only a handful of Maghrébin or non-Whites in their elite universities, such as Sciences Po, or professional workplaces. Rawls and Duck write that, »[t]here is no place in White American society where a Black American, however accomplished, can count on having their competence and qualifications recognized« (2020: 23). This is also the case for middle-class racial and ethnic minorities in France (and not just Maghrébin-origin individuals). My interlocutors also reported their actions and behaviors doubly scrutinized and their deservingness continually questioned in the workplace relative to their White counterparts.

Moreover, these children of Maghrébin immigrants have to continually imagine their locations within French society through the lens of how their White counterparts view them. Because the French state routinely disavows categories based on Race and ethnicity, these individuals are continually regarded as not French, or as foreigners or immigrants, because they are non-White. My interlocutors would report how other French people would ask them, »where are you *really* from?«, when they would initially respond to questions of origin with their town or region in France where they grew up. Relatedly, they often experienced being called ethnic slurs or being told to go back to their country by White counterparts as children. To relate to Rawls and Duck, this suggests that there exist rules to interracial interaction in French society, and a commonly agreed upon racial grammar which reinforces a racial order in this seemingly non-racial and anti-racial society.

Rawls and Duck situate the racial interaction order in the US as dating from slavery and its related construction of racial categories. While the French context is different historically, a consideration of France's colonial rule (including its own history of colonial slavery) and subsequent migration to the metropole in the postcolonial period reveals the roots of France's racial grammar. France's colonization of the Maghreb, West Africa, Vietnam, and parts of South America and the Caribbean (including Guadeloupe and Martinique which are presently overseas *départements* of France), was part of its civilizing mission to spread its ›values‹ around the world. While French Republican ideology does not recognize identity-based categories, including Race and religion (Chapman/Frader 2004), France's colonial empire relied on a differential construction of populations seen as ethnically different (Kastoryano/Escafré-Dublet 2012). In this way, racial and ethnic distinctions are made in the absence of official state categories. Such distinctions did not end when French colonial rule ended. As individuals from these former colonies migrated to the metropole (France actually has a long history of immigration, but World War I and the end of colonial rule saw an increase in the numbers of migrants), settled and raised children, France was continually forced to confront its ugly colonial history, as Maghrébin and Black individuals were often visible reminders of France's colonial empire that it would prefer to ignore in the postcolonial period. This relates to what anthropologist Ann Stoler (2011) terms France's »colonial aphasia«, as an alternative to the terms »forgotten history« or »colonial amnesia« in that it emphasizes the occlusion of knowledge. This erasure of the colonial leads to a »panic« of the postcolonial. And interracial or interethnic interactions exemplify this »panic«, as France struggles to promote its narrative of national cohesiveness in multicultural society. Reckoning with Europe's history of colonial and imperial rule moves us beyond solely an immigrant-focused lens to grappling with how actual citizens are marginalized in France – and across Europe – because of their Race and ethnic origin. So ›interaction orders of Race‹ are not new in France, but rather have been established during France's colonial rule.

Moreover, contemporary patterns of policing in France, particularly towards Black and Maghrebin-origin individuals, reveal ongoing colonial logics in the postcolonial period. As Rawls and Duck use »submissive civility« to explain the expected behavior of Black men in the face of White police officers, this ›submissive civility‹ is also applicable in the French context, as police officers perform identity checks, or *les contrôles d'identités*, disproportionately targeting Black and Maghrebin-origin individuals (Fassin 2013; Jobard/Levy 2009). Many of the interlocutors in my research perceive these checks as reinforcing that they do not fully belong in French society. Some identity checks lead to deaths, such as the case of Zyed Benna, a 17-year-old of Tunisian origin, and Bouna Traore, a 15-year-old of Malian origin, whose deaths in an electricity substation as they fled police in the *banlieue* of Clichy-sous-Bois, led to uprisings in *banlieues* throughout France. This police violence reinforces a second-class citizenship or status for these minority populations. Such a racial grammar and second-class status is an extension of the racial order between French police and colonized peoples in Algeria or Senegal or Guadeloupe. It is an extension of the violence present in France's colonial empire.

Finally, I want to discuss the issue of transatlantic comparison related to Race and racism, which remains a debate in academia as scholars must simultaneously pay attention to local specificities and contexts while comparing societies. In the case of France, this is particularly fraught as mention of Race and racism easily invokes accusations of importing Anglo-American concepts and frameworks. As France is both anti-racial and non-racial, it is complicated for scholars, both within the French academy and outside of it, to analyze and discuss racism in France, tacit or otherwise. Critiques abound of the multiple differences between France and the United States in terms of their racial and colonial histories, among other phenomena. Yet these discussions are not new. From the Nardal sisters and other Negritude thinkers and their salons in Paris with African-American expatriate Harlem Renaissance figures, including Langston Hughes and Claude McKay, to the present global anti-racist mobilization against police violence, encompassing both the United States and France, what becomes clear is that this racial grammar is not just locally specific, but also global or transnational.

And this brings us back to James Baldwin. As a Black woman who has studied Race in France for over a decade, I am repeatedly asked or reminded of the history of African-American expatriates to Paris – those individuals like Josephine Baker or Chester Himes who seemingly fled a racist United States for a more racially inclusive and accepting French society. Yet as Baldwin reminds us, this narrative is much more complicated. Rather, as Baldwin writes of how his US passport proclaimed that he was not »to be treated as one of Europe's uncivilized, Black possessions«. It makes one wonder why we are still in a position to ask if racism exists or is institutionalized in interaction in France, when the answer is clearly a resounding yes.

Ethnomethodology, Tacit Racism, and Modernity

Giolo Fele

The contribution by Anne Rawls and Waverly Duck on tacit racism is an important essay for three reasons: two are theoretical, one methodological.

The first reason concerns a theoretical innovation in their approach, and regards the fundamentals of social action. The essay provides a fresh perspective on the fundamental basis of sociality and social belonging. In short, the authors' approach to the study of social life is based neither on individuals nor on large structures (such as political power, economic institutions, or social classes). The authors rely instead on what they call an analysis of *social interaction*. The theme of tacit racism is studied not from a social psychological perspective, such as when stereotypes are analysed, nor from a structural, institutional perspective, in which racism is the result of unjust laws, political power, or economic systems. Those are clear forms of racism. However, what interests the authors is the study of the sly and persistent forms of racism, even in situations where racism is denied. Even seemingly liberal and democratic people are imbued with those prejudices that govern relations between people of different cultural background. From this point of view, the novelty of the authors' approach seems to me evident, representing a break with approaches based on psychological-social or institutional explanations. The authors wish to examine the structure of expectations in interactions between Whites and Blacks. They are interested in what people actually do, aside from their intentions or opinions. The peculiar focus of their approach is on the plane of normality that constitutes social life: paraphrasing Wittgenstein (1958: 129), their focus is on the things that are »hidden because of their simplicity and familiarity«, which are »always before our eyes« and for that simple reason we are »unable to notice« them. In this way, they are trying to lift the veil on reality before our very eyes. This is a genuine paradigm change in theoretical thinking. The authors are indicating where social life should be observed, not inside ourselves or far away in ›grand structures‹, but in its most open, obvious, everyday workings; they are inviting us to explore what happens around us regularly in the many exchanges we have with other people.

The second reason is methodological. In order to study social life closely, as it organizes itself before our eyes, the authors invite us to closely analyse social interaction in detail. The point that is highlighted by the authors is that we need to know what *really happens* in social interactions, without relying only on what we imagine might be happening. It is from this point of view, which may appear positivistic, but is, in fact, phenomenological and ethnomethodological, that the mechanisms of social interaction are revealed. This approach throws light on behaviour that is often unwanted and that lies outside consciousness and explicit awareness. The article divides the social interactions that make up daily social life into three categories: ›introductory sequences‹, ›fractured reflections‹, and ›submissive civility‹. For instance, the third, ›submissive civility‹ is based on a close examination of a video recording of an encounter between a Black individual and a policeman. The video recording allows us to precisely observe those delicate and volatile aspects of the interaction that cannot be noticed or remembered. The first, ›introductory sequences‹, is based on a small experiment (vom Lehn 2019) that consisted of a group of strangers introducing each other. The authors invited female students, who did not know each other, to introduce themselves. The second, ›fractured reflections‹, consisted of subjects remembering details of their past personal experience. All three analytic strategies represent a working method for social research that I would call fundamental because they analyse the fundamentals of social life. As such, this method is particularly important and should be followed by all those who study social processes.

The third reason is again theoretical. In the article a theory of modernity clearly emerges that ultimately rests on an innovative reinterpretation of the work of Durkheim, especially on Durkheim's *De la Division du Travail Sociale* (Durkheim 1893), which Anne Rawls has been carrying out for many years. Modernity has brought a radical change in human cohabitation: We live in a world where the movement of people in social space, in accelerated time, produces completely new situations, even compared to the recent past. More occasions arise in which we meet more and more different people in public spaces. Faced with these characteristics of modernity, social theory seems to have fallen behind. Contemporary sociological theories seem to base the ordering of our collective lives on the sharing of norms and values. Through an original reinterpretation of Durkheim's notion of mechanical and organic solidarity, Rawls and Duck introduce the distinction between societies based on consensus and societies based on practice. Modern society is a practice-based society, whereas traditional societies are based on substantial consensus on the fundamental values of a society – the model is of course more nuanced, and the authors are right to hasten to add that »all societies have some consensus and some self-regulation. The difference is in the proportion«. This position has important consequences: Social competence in modern society requires the ability to interact with people who do not necessarily share the same horizon of values. The social order derives from local and settled competences in which people come to understand each other »through seeable, hearable sounds and motions that occur in time and space«. The theoretical approach and methodological orientation that we briefly examined above becomes an essential tool for any social theory that aims to tackle the challenges of modernity, not to mention the theme of tacit racism.

Some final considerations: As an example of militant social analysis, the essay is characterized by a committed political orientation. Throughout the essay there is a strong commitment towards certain ideals about the way we should be, what we would like society to become. Throughout the essay one perceives not only the academic analysis, but the commitment to change, which is considered important in order to overcome the current state of social relations – in this case Race-based. The fact that commitment to societal change and scientific analysis are not separate, but are closely intertwined, is commendable, but at the same time it runs the risk of positioning this perspective above and beyond the pledge of adherence to the facts of social life. For example, the omni-relevance of racial categories (»racism shapes literally everything«) makes us view every interaction from this perspective. This perspective thus becomes a theoretical framework, an assumption that hinders our taking into account other aspects. When institutional interactions are analysed, for instance, I do wonder if what is relevant on these occasions is not the categories of ›Black‹ and ›White‹ man but rather policeman and citizen. Moreover, it sometimes appears that the analysis and *description* of how social interactions are structured gives way to the *explanation* of that behaviour. For example, from analysing how unacquainted people exchange greetings or how the police question a suspect on particular occasions to explaining that these certain interactional routines are in place for a certain reason – in this case, because of Race, people behave this way *because* they are ›Black‹ or ›White‹ . I found this transition from the *how* to the *why* a difficult shift and not always grounded in the data at hand. This is perhaps an old story in ethnomethodological conversation analysis – for example on the debate of the relevance of the category of gender in interaction (cf. Speer/Stokoe 2011). On the one hand, there is an exclusive concern oriented towards analysing the local structures of social interaction, but occasionally the overarching relevance of membership categories is missing; on the other hand, there is a strong commitment over the omni-relevance of some of these categories, and the fact that the analysis cannot be ›technical‹, neutral, and blind toward this matter of fact. Regarding this paper, my only fear is that to argue that everything is racial in social life can limit the ways in which other social or institutional constraints impinge on the phenomena under examination. Taking sides on one issue can make us less attentive toward other possible phenomena that need to be analysed and taken into consideration.

However, the research program on which this article is based has been successful in offering important food for thought on the ways Race is realized in social interaction. It extends and challenges previous studies in the field and it should be considered as a source of inspiration for all researchers studying the production of social order.

Islamophobia after Passing »the Dinner Table Test« – or How the Racialization of Muslims Becomes Tacit

Martijn de Koning

According to Baroness Sayeeda Warsi, in 2011, in the UK, Islamophobia had already passed the »dinner table test« (Batty 2011). Certain expressions and manifestations of anti-Muslim racism had become socially acceptable and their utterance no longer disrupted conversational civility at the dinner table, such as »not to worry, he's only fairly Muslim«, »the family next door is Muslim, but they're not too bad«, and, with reference to women wearing a face veil, she is »either oppressed or is making a political statement« (ibid.). Sometimes Islamophobic expressions are dressed up to look like forms of Islamic criticism. Sometimes they serve as to turn a blind eye towards (or even of making a justification for) forms of aggression: Why do Muslims behave as if they are the victims when they themselves perpetrate terrorist attacks? In this form it appears as if it is not ›we‹ who are marginalizing ›them‹, but rather that ›we‹ are merely being critical, or simply want to find out who this other person is, for he/she belongs to a group that is causing so many problems. Islamophobia then becomes almost unrecognisable as such and can even sound reasonable and realistic, as Van Baar explains in regard to another form of racism: antiziganism (Van Baar 2014).

All these forms of racism are integral parts of mainstream culture and occur regularly in everyday interactions; they may even form part of the structures of anticipated and accepted modes of interaction. However, such forms, and the processes through which they become unrecognisable, are difficult to detect and analyse. It is here that Anne Warfield Rawls and Waverly Duck's book *Tacit Racism* (2020), and their opening statement for this debate, became highly relevant and inspiring, concentrating as they do on explaining and analysing the everyday racism of interactions in the USA with the aim of showing how interaction orders are institutionalized. The book is particularly strong, in my view, when concrete interactions are analysed in detail.

In teasing out the connection between tacit racism in Europe and the US, it is worthwhile to have a look at anti-Muslim racism. In my work on anti-Muslim racism and racialization in the Netherlands, I have been inspired by various authors who have conceptualized Islamophobia as a form of racism (Sayyid/Vakil 2010; Van der Valk 2015), by authors who have analysed how people respond to racism and oppression (hooks 1989), and how historical and contemporary perceptions of alleged ›Islamic threats‹ related to the representation of Islam as a sexist religion bent on oppressing women (Rashid 2016).

Terms such as anti-Muslim racism and Islamophobia are not easy to work with. The term Islamophobia in particular is contested inside academia and elsewhere (Halliday 1999). The arguments against the term Islamophobia and the interpretation of it as racist (including but not limited to hostility and discrimination) against Muslims and Islam are usually built upon the claim that Islam is a set of ideas to which people can freely subscribe (and, therefore, dissent from), making anti-Islam antagonism different from hostility and oppression based on racial and gender categories. In some cases, this argument is expanded to argue that, because Islam is different from race and gender, taking action against Islamophobia would amount to threatening free speech, which would feed into the discourses and practices of Islamists and could be a justification for individuals to commit intolerant (violent) acts in the name of Islam (Meer/Modood 2009). Yet, many authors point to the historical hierarchies, determinism, and essentialism that make up the discourses and identities that are ascribed to, and imposed upon, Muslims by a variety of actors, such as state institutions, politicians, and companies (Bravo López 2011). It is therefore crucial to understand the historical trajectories of race and racism in each country, as Anne Warfield Rawls and Waverly Duck rightfully point out. It is therefore puzzling that the authors also argue that »English colonies in North America developed a Black/White Race binary while Spanish and Portuguese colonies did not«, because of the fact that »[r]ace was invented to support the system of colonial labor in the American colonies when it confronted a sudden scarcity of unfree English/Irish labor«.

Although not exactly the same as the Black/White binary mentioned by Anne Warfield Rawls and Waverly Duck, ideas about race did exist in the Spanish Empire, both in and outside of Europe – ideas which continued to develop in Europe even during and after the Spanish, Dutch, French and British colonisers built their empires, as, for example, Heng (2018) persuasively argues. Throughout the history of Europe, religion, culture, history, and territories were characterized and interpreted in a manner that served to differentiate between Europeanness and non-Europeanness (Sayyid 2018). The construction of racial categories mainly pertained to Jews, Muslims, and Black people as racial Others (Jansen/Meer 2020; Topolski 2018).

This, of course, does not mean that the approach set out by Anne Warfield Rawls and Waverly Duck is not relevant to Europe. I would argue that it is in fact relevant. As they demonstrate, each country has its own issues and trajectories of racism and racialization such that focusing on the intricacies of interaction could indeed make the implicit manifestations of race, racism, and racialization much more visible.

This kind of focus could also provide us with insight into how racism goes ›underground‹ or, in the case of Islamophobia, how Islamophobia becomes normalised in politics and policies. For example, through those discourses that are based upon on the almost self-evident necessity of integration and security and which are meant to safeguard ›our way of life‹, while, at the same time, defending secular freedoms as well as the Judaeo-Christian tradition (Van Den Hemel 2014; Vieten 2016; De Koning 2020). If Islamophobia is almost undetectable as a mode of racism, do other ways of thinking and/or opposing anti-Muslim racism then become deviant and abnormal?

In this regard, it is interesting that one of the most innovative contributions to anti-Islamophobia research, and one that reveals the process of Islamophobia normalisation in the Netherlands, was carried out by the Dutch anti-racism NGO *Meld Islamofobie*

(Report Islamophobia). Through exploratory research, they showed how political rhetoric in media and in parliament trickles down into people's lives in a myriad of ways (Meld Islamofobie 2019). Take, for example, those kinds of assumptions imposed upon Muslims and migrants that render them ›not really from here‹, or the examples mentioned at the beginning of the article. Importantly, people are often not entirely sure about how to interpret such an interaction, as I have also noticed in my own work. For example, in my work with Muslim militant activists (some of whom went to Syria to join IS or Al Qaeda from 2012 onwards) many recounted to me these kinds reoccurring experiences at school. One man told me:

»It was the day after 9/11. We talked about it in class and our teacher showed the video with George W. Bush saying: ›you are either with us or against us‹. Then the teacher stood up, pointed at me and asked ›And AA, where do you stand?‹. I didn't know. But I knew I wasn't with the Americans«.[19]

I have described elsewhere (De Koning 2019) how this remark reveals a sense of misrecognition and alienation. Yet, my conversations with him and many of his friends inside these militant circles, but also with other Muslims, for example in anti-racism organisations, show that people are often uncertain about how to understand a particular question or remark. Many recount such experiences but also pose questions to each other such as: »Are you sure you understood it well? Are you sure it was not just an innocent question?« It is important to not take for granted such ambiguities in people's experiences as they are manifestations of moral reasonings, of how they try to make sense of the world and of other people, their perceptions of them and, perhaps, of attempts to translate them into action. It is in this moment of ambivalence where a lot of reflection (sometimes inattentively, sometimes deliberately) takes place as to what the exact meaning of the interaction might be, and how best to respond to it. It would be useful to explore these moral reasonings and moments of ambivalence at greater depth and to investigate the processes by which racism becomes tacit.

As I have shown in my work on the Dutch anti-Islamophobia initiatives, these initiatives create spaces for discussing Islamophobia and to raise awareness about everyday and institutionalized forms of Islamophobia (De Koning 2016). Although the research project undertaken by *Meld Islamofobie* was exploratory and based on an online questionnaire. Research of this sort may help to explain how particular events and rhetorical gestures in politics become part and parcel of the everyday ›interaction order‹. Work by colleagues in Spain in critical discussion groups (with different objectives) may also contribute to make such events visible (Lems 2020; Moustaoui Srhir 2020). This is similar to what Garfinkel (1940) has shown (also mentioned by Anne Warfield Rawls and Waverly Duck) with regard to the concealed social structures of Jim Crow and how they were exposed once two Black bus passengers refused to ›play the game‹, or, given the limits of such interference, to small acts of lesser disruption which can also highlight ongoing processes of normalisation. The kind of work done by *Meld Islamofobie* can be seen as ›breaching experiments‹ which cause disruption and perhaps interrupt the way in which the everyday order of things is taken for granted. In this way they become »diagnostic events« (Moore 1987) which reveal how tacit understandings are embedded in the moral orders. Following up on the work done by Anne Warfield Rawls and Waverly Duck would, therefore, also be a promising avenue for scholarly activism in Europe.

19 My interlocutor probably mixed up different things here in his memory as Bush did say these words, but he did so on 20 September, 2001 and not 12 September, 2001. This is less relevant here as the focus of my work is on how people give meaning to particular events. See The White House/President George W. Bush (2001).

Racialization in Action: The Ethnomethodological Perspective on Race and Racism

Christian Meyer

The initiative presented by Anne Rawls and Waverley Duck to study tacit everyday interactional practices that are implicitly or explicitly racist is timely and a welcome lead to advancing current debates about racism in the social and cultural sciences. Most current research focuses either on structural factors that produce racialized and, simultaneously, racializing inequalities, or on racist psychological attitudes. Instead, the authors study the realization of Race as a social object and racism in the unfolding dynamics of the here and now of interactional practices as they are directly empirically accessible.

The particular approach that the authors present takes »interaction order« as a starting point, claiming that systemic or structural racism is institutionalized »in the taken-for-granted practices of everyday interaction«, ultimately leading to the situation in which »ordinary people are constantly doing racist things without being aware of it«.

According to the authors, the most important moment whereby racism is institutionalized in the interaction order is the »interactional expectations« of the co-participants in social situations. These expectations, especially when they are shared, represent the »structures of racism«, and »acting on these structures produces racist outcomes – *in what people do* – regardless of individual intent or awareness« (emphasis in the original).

Expectations are constitutive of the social objects and meanings they produce. The authors compare them to »rules of a game«. Co-participants in interactional practices, as the authors put it, must necessarily orient themselves to the same expectations or rules and use the same definition of the situation. In doing so, they must presuppose that other participants are competent and confirm their competent interactional work. All of this, however, »occurs at an unconscious level of taken-for-granted, and thus largely hidden, practices«. This is why the authors call their topic »tacit racism«.

Interactional expectations can be understood as a constitutive grammar of interaction. They belong to social situations »such that they are ›constitutive‹ of *the recognizability of an action as action* of a particular sort« [emphasis in the original]. This is true at least for those people who share those expectations (called »members« by Garfinkel 1967: vii).

Therefore, interactional expectations are fundamental to the procedural production of intersubjectivity, action coordination, and social order in general and Race is inextricably embedded in this: »When actions do not meet the constitutive expectations of others, those others cannot recognize what has been done, or said«. According to the authors, cultural and racial biases and culturally and racially biased social categories in the form of Black/White binarity are »coded into the interactional expectations«. Thus, social order and racial order are fundamentally intertwined and the abandonment of one would inescapably also disturb, or even demolish, the Other – the social contract, in other words, is a racial contract (Mills 1999).

The intention of the authors is thus to present an approach to Race (and racialization) that does not focus on stable mental concepts or psychic attitudes, or on comprehensive symbolic systems of a society, but rather on *how* social categories are created and used in situ, in the here and now of a particular situation through interactional practice. Inspired by conversation and embodied interaction analysis, their approach focuses on the »order properties« of sequences of social action that people tacitly constitute and constantly adjust in making sense together. This is where the greatest benefit of their approach lies and where their empirical analyses produce important insights. They demonstrate that racialization is already interactionally accomplished when Americans first meet one another and start a conversation, or that class differences are equally racialized, as when high status Black Americans are not treated in accordance with their actual class positions.

The approach that the authors present captures important dimensions of racialized and racializing interactional practices. Further and complementary ethnomethodologically informed research should address in even more detail *how* co-participants select in the here and now of a social situation among a multitude of possible shared expectations those which are relevant for, and applicable in, the situation at hand in order not to transgress the fine line between creative and innovative (»artful«, Garfinkel 1967: vii) social action and the breaching of background expectancies that in social situations would lead to troubles of both cognitive understanding and normative evaluation. While co-participants in a social situation and members of a collectivity in general can orient themselves to, and thereby establish, shared rules in an infinite number of acceptable ways and, in doing so, »innovate endlessly«, they will typically be troubled by breaches in the constitutive rules, and »assign motive/blame to the individual who has done the unexpected thing«, as the Rawls and Duck say in reference to Garfinkel (1963). However, because breaches are typically attributed in interactions to the cooperative stance of the co-participants and not to the fragility of social order itself, the »immortality« (Garfinkel 1988) of social and, as entailed, racial order – as a fiction and continuing presupposition for further interactions – is guaranteed.

Therefore, an analysis of racism in action needs to investigate how the fiction and presupposition of the sharedness of those dimensions that constitute a racialized social order – such as expectancies, rules, codes, categories, the Black/White binarity – are established and continuously maintained, achieved, and accomplished in interactional practice. To take these dimensions for granted as (possibly shared) *a priori* elements fed into interactions would again imply a mentalization even if they are investigated as manifested in the course of interaction. I therefore propose to return to Garfinkel's *Studies in Ethnomethodology* (1967):

> »The activities whereby members produce and manage settings of organized everyday affairs are identical with members' procedures for making those settings ›account-able‹. The ›reflexive‹, or ›incarnate‹ character of accounting practices and accounts makes up the crux of that recommendation. When I speak of accountable my interests are directed to such matters as the following. I mean observable-and-reportable, i.e. available to members as situated practices of looking-and-telling« (Garfinkel 1967: 1).

If we want to find out how racializing expectations, rules, codes, and categories are co-constituted and shared – procedurally and always preliminarily – in the here and now of social situations, we need to focus on how they are embedded and made available in situated practices of looking-and-telling. We need to investigate the pre-institutional, pre-codified, and pre-semiotic dimensions of Race and racialization inherent in these practices.

In the latter works mentioned above, Garfinkel (2002; 2007; Garfinkel/Livingston 2003) has developed a vocabulary to grasp the interconnectedness of looking and telling, of procedures which »produce and manage settings of organized everyday affairs« and which »make those settings ›account-able‹« (Garfinkel 1967: 1). He calls the organizational details of coherent social objects (such as Race) »phenomenal field properties« and conceptualizes them as being endogenously accomplished in practices that co-participants contribute to the scenery. These details mutually point to and elaborate one another, thus establishing what Garfinkel (1967: 40; 2007: 43–47) calls the »essential indexicality« of social phenomena. In this way, a scenery familiar to members is created and practically interpreted beyond itself as a »document for« all kinds of further social phenomena. A scenery is familiar when situated practices of looking and telling fall into one.

In recent years, a number of studies were published which analyze racialized and racializing practices of looking-and-telling in social situations as well as the racialized and racializing reflexive and incarnate character of accounting practices from a phenomenological perspective, partly referring to Frantz Fanon's (1952) ground-breaking work in *Black Skin, White Masks* (Ahmed 2007; Alcoff 1999; Al-Saji 2014; Bloul 2013; Tullmann 2020; Yancy 2008). They help clarify the incremental and ever-changing phenomenal field properties of the social object Race and their effects on racializing social sceneries and situations. While they do not take video-recorded data of embodied interaction as evidence, they present autoethnographic accounts of racialized and racializing interaction.

In particular, these studies show that Du Bois' »double consciousness« can, in practice, also be viewed as ›double membership‹, in the ethnomethodological sense, of Black Americans in American society. This double membership burdens them with the double competence to participate in an incarnate and reflexive manner in both worlds, a burden that White Americans do not share, in spite of some self-descriptions: For one, they are able (and, for reasons of intelligibility and normative pressure, often forced) to participate competently in the racialized and racializing practices of wider American collectivity, in which the Black body is »a battleground« that

> »has been historically marked, disciplined, scripted and materially, psychologically and morally invested in to ensure both white supremacy and the illusory construction of the white subject as a self-contained substance whose existence does not depend upon the construction of the Black qua inferior« (Yancy 2008: 844).

Secondly, they competently participate in familiar practices of Black collectivities where their bodies are unproblematic, taken-for-granted, and in no need to become »hypervigilant« (ibid.: 857) as in encounters with White Americans, where they are forced to pay:

> »almost neurotic attention to my body movements, making sure that this ›black object‹, what now feels like an appendage, a weight, is not too close, not too tall, not too threatening. ›Double layers of self-awareness must interrogate the likely meanings that will be attributed to every utterance, gesture, action one takes‹. So, I genuflect, but only slightly, a movement that somewhat resembles an act of worship. I am reminded of how certain postures – ›bowing and scraping‹ – were carried over generations through the movement, sometimes no doubt unconscious, of the Black body« (ibid.: 858).

Once again applauding Rawls and Duck for their endeavor to approach Race and racialization from an ethnomethodological and embodied interaction perspective, I suggest complementing their perspective with phenomenological inquiries into the »phenomenal field properties« of racialized embodiment and perception.

Are Turks Black and What Does it Matter?

Levent Tezcan

The following article examines to what extent, and in what ways, the concept of ›tacit racism‹ ,proposed by authors Rawls and Duck, can be productively applied in Germany. It is a response to an invitation that was issued by the authors with the following caveat: that the focus on »systemic racism embedded in social interactions« should take into account »that the conceptions of Race and the tacit structures of interaction involved will not be the same across countries (or even regions)« (Rawls/Duck 2020: 2). I intend to take this caveat into consideration in asking the question »Are Turks Black?« The answer is clearly: no, they are not Black and this has consequences for the researcher. The thesis, to which I subscribe, is as follows: certain problems should be considered in conjunction with the concept of ›systemic racism‹. Otherwise, one runs the risk of equating with racism the assorted frictions in interethnic relations, for which other modes of description may be better suited. As such, the focus should be on the issue of how »processes of figuration for societies of migration« (Hüttermann 2018) can be appropriately observed in their multiplicity.

The Lack of Slavery and Colonialism

Before exposing the specificity of interethnic relations in Germany, as compared with Black/White figurations in the USA, I shall give a brief summary of the authors' thesis. In its present version, the concept of ›tacit racism‹ is offered as an alternative to two other perspectives. It is distinguished, on the one hand, from ›microaggressions theory‹ (Sue 2010), which is equally concerned with the hidden structures of day-to-day racism, and which takes as its focus the individual and its structures of perception. It is also distinct from ›institutional racism‹ in so far as it focuses neither on legal documents nor formal structures. Hence, its unit for observation is constituted neither by the individual of the first theory nor the institution of the second. It is, rather, interactions that come to the fore. That racism is thereby embedded in material social-structures is particularly instructive: it was not until the White labour force was replaced by slaves that racism first took shape as a regulatory principle, with broad sections of the White population adapting to/taking advantage of the new order. This order of racism, profoundly anchored in social structures, is of fundamental importance for any further analysis; without it, the hierarchies at work in the interactions between White and Black people, whether explicit or concealed, cannot be understood. Though these hierarchies can be observed throughout the USA, they do not always appear in the same guise. As such, the authors turn to the sociology of Durkheim for support: wherever social solidarity is based on consent (collective consciousness), such as in the Southern United States, racism has consistently appeared openly. In areas with a greater division of labour, on the other hand, racism is less visible. In terms of observing relations, it is under the conditions of the latter case that ›tacit racism‹ – for which the authors avail of ethnomethodological tools as proposed by Garfinkel – is particularly well suited.

The Turks, in this case, stand for a particular – and historically specific – type, namely the migrant who is not of European descent, but rather who migrates, ideally, from Europe's boarders, without thereby becoming ensnared in a colonial history of dependence. Regardless of whether or not they are the object of racially-motivated hostility, which they undoubtedly are, it is crucial to grasp that the relations of figuration, into which migrants of Turkish descent enter with local Germans, are not in the least characterised by the same history of slavery as there are in the US. This is due to the fact that they were neither enslaved nor colonised, plain and simple. There is no such history of subjugation and humiliation informing day-to-day encounters. History, if anything, offers the chance of mobilising the historical image of the Muslim ›Turkish danger‹ in order to stoke fears, not unsuccessfully, of the Turkish-Muslim migrant. Hence, what is means to have experienced slavery – or not, as is the case here – and its poisonous effects for the spirits of both parties is of critical importance. It was the fight against this phenomenon to which

Franz Fanon dedicated his life. In *Black Skin, White Masks* (1952), Fanon rejects any attempt to explain the situation of former slaves with abstract theories – such as the contemporary concept of ›Othering‹ – that do not take specific *existences* into account. To other someone certainly involves hostility, but there is still an acknowledgement of the Other as an Other. This acknowledgement was denied slaves who, in the entirety of their being, were reduced to mere objects. This distinction, I might add, is rarely questioned by more recent forms of contemporary critical Race theory when it applies the lens of racism to interpret any halfway negative depiction of the ther by the majority. If my understanding of Fanon is accurate, neither racism nor slavery are odious because they engage in a politics of Othering, but rather because they deny the slave the very status of the Other. If we take Rawls' and Duck's main premise seriously, that is, that the history of slavery is foundational for the further efficacy of racism in interactions, then this foundation, as applied to (in this case, specifically: Turkish) migrants in Germany, is entirely absent. This is a warning to tread carefully with any comprehensive application of ›tacit racism‹. Of course, this does not mean that either the existence of racism or any of the diverse forms of discrimination are irrelevant. Rather, it expresses a scepticism for any potential attempts to account for interethnic relations primarily by way of this concept. By contrast, researching the meaning and effects of racism as a specific form of positioning in its diverse interactions makes a great deal of sense.

The situation of migrants can be observed from the beginning of the recruitment of guest workers. Guest workers were not engaged in forced labour. They were not forced, against their will, and under abhorrent conditions, onto ships. Instead, they took the road voluntarily and full of hope. They were not subject to the slave trader's desire to subsume them into a faceless mass, by classifying them as Black on the sole basis of their skin colour, and creating for them the single category ›African‹, for what was, in fact, a diversity of peoples. Even racial slurs such as ›Makkaroni-Fresser‹, ›Kümmel-Türken‹, ›Jugos‹ or ›Ithakas‹ afford some degree of esteem to those addressed, in so far as they register the specific belonging, which each group would ascribe to itself (that is, Italians, Turks, Yugoslavs, Greeks and so on). That they did not belong was not the consequence of racial subjugation, but rather a result of the fact that owing to their immigration or descent, they simply did not belong. They each brought with them their own sense of belonging, which they maintain to this day. Indeed, once the illusion of the guest worker had evaporated, that is, once the ideas of returning had subsided, the lack of a colonial experience for Turkish migrants would come to be of particular importance for the psychosocial effects of the relations of figuration. Once again, this does not mean that they were spared any experience of racism. They were undoubtedly the object of discrimination, both day-to-day and institutional, codified in the Foreigners Act. However, their historically-specific background may well have numbed them against such personal attacks somewhat. Ultimately, even the poorest ›Hanswurst‹, suffering the most serious identity crisis, can engage in an imaginative act of self-healing by asserting that »our ancestors once put the fear of God into the Europeans«. This could equally be said to differentiate their experiences from those of the descents of former slaves.

This point can be expanded to include one further aspect. Not only are the Turks not Black, they cannot even claim the status of people of colour. At this juncture, it is worth briefly examining this dubious term. Fundamentally, it brings together distinct ethnic groups under one category of supposed belonging, which otherwise does little to unite them, and may indeed do more to separate them. What do the Turks of today (and, to an extent, those of the past) have more in common with Arabs, Chinese, Indians and

Vietnamese – and what, indeed, do these groups all have more in common with one another – than they do with Germans (and vice versa)? What they have in common is undoubtedly that *they are not Germans*, and that, in Germany, is not insignificant. But does this justify raising this single distinction to the central category of a negative, concrete belonging? This is a category that was created as a critique of racism, the distinguishable characteristic of which is that it constitutes a counter position, that is, it can only be negatively affirmed. Black, as a category, first violently implemented by Whites, and subsequently adopted by African-Americans toward self-description, has its historical site within the White/Black figuration of slavery. The category ›people of colour‹, by contrast, is divorced of any such practical and experiential context. It generalises an historically-specific figuration by translating it into an abstract dichotomy in order to construct a felt sense of belonging. Some attempts have been made by some Turks to expand this notion to include Turkish people in Germany, who like other people of colour belong to the group of young educated migrants. But they're missing the experiential foundations.

The Germans have never been White for the Turks (nor, evidently, have they ever been so for the Kurds or other ethnic groups). Similarly, the Turks are neither White nor Black. The Black/White dichotomy is equally unsuited for the descriptions of self and Other in which Europeans are involved. Instead, it is the ›European/Westerner/Christian‹ that constitutes the other for the Turks, Kurds, Arabs and so on. Whoever wishes can throw together an ›illustrious‹ history of successfully defending against the ›crusaders‹. Indeed, levels of nationalism and fascism among migrants are far from trivial.

With regard to German-Turkish figuration, two particular features are now clearly discernible: both the lack of any history of colonialism or slavery on the one hand, and the fact that migration (temporary at first, then de facto long-term) was voluntary, on the other, fundamentally distinguish the existence of Turkish migrants in Germany from the Black population in the United States.

The thesis of »submissive civility«, which is ascribed by the authors to African-Americans, cannot be readily applied to migrants in Germany. It is certainly true of the German case that undemocratic, fundamentalist and nationalistic orientations can be widely observed among the migrant population (Tezcan 2002). And this regardless of the extent to which the dichotomy of ›White strong man‹, on the one side, and ›submissive man‹ (Black), on the other, is relevant for the foundation of American democracy. In any case, the Turkish referendum of 2017 saw a significant portion of Turkish migrants in Europe vote to extend the powers of a dictator. In relation to this, we might also ask whether this intimate transnational bond to the nation states of the countries of origin does not also constitute a further distinction to the situation of the Afro-Americans in the US.

Alternative Models?

Research projects on the dynamics of interethnic relations in Germany, which do not explicitly rely on analyses of racism, are already available in Germany, and they have produced important findings. The existence of racism is in no way denied thereby. But the dynamics of interaction are far too diverse as to be adequately captured through the lens of racism. Process-sociological analyses, primarily produced by Jörg Hüttermann (2018), provide us with an elaborate model in this regard, one which is based on several empirical studies.

This sophisticated model links the inter-group relations to the socio-economic circumstances, without reducing either aspect to the Other. As such, it is similar to the approach taken by Rawls and Duck. Different stages in the presence of migrants correspond to a particular, dominant pattern of figuration, which consists of corresponding roles. For the ›foreign guest‹, confronted with the ›ushering host‹, relations are essentially governed by the right to hospitality. The later ›peripheral foreigner‹ establishes another relation of figuration, together with the ›usher‹. Though the former more frequently operates in communal life worlds, he does so in the absence of social ›lawyers‹ to act in his favour. The ›advanced foreigner‹, to which Hüttermann attaches a further figuration, no longer holds to the normative power of the right to hospitality, which had previously served as orientation for guest workers. Hüttermann adds further figurations involving ›culture subjects‹ and more individualised ›someones‹, the latter referring to a positionality around functional roles. We have here a dynamic model of interaction that links roles to both material contexts and social positioning. It is duly grounded while remaining sufficiently open. Above all, the model is particularly useful in examining interactions between the most significant minority groups and German locals as these are informed neither by a history of slavery nor one of colonialism.

The concept ›systemic/tacit racism‹ could certainly enrich the more ample model of sociological figuration, with a view to seeing figurations characterised by racism in greater detail. If it were the primary model, however, it would likely narrow our view of the diverse dynamics of relations of figuration described here. These simply cannot be adequately apprehended with the concept of racism.

Translation from German: Michael Dorrity.

Response to Contributors to the Debate

Anne Warfield Rawls and Waverly Duck

In our book *Tacit Racism*, and our article for this debate, we explain our approach to exposing systemic racism in social interaction through detailed studies of language and interaction and then address the question whether and how this new approach to Race and racism – based as it is on research in the US – could be a fruitful approach in Europe and elsewhere. Many countries in Europe claim not to have a problem with racism, talking instead about their difficulties with refugee and immigrant populations in terms of ›democracy‹, ›assimilation‹, ›inter-ethnic relations‹ and ›post-colonialism‹. However, such issues are often ›racialized‹ in ways that are obscured by approaches that focus more on »the assorted frictions in interethnic relations«, as Tezcan puts it, »for which other modes of description [than Race] may be better suited«. The danger is that categories of ›ethnicity‹, ›religion‹ and ›immigrant‹ may have been ›racialized‹ in ways that lead to an experience of exclusion best seen as racism. The problem we confront in discussing Race is that racism finds many ways of hiding in plain sight, and a focus away from racism toward categories not typically associated with Race is one of those ways.

While the particular processes and categories related to Race, racism and racialization in the US may be different from those elsewhere (or not), essential problems associated with what is being called ›ethnic‹ and ›inter-ethnic‹ relations and ›immigration‹, are very likely more properly viewed in racial terms, as a number of young scholars in the US and Europe argue (Garcia 2017; Husain 2017; Castañeda 2018; Beaman 2017). Making this adjustment requires rethinking how ›immigrant‹, ›Illegal‹, ›Turk‹, ›Muslim‹, etc., are social categories assigned on the basis of ›appearance‹ in ways that are determined by majority persons during interaction – just as Race is – and that such categories can thus be ›racialized‹. As Garfinkel (2012[1947]) noted, in such cases the person being categorized has no say in the matter. The consequence is that fourth generation citizens are often categorized as immigrants, and Christians and Hindus as Muslim.

Overall the contributors have been receptive to our recommendation to look for tacit systemic racism in ›interaction order‹ expectations; pointing out that existing research has focused either on formal structures (like formal laws/policies), or on individual prejudice (often tied to beliefs and values), with the result that the domain of racism in interaction we focus on has been overlooked.

Focusing as we do on social interaction as process, our research is detailed. As Meyer notes, »the authors study the realization of ›Race‹ – as social object – and racism in the unfolding dynamics of the here and now of interactional practice as it is directly empirically accessible«. While others focus on individual and/or formal structures, we take the focus away from racists, laws, and roles/identities, because treating racism as inherent in persons, institutions and/or identities is both limiting and easily defeated by denials of intent to discriminate. We focus instead on forms of *racism* as interactional processes that do not require racist intent.

Our argument that systemic racism has become embedded in social interaction combines the idea that Interaction Orders organize everyday interaction (Goffman 1983; Rawls 1987), with the finding that social expectations can develop in response to oppression to produce what we call ›interaction orders of Race‹ (Rawls 2000). Focusing on interaction as process makes it possible to separate tacit systemic racism from other forms of discrimination and empirically document just how processes that support racism have become embedded in our most familiar daily actions.

The principal question raised in this debate is the extent to which an approach based on aspects of Race grounded in US history can be useful in the context of problems in Europe and elsewhere more commonly discussed in terms of ›immigration‹, ›ethnicity/religion‹ and/or ›colonialism‹. We suggest the answer is to be found in rethinking the categories that dominate the discussion in Europe in the context of a contrast between the positions of Franz Fanon (1952) and W.E.B. Du Bois (1904). While Fanon described negative effects of attempts to assimilate, to the extent that people are excluded from participation and blocked from assimilating on the basis of *surface appearances* that they cannot hide (and which may bear no relationship to their actual social status), they are likely to experience a consciousness of Race described by Du Bois as »double-consciousness«. Researchers in both the US and Europe are now reporting this kind of experience in conjunction with identities that have not historically been considered ›racial‹. Garcia (2017), for instance, argues that immigration has been racialized, which she calls »racializing illegality«, while Husain (2017) refers to »using religion as a starting point for understanding racialization today«. Castañeda (2018) describes the ›racializing‹ of various ›Hispanic‹ migrant populations. It is easy to forget that ›immigrant‹ and ›religion‹ are not visible – and that people use appearance, dress and speech as proxies for such categories in interaction in a way that can ›racialize‹ their use.

While some contributors doubt that Race and racism are prevalent in Europe, particularly in the context of what are being called »voluntary« immigrants and guest workers, current research suggests that processes of racialization are much more prevalent in Europe than Majority Europeans and many immigrants would like to believe – and that this racialization is being hidden by the current focus on ›religion‹, ›ethnicity‹ and the potential for ›assimilation‹ into a ›democratic‹ society. Beaman (2017) and Castañeda (2018) point out that processes of exclusion in France, can occur (and be felt) much the same way racism is in the US, which Beaman suggests is likely to have complex tacit counterparts that are being overlooked. Both maintain that the tendency in France to insist that their society is not caught up in racism, makes it difficult to even talk about racism and how it works there – and the same is likely true for other countries in Europe. Beaman concludes that looking at tacit aspects of racism might be helpful in showing how racism is present in French society.

Before Trump most Americans also denied not only that they were racist, but that there was any significant racism in the country. This state of denial made it difficult to talk about Race or get research on racism taken seriously, while also marginalizing the work of minority scholars. Ethnicity was a more popular focus and research often focused on Irish, Italian and African ›immigrants‹ and their ›cultures‹ as if the processes involved were equivalent. The overt racism of the Trump years (including racial disparities exposed by COVID-19), in conjunction with police executions of George Floyd, Breonna Taylor (and many other Black Americans), BLM protests, and the current struggle over voting rights have made racism more obvious. Nevertheless, many still deny it. Discussions of tacit racism have been a powerful tool in overcoming denial of racism in the US and could do the same in Europe.

Like de Koning and Tezcan we think the common practice of referring to Race as a process of Othering, in other words, as just one among many processes of Othering (and intersectionality), may be part of the problem – and that our approach might be useful in addressing this tendency. Certainly, Othering is going on, and intersectionality is an important contributing factor. But, racism and racialization rise to another level of exclusion in ways that require taking tacit racism into account on its own terms. The problem is not merely that people are constructed as ›Other‹, but is rather, a deeper failure to recognize them as human members of society, which leads in turn to creative survival responses that change the dynamics of interaction order expectations.

In assessing the relevance of our research in the German context, Tezcan emphasizes the essential role of slavery in the formation of the US Black/White binary and asks, »are Turks Black?« While it is true that the categories Black/White developed in the context of US slavery, Europe also participated in the slave trade and the rush to colonize the countries it destabilized. Still, none of that answers the question whether »Turks are Black«, or whether they experience racism in Germany. The experience of ›Blackness‹ and racialization are not limited to those who are categorized or self-identify as Black. Rather, the question involves social definitions and experiences of exclusion and interaction order differences that are constantly evolving. In asserting that »The answer is clearly: no, they are not Black and this has consequences for the researcher«, Tezcan assumes the question has a definite answer, going on to suggest that the problem in Germany is more complicated than Race and racism, and expressing concern that our focus on tacit racism, while important, would be problematic if it became the main approach.

We take the position that NOT recognizing the importance of Race/racialization as social process is the problem. Race is not something ›real‹ that people actually have or do not have. Race is socially defined, and actualized through tacit practices in social interaction – which the recipient of the category has no control over. What matters is whether a category excludes in ways that produce the experience of exclusion that accompanies Race and/or whether persons in the category still look forward to being assimilated.

That exclusion occurs in Germany to persons of Middle-Eastern background in terms best described as racial is indicated by a March 30, 2021 (dw.com) report on the racism experienced by a Syrian candidate for parliament in Germany: »On Tuesday, Tareq Alaows, a 31-year-old Damascus-born Syrian refugee and human rights activist, announced that racist attacks and personal threats had forced him to withdraw what had been billed as a historic political candidacy for Germany's parliament, the Bundestag«. Alaows described his own experience in racialized terms, saying that he was »exposed to ›massive racism‹ during [his] short candidacy«.

In keeping with current research on how social categories can be racialized, we argue that it is likely that the social categories ›Turk‹, ›Middle-Eastern‹, ›immigrant‹, ›Muslim‹, etc., are all currently being racialized in Germany, as Beaman and Castañeda argue they have been in France. To the extent such categories are assigned on the basis of ›appearance‹ or ›language‹, in ways that *block attempts to assimilate*, as in Alaows' case, they likely produce the experience of »Race consciousness«.

Our point in explaining the origin of Black/White Race categories in US slavery was that they are social constructions that racialized identities that were not previously considered in racial terms. Categories related to immigration in Europe are being racialized much the same way »illegal« has been racialized in the US (Garcia 2017). Racialization is a fluid process. As a Turkish researcher recently told us, she has developed a consciousness of Race she never had before coming to the US (Ringen Firat). The same thing has happened recently for Asian Americans, many of whom have remarked on a new »Race consciousness« that conflicts with their prior (typically frustrating) efforts to assimilate. These experiences of Race consciousness are not determined by whether people are identified as Black, but rather, by the degree of exclusion they are subjected to and how they experience it.

The question then is not, as Tezcan puts it, whether certain people ›are‹ Black or White in Germany, or live in a country with a history of slavery. The question is whether the categories they are subjected to, and the exclusion enacted through those categories is experienced such that they develop a »Race consciousness« – in which case these categories and people have been ›racialized‹ – *and that is an empirical question* that involves what happens in social interaction.

It is our position that widespread development of such Race consciousness is ultimately a good thing. Bonilla-Silva (2003), in writing about color-blind racism, argued that the possibility of assimilating (or believing in the possibility), combined with a denial of being either Black or People of Color had led lighter skinned Latino/a people to side with White Americans against Black Americans. If it is the possession of Race consciousness that leads to awareness of inequality and the embrace of more democratic ideals – as Du Bois maintains – then the more people who develop such a consciousness the stronger the democratic heart of a people will be. Currently in the US, it is all but impossible for those not unequivocally ›seen‹ as White to avoid such an awareness. This likely explains the recent political shift of many Latino/a and Asian Americans in a more inclusive direction. It is also the principle behind our advocating the development of what we call a »White double-consciousness«. Ironically, pressure to assimilate works against this development and its corollary: an increased appreciation for democracy.

In this regard, fine points of difference between Fanon and Du Bois on the issue of oppression and assimilation matter. Fanon's concern is with conflicts for those who experience exclusion but are still trying to assimilate, which could be more likely under European conditions, whereas in the US the impossibility of assimilating is likely to lead to development of Race consciousness and the more democratic standards and expectations that come with it. This, Du Bois argued, is what enabled Black Americans to use Race to transcend Race – while in social contexts where assimilation is possible (or seems possible), pressure to assimilate tends to force people to continue trying to meet conditions that can lead to self-hatred and low self-esteem.

Assimilation is now a negative force that asks people to give up who they are, which includes both cultural practices and identities. It presumes that the majority society is best and has nothing to learn from incoming minorities. If we believe a modern society is strengthened by diversity, then we *should be able to see* that assimilation works against that diversity. What we should want, according to Castañeda (2018: 2f.) is ›integration‹ without loss of culture – a multicultural ideal. Progress requires constant change that maintaining cultural homogeneity works against. To what extent Europe will tend toward Fanon's end of the scale and away from Du Bois' will depend in part on the degree to which members of excluded groups believe assimilation is possible, or begin to develop a Race consciousness. This may be rapidly changing at present as Alaows' case indicates.

Beaman relates tacit racism to what she calls a »racial grammar«, in the Wittgensteinian sense. Referring to the roots of a racial grammar in France, she relates that development to colonialism, arguing that »France's colonization of the Maghreb, West Africa, Vietnam, and parts of South America and the Caribbean (including Guadeloupe and Martinique which are presently overseas *départements* of France), was part of its civilizing mission to spread its ›values‹ around the world,« and that »While French Republican ideology does not recognize identity-based categories, including race and religion (Chapman/Frader 2004), France's colonial empire relied on a differential construction of populations seen as ethnically different (Kastoryano/Escafré-Dublet 2012)«. In other words, such »racial grammars« enable racial and ethnic distinctions to become essential in ordinary interaction even »in the absence of official state categories«. The tacit character of such racialization – and the development of related racialized grammars that avoid mentioning Race – such as those involving ›illegals‹, ›Turks‹ and ›Muslims‹ – all work to hide racism from view.

Citing James Baldwin's experience in Paris, Beaman notes that, as in our book we »use ›submissive civility‹ to explain the expected behavior of Black men in the face of White police officers in the US, this ›submissive civility‹ is also applicable in the French context, as police officers perform identity checks, or *les contrôles d'identités,* disproportionately targeting Black and Maghrébin-origin individuals (Fassin 2013; Jobard/Levy 2009)«. Beaman notes that an American accent can modify treatment of Black and Muslim people, suggesting that the racialization of these categories is very complex. »What becomes clear« Beaman says, »is that this racial grammar is not just locally specific, but also global or transnational«, which would suggest its significance throughout Europe. The tacit character of this racialization, »[t]his erasure of the colonial« and the work that goes into hiding it behind other factors, Beaman argues: »leads to a ›panic‹ of the postcolonial«.

De Koning notes that, »the kind of assumptions imposed upon Muslims and migrants which render them ›not really from here‹« also render particular interactions »›diagnostic events‹ (Moore 1987), which reveal how tacit understandings are embedded in the moral orders«. Such diagnostic events, we argue, are essential to the work of revealing tacit racism – and we rely heavily on them. After describing a classroom scene after 9/11 in which the teacher pointed at a Muslim student and asked »are you with us or against us?«, de Koning says, »[i]t is important to not take for granted such ambiguities in the experiences of people as they are manifestations of moral reasonings that pertain to how people try to make sense of the world, trying to make sense of other people and their perceptions of them and, perhaps, translate them into action«.

These moments of moral reasoning are often analysed without mentioning Race, even though such ›events‹ are often based on appearance, and thus require a context of racialization to make sense of in the first place. Thinking of racism as both tacit and systemic, and focusing on what Beaman calls a »grammar« of racism and de Koning calls »moral reasonings«, should help make better sense of such questions. Ethnomethodology explores the way people make sense together – their moral reasoning as it is exposed by interactional trouble – which is one way, as de Koning concludes, that showing how »racism becomes tacit would be useful« and »a promising avenue for scholarly activism in Europe«.

In doing this research, it is essential, as Meyer and Fele underscore, to do detailed empirical observation of how actual interactions take place, which makes ethnomethodology and conversation analysis fruitful additions to ethnographic and interview approaches to racism and racialization.

Additionally, as Fele notes, there is a new theory of modernity involved in our approach that builds on novel interpretations of Durkheim and Du Bois to emphasize the importance of tacit practices that are constitutive of racism, and argue that reciprocity and equality are needed to support these practices in diverse modern social spaces where stranger/stranger interactions predominate (Rawls 2019). This theory posits that diversity is not only a strength of modernity – diversity is necessary for progress in science and occupations – and that it cannot succeed without equality and reciprocity. The consequence is that assimilation is anti-modern; while integration and multiculturalism are modern.

Lastly, we respond to Fele's concern »that to argue that everything is racial in social life can limit the ways in which other social or institutional constraints impinge on the phenomena under examination«. This is an important concern that is likely to be repeated by others. Therefore, it is important to point out that we are *not arguing that everything is racial*, or that people are aware of these effects of Race; but rather, that without the White majority being aware of it *Race has gotten into everything and many social categories have been racialized*. This is something the excluded are often aware of – while the White majority remain unaware.

In a world in which Race categories have been allowed to organize political, economic, and social spaces for hundreds of years – the effects of Race will turn up all over the place – in aspects of social life that are in no way about Race. Trying to confine studies of Race to parts of social life that are *about* Race has the unfortunate effect of turning attention away from Race and scholars of Race, when what we need is to focus on them more. The result has been that Black and marginalized scholars, like Du Bois and Eric Williams (1943), who long ago pointed out the wide-ranging effects of slavery and the resulting racial binary, have been treated as ›merely‹ scholars of Race, while the study of Race and racism has been confined to marginal spaces and treated as if it concerned only racial minorities. *This has been a huge mistake.*

Fele is of course right that the shift from ›how‹ to ›why‹ is »a difficult shift, not always entirely grounded in the materials at hand«. It is a theoretical shift, but one in which we keep as close as possible to the intersection between the writings of racialized scholars like Du Bois and our own empirical research. Not to make this shift, however, would be to remain within the mainstream White dominated form of reasoning that enables racism to remain hidden.

We maintain that the »moral authority« of Whiteness controls public expectations – including the reasoning of mainstream researchers – to such an extent that categories of people who have been racialized not only have trouble getting their voices heard, but often have difficulty being recognized as human. There are no social roles that neutralize Race: even powerful roles such as ›President of the US‹, ›Police Officer‹, or ›Company Vice President‹. This problem permeates every aspect of daily life in the US and we suspect elsewhere. Therefore, centering Race and its attendant issues – and refusing to subordinate them to other concerns – is a critical issue for theory and research. We do not think the danger is that focusing on tacit racism will obscure the complex nuances of inter-ethnic relations. In fact, we believe the reverse is the case and that talking about these issues without mentioning Race is obscuring racism. Recognition of the centrality of Race to social, economic and political issues worldwide is long overdue, and we maintain that the possibility of true democratic social action awaits this recognition.

In Europe as in the US, tacit racism will likely be difficult to expose, because it is well hidden and it's non-existence is taken-for-granted. It will also be difficult for the Majority to accept because acceptance means giving up cherished beliefs about the fairness and democratic character of a given society and the positive value of assimilation into it. Tacit racism can be found by close examination of social interaction, because that is where racism is enacted in daily life. Failure to document how this works will leave societies believing they do not have a Race problem, when they do, and thus unable to deal with it – or even to talk about it.

When researchers do find racism embedded in interaction they can work *backward* from what they find to how it might have emerged, bringing that history and the marginalized scholars who have likely already written about it to the forefront. The process can also work *forward* to implications for improving the current situation. This would be an important addition to our understanding of Race and racism in Europe that will not come from conventional studies of ›ethnicity‹, ›inter-ethnic relations‹, ›religion‹, ›immigration‹, etc.

Literature

Ahmed, Sara (2007): »A Phenomenology of Whiteness«. In: *Feminist Theory* 8: 2, 149–168.

Alcoff, Linda M. (1999): »Towards a Phenomenology of Racial Embodiment«. In: *Radical Philosophy* 95, 15–26.

Alexander, Michelle (2016 [2011]): *The New Jim Crow: Masseninhaftierung und Rassismus in den USA*, translated by Gabriele Gockel and Thomas Wollermann, München: Kunstmann.

Allen, Jafari Sinclaire/Jobson, Ryan Cecil (2016): »The Decolonizing Generation: (Race and) Theory in Anthropology since the Eighties«. In: *Current Anthropology* 57: 2, 129–148.

Allen, Theodore (1994): *The Invention of the White Race, Volume One: Racial Oppression and Social Control*, London: Verso.

Allen, Theodore (1997): *The Invention of the White Race, Volume Two: The Origin of Racial Oppression in Anglo-America*, London: Verso.

Al-Saji, Alia (2014): »A Phenomenology of Hesitation: Interrupting Racializing Habits of Seeing«. In: *Living Alterities: Phenomenology, Embodiment, and Race*, ed. by Emily S. Lee, Albany: State University of New York Press, 133–172.

Amjahid, Mohamad (2021): *Der weiße Fleck. Eine Anleitung zu antirassistischem Denken*, München: Piper Verlag.

Amjahid, Mohamad (2017): *Unter Weißen. Was es heißt, privilegiert zu sein*, Berlin: Hanser.

Anderson, Carol (2016): *White Rage: The Unspoken Truth of Our Racial Divide*, London: Bloomsbury Publishing.

Anderson, Carol (2018): *One Person No Vote: How Voter Suppression Is Destroying Our Democracy*, London: Bloomsbury Publishing.

Arndt, Susan (2005): »The ›Racial Turn‹. Kolonialismus, *weiße* Mythen und Critical Whiteness Studies«. In: Marianne Bechhaus-Gerst, Sunna Gieseke & Reinhard Klein-Arendt (ed.): *Koloniale und postkoloniale Konstruktionen von Afrika und Menschen afrikanischer Herkunft in der deutschen Alltagskultur*, Frankfurt/M., Peter Lang, 12–25.

Baldwin, James (1955): *Notes of a Native Son*, Boston: Beacon Press.

Balkenhol, Markus/Schramm, Katharina (2019): »Doing Race in Europe: Contested Pasts and Contemporary Practices«. In: *Social Anthropology / Anthropologie Sociale* 27, 585–593.

Batty, David (2011): »Lady Warsi claims Islamophobia is now socially acceptable in Britain«. In: *The Guardian*, 20.01.2011, https://www.theguardian.com/uk/2011/jan/ 20/lady-warsi-islamophobia-muslims-prejudice (21.03.2020).

Beaman, Jean (2017): *Citizen Outsider: Children of North African Immigrants in France*, Oakland: University of California Press.

Bell, Derrick (1973): *Race, Racism, and American Law*, Boston: Little and Brown.

Bittner (1967): »The Police on Skid-Row: A Study of Peace Keeping«. In: *American Sociological Review* 32 (5): 699–715.

Bittner (1970): *The Functions of the Police in Modern Society*, Chevy Case: National Institute of Mental Health, Center for Studies of Crime and Delinquency.

Bloul, Rachel (2013): »Do I look Jewish in This? A Phenomenological Approach to Intercorporality and Racism«. In: *Identities* 20: 5, 522–543.

Bolden, Galina/Robinson, Jeffrey (2011): »Soliciting Accounts with Why-Interrogatives in Conversation«. In: *Journal of Communication* 61 (1), 94–119.

Bonilla-Silva, Eduardo (2003): *Racism without Racists*, Lanham: Rowman and Littlefield.

Bravo López, Fernando (2011): »Towards a Definition of Islamophobia: Approximations of the Early Twentieth Century«. In: *Ethnic and Racial Studies* 34, 556–573.

Bui, Pipo (2003): *Envisioning Vietnamese Migrants in Germany. Ethnic Stigma, Immigrant Origin Narratives and Partial Masking*, Forum Europäische Ethnologie, Münster: LIT-Verlag

Butler, Paul (2017): *Chokehold: Policing Black Men*, New York: The New Press

Cankaya, Sinam/Mepsche, Paul (2019): »Facing Racism: Discomfort, Innocence and the Liberal Peripheral Side of Race in the Netherlands«. In: *Social Anthropology / Anthropologie Sociale* 27, Special Issue on »Doing Race in Europe«, 626640.

Castañeda, Ernesto (2018): *A Place to Call Home: Immigrant Exclusion and Urban Belonging in New York, Paris, and Barcelona*, Stanford: Stanford University Press.

Chapman, Herrick/Frader, Laura L. (Eds.) (2004): *Race in France: Interdisciplinary Perspectives on the Politics of Difference*, New York/Oxford: Berghahn Books.

Chevigny, Paul (1969): *Police Power: Police Abuses in New York City*, New York: Vintage Books.

Crenshaw, Kimberlé/Gotanda, Neil/Peller, Gary/Thomas, Kendall (ed.) (1995): *Critical Race Theory: The Key Writings That Formed the Movement*, New York: The New Press.

De Koning, Martijn (2016): »›You Need to Present a Counter-Message‹. The Racialization of Dutch Muslims and Anti-Islamophobia Initiatives«. In: *Journal of Muslims in Europe* 5, 170–189.

De Koning, Martijn (2019): »Routinisation and Mobilisation of Injustice: How to live in a Regime of Surveillance«. In: *Radicalization in Belgium and the Netherlands – Critical Perspectives on Violence and Security*, ed. by Nadia Fadil/Martijn De Koning/Francesco Ragazzi, London: IB Tauris.

De Koning, Martijn (2020): »The Racialization of Danger: Patterns and Ambiguities in the Relation between Islam, Security and Secularism in the Netherlands«. In: *Patterns of Prejudice* 54, 1–13.

Delgado, Richard/ Stefancic, Jean (1995): *Critical Race Theory: An Introduction*, New York, London: New York University Press.

DiAngelo, Robin (2018): *White Fragility: Why It's So Hard for White People to Talk About Racism*, Boston: Beacon Press.

Du Bois, W.E.B. (1890): *The Submissive Man*, Harvard University Commencement Address, The Du Bois Archive.

Du Bois, W.E.B. (1940): *Dusk of Dawn: An Essay Toward an Autobiography of a Race Concept*, New York: Harcourt, Brace and Company.

Du Bois, W.E.B. (1994 [1903]): *The Souls of Black Folk: Essays and Sketches*, Mineola, New York: Dover Publications.

Du Bois, W.E.B. (2003 [1903]): *Die Seelen der Schwarzen,* translated by J. and B. Meyer-Wendt, Freiburg: orange press.

Duck, Waverly (2015): *No Way Out: Precarious Living in the Shadow of Poverty and Drug Dealing*, Chicago: University of Chicago Press.

Duck, Waverly (2016): »Becoming a Drug Dealer: Local Interaction Orders and Criminal Careers«: In: *Critical Sociology* 42: 7-8, 1069–1085.

Duck, Waverly (2017): »The Complex Dynamics of Trust and Legitimacy: Understanding Interactions between the Police and Poor Black Neighborhood Residents«: In: *The Annals of the American Academy of Political and Social Science* 673:1, 132–149.

Durkheim, Émile (1893): *De la Division du Travail Social*, Paris: Félix Alcan.

Durkheim, Émile (1925). *Moral Education*, Mineola: Dover Publications.

Durkheim, Emile (1992 [1893]): Über soziale Arbeitsteilung. Studien über die Organisation höherer Gesellschaften, translated by Ludwig Schmids, Frankfurt/Main: Suhrkamp.

dw.com (2021): »Syrian refugee withdraws bid for German parliament seat after threats«, https://www.dw.com/en/syrian-refugee-withdraws-bid-for-german-parliament-seat-after-threats/a-57051621 (30.06.2021).

Eickhof, Ilka (2010): *Antimuslimischer Rassismus in Deutschland.* Theoretische Überlegungen, Berlin: Wissenschaftlicher Verlag Berlin.

El-Mafaalani, Aladin (2021): *Wozu Rassismus? Von der Erfindung der Menschenrassen bis zum rassismuskritischen Widerstand*, Köln: Kiepenheuer und Witsch.

El-Tayeb, Fatima (2001): *Schwarze Deutsche: Der Diskurs um Rasse und nationale Identität 1890-1933*, Frankfurt am Main: Campus.

El-Tayeb, Fatima (2016): *Undeutsch. Konstruktion des Anderen in der postmigrantischen Gesellschaft,* Bielefeld: Transcript.

Essed, Philomena (1990): *Everyday Racism*, Newbury Park/ London/ New Delhi: Sage Publications.

Fanon, Frantz (1952): *Black Skin, White Masks*, New York: Grove Press.

Fanon, Frantz (1952): *Peau noire, masques blancs*, Paris: Éditions du Seuil.

Fanon, Frantz (1985 [1952]): *Schwarze Haut, weiße Masken*, translated by Eva Moldenhauer, Frankfurt/ Main: Suhrkamp.

Fanon, Frantz (2016): *Schwarze Haut, Weiße Masken*, Wien, Berlin: Verlag Turia + Kant

Fassin, Didier (2013): *Enforcing Order: An Ethnography of Urban Policing*, Cambridge and London: Polity Press.

Fassin, Didier (2016): »Vom Rechtsanspruch zum Gunsterweis: Zur moralischen Ökonomie der Asylvergabepraxis im heutigen Europa«. In: *Mittelweg 36. Zeitschrift des Hamburger Instituts für Sozialforschung* 25, 62–78.

Fassin, Didier (2021): *Death of a Traveller*, Cambridge, UK und Medford, MA: Polity Press.

Feagin, Joe (2009): *The White Racial Frame: Centuries of Racial Framing and Counter Framing*, New York: Routledge.

Foroutan, Naika (2019): *Die postmigrantische Gesellschaft: Ein Versprechen der pluralen Demokratie*, Berlin: Aufbau.

Gabbidon, Shaun (2007): *W.E.B. Du Bois on Crime and Justice: Laying the Foundations of Sociological Criminology*, Hampshire, Burlington: Ashgate Publishing.

Garcia, San Juanita (2017): »Racializing ›Illegality‹: An Intersectional Approach to Understanding How Mexican-Origin Women Navigate an Anti-Immigrant Climate«. In: *Sociology of Race and Ethnicity* 3(4), 474–490.

Garfinkel, Harold (1940): »Color Trouble«. In: *Opportunity*, May 1940. Reprinted in *Best Short Stories* of 1941 and *Primer for White Folks* in 1945.

Garfinkel, Harold: (1949 [1942]): MA Thesis »Inter-Racial and Intra-Racial Homicide in Ten Counties in North Carolina, 1930–1940«. Shortened version in: *Social Forces* 27, 370–381.

Garfinkel, Harold (1956): »Conditions of Successful Degradation Ceremonies«. In: *American Journal of Sociology* 61:5, 420–424.

Garfinkel, Harold (1963): »A Conception of and Experiments with Trust as a Condition of Stable Social Actions«. In: *Motivation and Social Interaction: Cognitive Determinants*, ed. by O. Harvey, New York: Ronald Press 2012Company, 187–238.

Garfinkel, Harold (1967): *Studies in Ethnomethodology*, Englewood Cliffs: Prentice Hall.

Garfinkel, Harold (1988): »Evidence for Locally Produced, Naturally Accountable Phenomena of Order, Logic, Reason, Meaning, Method, etc. in and as of the Essential Quiddity of Immortal Ordinary Society (I of IV): An Announcement of Studies«. In: *Sociological Theory* 6: 1, 10–39.

Garfinkel, Harold (2002): *Ethnomethodology's Program. Working Out Durkheim's Aphorism*, ed. by Anne W. Rawls, Lanham: Rowman and Littlefield.

Garfinkel, Harold (2002): *Seeing Sociologically: The Routine Grounds of Social Action*, Boulder: Paradigm Publishers.

Garfinkel, Harold (2007): »Lebenswelt Origins of the Sciences«. In: *Human Studies* 30: 1, 9–56.

Garfinkel, Harold (2012 [1947]): »The Red as an Ideal Object«. In: *Etnografia e Ricerca Qualitativa* 5(1), 19–34.

Garfinkel, Harold (2020 [1967]): *Studien zur Ethnomethodologie*, ed. by Erhard Schüttpelz/Anne Rawls/Tristan Thielmann, translated by Brigitte Luchesi, Frankfurt/Main, New York: Campus.

Garfinkel, Harold/Livingston, Eric (2003): »Phenomenal Field Properties of Order in Formatted Queues and Their Neglected Standing in the Current Situation of Inquiry«. In: *Visual Studies* 18: 1, 21–28.

Goffman, Erving (1961): *Asylums: Essays on the Condition of the Social Situation of Mental Patients and Other Inmates*, New York: Anchor Books.

Goffman, Erving (1973 [1959]): *Wir alle spielen Theater. Selbstdarstellung im Alltag*, translated by Peter Weber-Schäfer. München: Piper.

Goffman, Erving (1983): »The Interaction Order: American Sociological Association, 1982 Presidential Address«. In: *American Sociological Review*, 48:1, 1–17.

Goffman, Erving (2010 [1963]): *Stigma: Über Techniken zur Bewältigung einer beschädigten Identität*, translated by Frigga Haug, Frankfurt/Main: Suhrkamp.

Goldberg, David T. (2006): »Racial Europeanization«. In: *Ethnic and Racial Studies* 29:2, 331–364.

Güler, Serdal (2009): *Die Konstruktion der Anderen. Rassistische Legitimations- und Herstellungspraktiken. Dipl-Thesis*, Social Sciences, Freie Universität Berlin.

Halliday, Fred (1999); »›Islamophobia‹ reconsidered«. In: *Ethnic and Racial Studies* 22, 892–902.

Haney-Lopez, Ian (2013): *Dog-Whistle Politics: How Coded Racial Appeals Have Reinvented Racism and Wrecked the Middle Class*, Oxford: Oxford University Press.

Hasters, Alice (2019): *Was weiße Menschen nicht über Rassismus hören wollen aber wissen sollten*, München: Carl Hanser Verlag.

Hasters, Alice (2020): »Mückenstiche mit System. Zum Umgang mit Alltagsrassismus«. In: *APUZ – Aus Politik und Zeitgeschehen* 40-42, 4–7.

Heinemann, Alisha M.B./Mecheril, Paul (2017): »Institutioneller Rassismus als Analyseperspektive. Zwei Argumente«. In: Heinrich-Böll-Stiftung (ed.): *Ideologien der Ungleichwertigkeit.* Herausgegeben von der Heinrich-Böll-Stiftung in Zusammenarbeit mit Weiterdenken – Heinrich-Böll-Stiftung Sachsen, 45–55.

HENG, Geraldine (2018): *The Invention of Race in the European Middle* Ages, Cambridge: Cambridge University Press.

HILL-COLLINS, Patricia (1990): *Black Feminist Thought*, New York: Routledge.

HOBBES, Thomas (1966 [1651]): *Leviathan oder Stoff, Form und Gewalt eines bürgerlichen und kirchlichen Staates*, Darmstadt/Neuwied: Luchterhand.

HOOKS, bell (1989): *Talking back: Thinking feminist, thinking black*, Boston: South End Press.

HUNOLD, Daniela/WEGNER, Maren (2020): »Rassismus und Polizei: Zum Stand der Forschung«. In: *APUZ - Aus Politik und Zeitgeschehen* 40-42, 27–32.

HUSAIN, Atiya (2017): »Retrieving the Religion in Racialization: A Critical Review«. In: *Sociology Compass*, https://doi.org/10.1111/soc4.12507 (30.06.21).

HÜTTERMANN, Jörg (2018): *Figurationsprozesse der Einwanderungsgesellschaft. Zum Wandel der Beziehungen zwischen Alteingesessenen und Migranten in deutschen Städten*, Bielefeld: Transcript.

JÄGER, Siegfried (1992): *Brandsätze. Rassismus im Alltag.* Diss-Studien, ed. by Duisburger Institut für Sprach- und Sozialforschung, https://www.diss-duisburg.de/Internetbibliothek/Buecher/Brandsaetze/Brandsaetze_web.pdf (15.01.2022).

JANSEN, Yolande/MEER, Nasar (2020): »Genealogies of ›Jews‹ and ›Muslims‹: Social Imaginaries in the Race-Religion Nexus«. In: *Patterns of Prejudice*: 1–14.

JEFFERSON, Gail (1979): »A Technique for Inviting Laughter and Subsequent Acceptance/Declination«. In: *Everyday Language: Studies in Ethnomethodology*, ed. by George Psathas, New York: Irvington, 79–96.

JOBARD, Fabien/LEVY, René (2009): *Profiling Minorities: A Study of Stop-and-Search Practices in Paris*, Paris: Open Society Institute.

KALPAKA, Annita/RÄTHZEl, Nora (1986): *Die Schwierigkeit, nicht rassistisch zu sein*, Berlin: Express Edition.

KALPAKA, Annita/RÄTHZEL, Nora/WEBER, Klaus (ed.) (2017): *Rassismus. Die Schwierigkeit, nicht rassistisch zu sein*, Hamburg: Argument Verlag.

KASTORYANO, Riva/ESCAFRÉ-DUBLET, Angéline (2012): »France«. In: *Addressing Tolerance and Diversity Discourses in Europe: A Comparative Overview of 16 European Countries*, ed. by Ricard Zapata-Barrero/Anna Triandafyllidou, Barcelona: Barcelona Centre for International Affairs, 27–47.

KASTORYANO, Riva/ESCAFRÉ-DUBLET, Angéline (2013): *Concepts and Practices of Tolerance in France*, Synthesis Reports, Retrieved from Cadmus, European University Institute Research Repository, http://hdl.handle.net/1814/23255 (30.06.21).

KOP – KAMPAGNE FÜR OPFER RASSISTISCH MOTIVIERTER POLIZEIGEWALT (ed.) (2021): *Chronik rassistisch motivierter Polizeivorfälle für Berlin von 2000 – 2021*, https://kop-berlin.de/files/documents/chronik.pdf (15.01.2022).

LEMS, Johanna M. (2020): »Staying Silent or Speaking Up: Reactions to Racialization Affecting Muslims in Madrid«. In: *Ethnic and Racial Studies*, 1–19.

MANNHEIM, Karl (1995 [1929]): *Ideologie und Utopie*, Frankfurt/Main: Vittorio Klostermann.

MAYER, Jane (2016): *Dark Money: The Hidden History of the Billionaires Behind the Rise of the Radical Right*, New York: Doubleday.

MAYNARD, Douglas/ZIMMERMAN, Don (1984): »Topical Talk Ritual and the Social Organization of Relationships«. In: *Social Psychology Quarterly* 47: 4, 301–316.

MECHERIL, Paul (2007): »Die Normalität des Rassismus«. In: *Überblick. Zeitschrift des Informations- und Dokumentationszentrums für Antirassismusarbeit in Nordrhein-Westfalen* 13, 3–9.

MEER, Nasar/MODOOD, Tariq (2009): »Refutations of Racism in the ›Muslim Question‹«. In: *Patterns of Prejudice* 43, 335–354.

MELD ISLAMOFOBIE (2019): *Alledaagse islamofobie in Nederland*, Den Haag: Meld Islamofobie.

METZL, Jonathan (2019): *Dying of Whiteness: How the Politics of Racial Resentment Is Killing America's Heartland*, New York: Basic Books.

MILLS, Charles W. (1999): *The Racial Contract*, Ithaca, London: Cornell University Press.

MOORE, Sally Falk (1987): »Explaining the Present: Theoretical Dilemmas in Processual Ethnography«. In: *American Ethnologist* 14, 727–736.

MORRIS, Aldon D. (2015): *The Scholar Denied: W.E.B. Du Bois and the Birth of Modern Sociology*, Oakland: University of California Press.

MOUSTAOUI SRHIR, Adil (2020): »Making Children Multilingual: Language Policy and Parental Agency in Transnational and Multilingual Moroccan Families in Spain«. In: *Journal of Multilingual and Multicultural Development* 41, 108–120.

POLANYI, Michael (1966): *The tacit dimension*, New York: Doubleday & Compagny.

POLANYI, Michael (1985): *Implizites Wissen*, Frankfurt a.M.: Suhrkamp.

POLANYI, Michael/PROSCH, Harry(1975): *Meanin,*. Chicago: Chicago University Press.

POMERANTZ, A. (1986): »Extreme Case Formulations: A Way of Legitimizing Claims«. In: *Human Studies* 9 (2-3), 219–229.

RASHID, Naaz (2016): *Veiled threats: Representing ›the Muslim Woman‹ in UK Public Policy Discourses*, Bristol: Bristol University Press.

RAWLS, Anne (1983): *Constitutive Justice: An Interactionist Contribution to the Understanding of Social Order and Human Value.* Unpublished Dissertation, Boston University.

RAWLS, Anne W. (1987): »The Interaction Order Sui Generis: Goffman's Contribution to Social Theory«. In: *Sociological Theory* 5:2, 136–149.

RAWLS, Anne (1989): »Language, Self, and Social Order: A Re–Evaluation of Goffman and Sacks«. In: *Human Studies* 12: 1, 147–172.

RAWLS, Anne (1990): »Emergent Sociality: A Dialectic of Commitment and Order«. In: *Symbolic Interaction* 13: 1, 63–82.

RAWLS, Anne (2000): »›Race‹ as an Interaction Order Phenomenon: W.E.B. Du Bois' ›Double Consciousness‹ Thesis Revisited«. In: *Sociological Theory* 18: 2, 241–274.

RAWLS, Anne (2018): »The Wartime Narrative in US Sociology 1940-1947: Stigmatizing Qualitative Sociology in the Name of ›Science‹«. In: *The European Journal of Social Theory* 59(1), 526–546.

Rawls, Anne (2019a): »Introduction to Garfinkel's ›Notes on Language Games‹: Language Events as Cultural Events in ›Systems of Interaction‹«. In: *The European Journal of Social Theory* 22(2), 133–147.

RAWLS, Anne (2019b): *Toward a Sociological Theory of Justice: Durkheim's Forgotten Introduction to The Division of Social Labor*, translated by Francesco Callegaro/Philip Chanial, Paris: Le Bord de l'Eau.

RAWLS, Anne W. (2019): *La Division du Travail Revisited: Vers une Théorie Sociologique de la Justice*, translated by Francesco Callegaro/Philip Chanial. Paris: Le Bord de l' Eau.

RAWLS, Anne (2021): Durkheim's Self-Regulating ›Constitutive‹ Practices: An Unexplored Critical Relevance to Racial Justice, Consensus Thinking, and the Covid-19 Pandemic«. In: *Durkheim & Critique*, ed. by Nicola Marcucci, London: Palgrave Macmillan.

RAWLS, Anne Warfield (2022): »Harold Garfinkel's Focus on Racism, Inequality and Social Justice: The Early Years 1939–1952«. In *The Ethnomethodology Program: Legacies and Prospects*, ed. by D. W. Maynard and J. Heritage, New York: Oxford University Press, 90–113.

RAWLS, Anne/DUCK, Waverly (2017): »›Fractured Reflections‹ of High-Status Black Male Presentations of Self: Non-Recognition of Identity as a ›Tacit‹ Form of Institutional Racism«. In: *Sociological Focus* 50:1, 36–51.

RAWLS, Anne/DUCK, Waverly (2019): *Developing a White ›Double Consciousness‹ of Race and Marginality: Implications of Du Bois and Garfinkel for the Scientific Awareness of Interaction Orders*, unpublished manuscript.

RAWLS, Anne/DUCK, Waverly (2020): *Tacit Racism*, Chicago: University of Chicago Press.

RAWLS, Anne/DUCK, Waverly/TUROWETZ, Jason (2018): »Problems Establishing Identity/Residency in a City Neighborhood during a Black/White Police-Citizen Encounter: Reprising Du Bois' Conception of Submission as ›Submissive Civility‹«. In: *City & Community* 17: 4, 1015–1050.

RAWLS, Anne/TUROWETZ, Jason (2019): »›Discovering Culture‹ in Interaction: Solving Problems in Cultural Sociology by Recovering the Interactional Side of Parsons' Conception of Culture«. In: *The American Journal of Cultural Sociology*, https://doi.org/10.1057/s41290-019-00079-6 (30.06.2021).

RAWLS, Anne/WHITEHEAD, Kevin/DUCK, Waverly (2020): *Black Lives Matter. Ethnomethodological and Conversation Analytic Studies of Race and Systemic Racism in Everyday Interaction*, A Routledge Freebook, https://www.routledge.com/go/black-lives-matter-an-ethnomethodology-freebook (30.06.2021).

SACKS, Harvey (1962): *On Understanding*. Unpublished manuscript, Garfinkel-Archiv.

SACKS, Harvey/SCHEGLOFF, Emmanuel/JEFFERSON, Gail (1974): »A Simplest Systematics for the Organization of Turn-taking in Conversation«. In: *Linguistic Society of America* 50: 4(1), 696–735.

SAYYID, Salman (2018): »Islamophobia and the Europeanness of the Other Europe«. In: *Patterns of Prejudice* 52, 420–435.

SAYYID, Salman/VAKIL, Abdoolkarim (2010): *Thinking through Islamophobia: Global Perspectives*, London: Hurst & Co.

SPEER, Susan A./STOKOE, Elizabeth (2011): *Conversation and Gender*, New York: Cambridge University Press.

SPILLERS, Hortense J. (1987): »Mama's Baby, Papa's Maybe: An American Grammar Book«. In: *Diacritics* 17:2, 64–81.

STOLER, Ann Laura (2011): »Colonial Aphasia. Race and Disabled Histories in France«. In: *Public Cultures* 23:1, 121–156.

SUE, Derald Wing (2010): *Microaggressions in Everyday Life. Race, Gender, and Sexual Orientation*. Hoboken: Wiley.

TERKESSIDIS, Mark (2004): *Die Banalität des Rassismus, Migranten zweiter Generation entwickeln eine neue Perspektive*, Bielefeld: Transkript.

TEZCAN, Levent (2002): Inszenierungen kollektiver Identität, Artikulationen des politischen Islam – beobachtet auf den Massenversammlungen der türkisch-islamistischen Gruppe Milli Görüs. In: *Soziale Welt* 53, 303–324.

THE WHITE HOUSE/PRESIDENT GEORGE W. BUSH (2001): »Address to a Joint Session of Congress and the American People«, https://georgewbush-whitehouse.archives.gov/news/releases/2001/09/20010920-8.html (17.03.2021).

TOPOLSKI, Anya (2018): »The Race-Religion Constellation: A European Contribution to the Critical Philosophy of Race«. In: *Critical Philosophy of Race* 6, 58–81.

TULLMANN, Katherine (2020): »The Contents of Racialized Seeing«. In: *Phenomenology and the Cognitive Sciences* (preprint), https://doi.org/10.1007/s11097-020-09674-2 (08.04.2021).

VAN BAAR, Huub (2014): »The Emergence of a Reasonable Anti-Gypsyism in Europe«. In: *When Stereotype Meets Prejudice: Antiziganism in European Societies*, ed. by Timofey Agarin, Stuttgart: ibidem-Verlag.

Van Den Hemel, Ernst (2014): »(Pro)claiming Tradition: The ›Judeo-Christian‹ Roots of Dutch Society and the Rise of Conservative Nationalism«. In: *Transformations of Religion and the Public Sphere*, ed. by Rosi Braidotti/Bolette Blaagaard/Tobijn De Graauw/Eva Midden, London: Palgrave Macmillan.

Van der Valk, Ineke (2015): *Dutch Islamophobia*, Zürich: Lit.

Vieten, Ulrike M. (2016): »Far Right Populism and Women: The Normalisation of Gendered Anti-Muslim Racism and Gendered Culturalism in the Netherlands«. In: *Journal of Intercultural Studies* 37, 621–636.

Vom Lehn, Dirk (2019): »From Garfinkel's ›Experiments in Miniature‹ to the Ethnomethodological Analysis of Interaction«. In: *Human Studies* 42: 2, 305–326.

Wacquant, Loic (1997): »For an Analytic of Racial Domination«. In: *Political Power and Social Theory* 11 (Symposium on »Rethinking Race« with Ann Laura Stoler, Patricia Dominguez, David Roediger, and Uday Singh Mehta), 221–234.

Williams, Bianca C. (2015): »Introduction #BlackLivesMatter«. In: *Cultural Anthropology*, Series on #BlackLivesMatter. Anti-Black Racism, Police Violence, and Resistance. https://culanth.org/fieldsights/introduction-black-lives-matter.

Williams, Eric (1944): *Capitalism and Slavery*, Chapel Hill: Univery of North Carolina Press.

Wittgenstein, Ludwig (1958): *Philosophische Untersuchungen. Philosophical Investigations*, Oxford: Blackwell.

Wollrad, Eske (2003): »Der Weißheit letzter Schluss. Zur Dekonstruktion von ›Weißsein‹«. In: *Polylog. Forum für interkulturelle Philosophie* 4, 1–21.

Woodward, Comer Vann (1955). *The Strange Casreer of Jim Crow*, Oxford: Oxford University Press.

Yancy, George (2008): »Elevators, Social Spaces and Racism«. In: *Philosophy & Social Criticism* 34: 8, 843–876.

Yildiz, Erol/Hill, Marc (ed.) (2014): *Nach der Migration: Postmigrantische Perspektiven jenseits der Parallelgesellschaft*, Bielefeld: Transcript.

Authors

ABRAHAMS, Lynn, Iziko Museums of South Africa, Curator, 25 Queen Victoria St, Gardens, Cape Town, 8001, ZAF, labrahams@iziko.org.za

ABITI, Nelson Adebo, M.A., University of the Western Cape, Department of History, Robert Sobukwe Rd, Bellville, Cape Town, 7535, ZAR, abdenel@gmail.com

BEAMAN, Jean, Prof. Dr., University of California Santa Barbara, Department of Sociology, CA 93106-9420, Santa Barbara, USA, jbeaman@soc.ucsb.edu

BRUS, Anna, Dr., Kunsthistorisches Institut der Universität zu Köln, Albertus-Magnus-Platz, 50923 Köln, DE, abrus@uni-koeln.de

DE KONING, Martijn, Dr., Radboud University, Department of Islamic Studies, Houtlaan 4, 6525 XZ Nijmegen, NLD, martijn.dekoning@ru.nl

DUCK, Waverly, Prof. Dr., University of California Santa Barbara, Department of Sociology, CA 93106-9420, Santa Barbara, USA, Waverly_Duck@ucsb.edu

FELE, Giolo, Prof. Dr., University of Trento, Department of Sociology and Social Research, Via Verdi, 26, 38122 Trento, ITA, Giolo.Fele@unitn.it

KNECHT, Michi, Prof. Dr., Universität Bremen, Institut für Ethnologie und Kulturwissenschaft, Enrique-Schmidt-Straße 7, 28359 Bremen, DE, knecht@uni-bremen.de

MBEWE, Mary, M.A., University of the Western Cape, Department of History, Robert Sobukwe Rd., Bellville, Cape Town, 7535, ZAR, mary.mbewe@mail.utoronto.ca

MEMEL-KASSI, Silvie, Dr., Directrice Générale de la Culture de Côte d'Ivoire, 32 Boulevard Carde, Abidjan, CI, silviememelk@yahoo.fr

MEYER, Christian, Prof. Dr., Universität Konstanz, Professur für Allgemeine Soziologie und Kultursoziologie, Fachbereich Geschichte und Soziologie, Universitätsstr. 10, 78464 Konstanz, DE, christian.meyer@uni-konstanz.de

MOURA, Sabrina, Dr., University of Campinas, IFCH – História, Rua Cora Coralina, 100 Campinas, BR, sabrinamoura@vastoart.org / sabrinamourad@gmail.com

MÜLLER, Bernard, Dr., Ecole Supérieure d'Art d'Avignon, 500 Chemin de Baigne Pieds, 84000 Avignon, FR, muller6691@gmail.com

RAWLS, Anne Warfield, Prof. Dr., Bentley University, Department of Sociology & Universität Siegen, Fakultät IV, School of Information, Hölderlinstr 3, 57068 Siegen, DE, arawls@bentley.edu

SIMÃO, Catarina, Artist and Researcher, lives and works between Maputo and Lisbon. Rua da Rosa no 170-1, 1200-390 Lisboa, PO, catarina.simao@gmail.com

SNOEP, Nanette J., Director Rautenstrauch-Joest Museum Kulturen der Welt, Cäcilienstraße 29–33, 50667 Köln, DE, nanette.snoep@stadt-koeln.de

TEZCAN, Levent, Prof. Dr., WWU Münster, Institut für Soziologie, Schlossplatz 2, 48149 Münster, DE, ltezcan@uni-muenster.de

TICHMANN, Paul, Iziko Museums of South Africa, Curator Social History, 25 Queen Victoria St, Gardens, Cape Town, 8001, ZAF, ptichmann@iziko.org.za

TOGUO, Barthélémy, Artist, lives and works in Paris and Bandjoun. Bandjoun Station B.P 52, Bandjoun, CMR, btoguo@gmail.com

TSOGANG FOSSI, Richard, Dr., Technische Universität Berlin, Institut für Kunstwissenschaft und Historische Urbanistik, Straße des 17. Juni 151/152, 10623 Berlin, DE, tsogangfossi@yahoo.fr

VERRAN, Helen, Prof. Dr., Northern Institute, Charles Darwin University, Ellengowan Drive, Casuarina NT 0810, AU, helen.verran@cdu.edu.au

ZILLINGER, Martin, Prof. Dr., Universität zu Köln, Institut für Ethnologie, Albertus-Magnus-Platz, 50932 Köln, DE, martin.zillinger@uni-koeln.de